Generative AI for the Medical Student

Campion Quinn

Generative AI for the Medical Student

Core Concepts to Clinical Practice

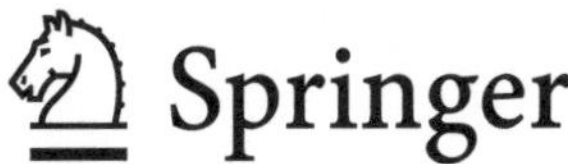

Campion Quinn
Rockville Medical, LLC
Rockville Centre, NY, USA

ISBN 978-3-032-01612-6 ISBN 978-3-032-01613-3 (eBook)
https://doi.org/10.1007/978-3-032-01613-3

© The Editor(s) (if applicable) and The Author(s), under exclusive license to Springer Nature Switzerland AG 2025

This work is subject to copyright. All rights are solely and exclusively licensed by the Publisher, whether the whole or part of the material is concerned, specifically the rights of translation, reprinting, reuse of illustrations, recitation, broadcasting, reproduction on microfilms or in any other physical way, and transmission or information storage and retrieval, electronic adaptation, computer software, or by similar or dissimilar methodology now known or hereafter developed.
The use of general descriptive names, registered names, trademarks, service marks, etc. in this publication does not imply, even in the absence of a specific statement, that such names are exempt from the relevant protective laws and regulations and therefore free for general use.
The publisher, the authors and the editors are safe to assume that the advice and information in this book are believed to be true and accurate at the date of publication. Neither the publisher nor the authors or the editors give a warranty, expressed or implied, with respect to the material contained herein or for any errors or omissions that may have been made. The publisher remains neutral with regard to jurisdictional claims in published maps and institutional affiliations.

This Springer imprint is published by the registered company Springer Nature Switzerland AG
The registered company address is: Gewerbestrasse 11, 6330 Cham, Switzerland

If disposing of this product, please recycle the paper.

To my wife Nancy, and our beloved children, Paige, Campion Jr., and Alannah

Your love fills my heart and strengthens my purpose. This book is for you.

Preface

Artificial intelligence has left the auditorium and entered daily rounds. The US Food and Drug Administration lists about 1016 AI or machine learning medical devices as of March 25, 2025, and roughly 9 more join the roster each month. Students and early-career clinicians must now decide when to trust, revise, or reject machine output during every step of patient care.

How This Book Is Organized

Part I: Foundations

You will diagram transformer layers, trace self-attention scores, and show classmates how a single prompt token changes an answer. Master these skills and you can explain any "black-box" result during bedside teaching.

Part II: Clinical Integration

You will design a pilot project, secure stakeholder support, insert legal and ethical checkpoints, and present results that speak to safety and equity. By the final page, you can defend or decline an AI tool with hard evidence, not hype.

Part III: Capstone Practice

Guided rubrics lead you through an AI journal club you can run on rotation. You will refine prompts with Plan-Do-Study-Act cycles and track accuracy, speed, or cost so the team sees measurable value.

Part IV: Professional Growth

Clear roadmaps connect micro-credentials, grant opportunities, and SMART goals to your residency timeline. A closing worksheet turns today's curiosity into tomorrow's expertise.

How You Will Learn

- **Quick-look questions** start each chapter and set the frame.
- **Mid-chapter quizzes** reveal gaps before they harden into habits.
- **Reflection prompts** tie new concepts to last week's patients.
- **Practical drills**—prompt tuning, bias audits, and PDSA cycles—convert theory into bedside routine.
- **Online notebooks, datasets, and a faculty guide** extend the experience beyond the printed page.

Every chapter follows the same reliable rhythm: objectives, concise theory, hands-on practice, takeaway tables, and a "Ready for Rounds" checklist. Sidebars flag regulatory changes, ethical dilemmas, and cautionary case reports. A glossary keeps jargon in check.

Your Guiding Question

Carry this question through every exercise: How will this tool improve patient-centered care where I practice? The answer will change as data shift, software updates, and policies evolve. Work through each quiz, prompt, and drill, and you will build the habit of continuous evaluation that defines responsible stewardship of clinical AI.

Thank you for investing your time and curiosity. May the skills you develop here deepen your clinical reasoning, strengthen teamwork, and, above all, improve the lives of the people who trust you.

New York City, USA
June 2025

Campion Quinn

Contents

Chapter 1
What Is Artificial Intelligence?

Learning Objectives

By the end of this chapter, students will be able to:

- Define artificial intelligence (AI), machine learning (ML), and deep learning (DL) in a clinical context.
- Distinguish between narrow AI, general AI, and augmented intelligence.
- Identify and evaluate current AI tools used in clinical documentation and decision support.
- Recognize common ethical challenges and trust-related concerns in clinical AI use.
- Reflect on the personal and professional implications of working with AI in medicine.

Clinical Vignette: "Assisted Judgment"

Thursday afternoon on the medicine ward, Anna, a third-year student, opens Mr. K.'s chart. The 67-year-old has decompensated heart failure and needs a discharge summary.

A pop-up appears: **"AI Summary Assistant: Auto-generate discharge summary?"** Her busy resident nods. Anna clicks. Within seconds, the draft pulls in medications, hospital course, labs, and yesterday's echo.

Then she spots a problem. The AI claims the ejection fraction "has steadily improved," yet a new echocardiogram, posted 2 h ago, shows it has fallen to 25%. No algorithmic malfunction occurred; the system had not ingested the freshest data, a documented risk in 11% of auto-generated notes [1].

© The Author(s), under exclusive license to Springer Nature Switzerland AG 2025
C. Quinn, *Generative AI for the Medical Student*,
https://doi.org/10.1007/978-3-032-01613-3_1

Rounds begin in 15 min. Anna must decide whether to start over or edit line by line and verify each detail. Speed tempts her, patient safety reminds her to slow down, and the clock keeps ticking.

Anna pauses. The technology is fast, but can it be trusted?

Big-Picture Takeaway: The Evolution of AI in Medicine

Artificial intelligence has already reached the patient's bedside. One public signpost is the Food and Drug Administration's (FDA's) AI/ML-Enabled Medical Devices list. This regularly updated spreadsheet tracks every algorithm cleared through the agency's 510(k), De Novo, or Premarket Approval (PMA) pathways. By April 2025, the list recorded 278 authorized products, most of which were in radiology, yet with an expanding share in cardiology, pathology, and critical care monitoring [2]. For you, a medical student, that number is not trivia; it is a reminder that AI tools you will use on the wards have passed a basic safety and effectiveness review, are tied to specific clinical indications, and must be monitored by the hospital for real-world performance.

So, what exactly is AI? In plain terms, it is software that performs tasks once associated with human thinking, such as identifying patterns in data or generating natural language. In the clinic, this looks like risk scores, draft notes, triage bots, and image classifiers that promise to save time and catch subtle findings. Speed and memory are the big advantages; a trained model can scan thousands of images or lab values in seconds, but that same speed comes with opacity because many models are so complex that their internal logic is difficult to audit.

AI in medicine did not start with today's neural networks. MYCIN, built in the 1970s, relied on fixed if-then rules to suggest antibiotics, proving that computers could assist reasoning but also showing the limits of rigid code [3]. Modern systems learn directly from large datasets, adjusting their parameters as new data arrive. The result is more flexible but also more complicated to govern.

For you, the lesson is clear: you do not need to program a neural network, but you do need to know that an FDA-cleared algorithm addresses a narrowly defined problem, that you remain responsible for clinical judgment, and that oversight mechanisms like post-market surveillance exist to catch drift or bias. The rest of this chapter gives you the vocabulary and critical questions that turn AI from a black box into a dependable partner in patient care.

The Emergence of MYCIN: A Pioneering Medical Expert System

One of the earliest and most influential applications of AI in medicine was the development of MYCIN, an expert system created in the early 1970s at Stanford University. Designed to assist physicians in diagnosing and recommending treatments for bacterial infections, particularly bacteremia and meningitis, MYCIN represented a significant advancement in the application of computer-based reasoning to clinical problems.

Development and Purpose

MYCIN was developed as part of the Stanford Heuristic Programming Project, with Edward H. Shortliffe leading the initiative under the guidance of Bruce G. Buchanan and others. The system aimed to emulate the decision-making abilities of infectious disease experts by using a knowledge base of approximately 600 rules derived from expert consultations.

How MYCIN Worked

The system operated using a backward-chaining inference engine, which started with potential conclusions and worked backward to determine if the available data supported those conclusions (see Fig. 1.1) MYCIN interacted with users through a series of questions about the patient's symptoms, laboratory results, and other relevant information. Based on the responses, it would generate a ranked list of possible pathogens and recommend appropriate antibiotic treatments, adjusting dosages according to patient-specific factors like weight.

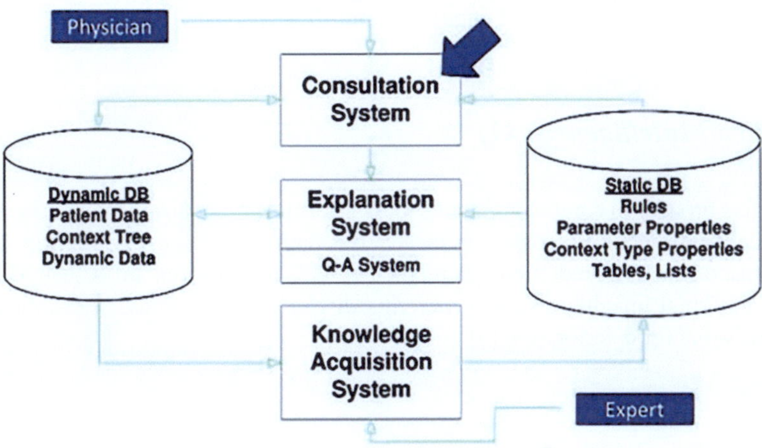

Fig. 1.1 MYCIN architecture

A notable feature of MYCIN was its use of "certainty factors" to handle uncertainty in medical decision-making. These factors quantified the confidence in a particular diagnosis or recommendation, allowing the system to weigh evidence and provide explanations for its conclusions. This approach enabled MYCIN to mimic the nuanced reasoning of human experts, who often deal with incomplete or ambiguous information.

Impact and Legacy

Although MYCIN was never implemented in routine clinical practice, primarily due to ethical, legal, and practical concerns, it had a profound impact on the field of medical informatics. The system demonstrated that computers could effectively replicate complex decision-making processes in medicine, paving the way for future developments in AI and expert systems.

MYCIN's architecture and reasoning methods influenced the design of subsequent AI systems, including the development of EMYCIN ("Essential MYCIN"), a more generalized expert system shell that could be adapted to various domains beyond infectious diseases. The principles established by MYCIN continue to inform the development of clinical decision support systems and AI applications in healthcare today.

Core Concepts in Context

Before using AI responsibly in clinical medicine, you need to understand what it is and what it is not. Although terms like "artificial intelligence," "machine learning," and "deep learning" are often used interchangeably, they represent different AI models with different levels of sophistication.

Artificial Intelligence (AI)

AI refers broadly to computer systems that perform tasks requiring humanlike intelligence. These include recognizing speech, translating languages, identifying visual patterns, or making predictions. In medicine, AI is used for functions such as flagging abnormal imaging results, generating discharge instructions, or estimating a patient's risk for deterioration [4].

Machine Learning (ML)

ML is a subset of AI. These algorithms learn patterns from data rather than following pre-written rules. In supervised learning, the model is trained on labeled data (e.g., chest X-rays marked "pneumonia" or "normal"). In unsupervised learning, the model finds patterns without labels, which helps identify hidden clusters or outliers in large datasets. Reinforcement learning, though less common in clinical practice, uses a feedback loop to optimize decisions over time [5].

Deep Learning (DL)

Deep learning is a specialized form of machine learning (ML) that utilizes artificial neural networks, mathematical systems inspired by the human brain. These models are particularly effective at tasks involving unstructured data, such as images, speech, or free text. DL models power many of the most advanced AI systems in radiology, pathology, and natural language processing [6].

Narrow AI Versus General AI

Most medical AI in use today is *narrow AI*. These models are trained to perform a single task, such as identifying pneumonia on a chest X-ray or predicting sepsis risk. They are fast and often highly accurate within their domain. However, they cannot generalize or reason beyond the data on which they were trained. *General AI*, that type of artificial intelligence capable of mimicking broad human cognition and potentially becoming our robot overlords, remains theoretical and is not used in clinical care [7].

Augmented Intelligence

In healthcare, the term *augmented intelligence* is increasingly preferred. It underscores that AI is a tool designed to support, not replace, clinicians [4]. For example, an AI model may highlight an abnormal CT finding, but the radiologist still interprets its relevance in the full clinical context. The best results are achieved when humans and machines work together.

Several key developments have marked the evolution of LLMs, they include the following:

- **GPT (Generative Pre-trained Transformer)**: Introduced by OpenAI, GPT was the first model to leverage the transformer architecture for natural language generation. GPT-1, released in 2018, demonstrated the power of pre-training a model on large amounts of text before fine-tuning it for specific tasks [8, 9].
- **BERT (Bidirectional Encoder Representations from Transformers)**: Developed by Google in 2018, BERT introduced a new approach to natural language understanding by training models to consider both the left and right context of words. This bidirectional training enhanced the accuracy of text comprehension tasks, such as question-answering and sentiment analysis [10].
- **Transformer Architecture**: The transformer model, introduced in 2017, revolutionized AI by replacing the sequential processing of previous models with parallel processing. This architecture utilizes self-attention mechanisms to assess the importance of words or phrases within a specific context, enabling faster training and more accurate predictions. It serves as the foundation for all subsequent large language models (LLMs), including specialized medical models such as Med-PaLM [8].

Why Transformers Have Revolutionized AI

Transformers have fundamentally changed the landscape of AI due to their ability to:

- **Process large datasets efficiently:** Unlike previous architectures, transformers can process entire sequences of text simultaneously, rather than word by word, thereby greatly improving speed and accuracy.
- **Understand complex context:** By using attention mechanisms, transformers can evaluate relationships between elements across an entire input, understanding the overall context.
- **Scale effectively:** The parallel processing capability allows for scaling to much larger datasets and model sizes than previous architectures, enabling the development of massive models like GPT-3, GPT-4, and Med-PaLM.

This parallel processing ability is particularly important in clinical applications where numerous data points—symptoms, diagnostic tests, and medications—must be considered simultaneously to generate coherent insights.

Attention Mechanisms: How Transformers "Pay Attention"

The key innovation of transformers is their use of attention mechanisms. Attention mechanisms allow models to determine which parts of an input are most relevant to understanding the overall meaning. In traditional AI models, input text was processed sequentially, word by word, making it challenging to capture long-range dependencies or complex relationships within the text. Transformers solve this problem by applying self-attention to the entire input simultaneously.

Think of self-attention as a high-speed highlighter. The transformer compares every word in a sentence with every other word and assigns a score that says "focus here" or "mostly ignore." In a clinical note, those scores bind together phrases like "chest pain," "dyspnea," and "electrocardiogram (ECG) changes" while giving little weight to filler words such as "the." The model then rebuilds the sentence so that high-scoring terms carry more influence. Because this weighting occurs for all words simultaneously, the algorithm maintains the entire clinical context in view, rather than working in short, disconnected chunks as older systems did [8].

Why does this matter to you? When you prompt a generative AI system, self-attention helps it pull the key symptoms, test results, and time cues out of your text. The summary or differential it produces is therefore more coherent and less likely to skip a critical finding. Knowing this mechanism reminds you to enter complete, well-structured information and to confirm that the output reflects every element you deem important.

How Large Language Models Are Trained

Training large language models involves processing enormous datasets through complex architectures, such as transformers [8]. This training process comprises two main phases: pre-training and fine-tuning [10]. To ensure clinical relevance, generative AI models must be trained on high-quality datasets, carefully curated to address the specific needs of healthcare professionals [11, 12].

Explanation of Datasets Used in Training

- **Public Sources:** Models like GPT-3 and GPT-4 are initially trained on vast amounts of publicly available text, including books, articles, websites, and other Internet-based content. This diverse data provides a broad foundational understanding of human language, grammar, semantics, and various domains of knowledge. However, general-purpose models may lack the specificity required for medical applications unless properly fine-tuned. Without specialized training, a model might misinterpret medical terminology or fail to provide clinically accurate recommendations.
- **Specialized Medical Datasets:** For clinical applications, training data must be curated to include clinical notes, research articles, clinical guidelines, medical textbooks, patient-physician interactions, and de-identified patient data. Specialized datasets enhance the model's ability to understand medical terminology, interpret clinical findings, and generate responses relevant to healthcare pro-

fessionals. High-quality, domain-specific data is essential to improve diagnostic accuracy, enhance decision-making support, and ensure clinical relevance. Med-PaLM, for example, is a medical-specific model fine-tuned using a combination of medical literature, clinical guidelines, and structured patient data. This process enables it to achieve higher accuracy in generating diagnostic suggestions and summarizing clinical notes.

Overview of the Training Process

Before a generative AI model can assist with clinical reasoning or documentation, it must undergo a structured training process that shapes how it understands and responds to language. This process occurs in two main phases—pre-training and fine-tuning—each of which plays a distinct role in preparing the model for safe and effective use in healthcare settings:

- **Pre-Training Phase:** During pre-training, the model is exposed to large datasets and learns to predict the next word or sequence of words within a given context. This unsupervised learning approach allows the model to develop a generalized understanding of language patterns, syntax, and context. This phase helps establish a broad foundational knowledge, but models trained on general datasets may lack clinical accuracy. Therefore, pre-training serves as a necessary but insufficient step for medical applications.
- **Fine-Tuning Phase:** Fine-tuning involves training the model on specialized, high-quality datasets to tailor its performance to specific applications. For healthcare, this phase includes training on clinical data to enhance accuracy and reliability in generating diagnostic information, summarizing clinical notes, or suggesting treatment recommendations. In clinical practice, fine-tuning ensures that models can generate clinically valid and reliable information. Fine-tuning using Health Insurance Portability and Accountability Act (HIPAA)-compliant datasets enhances the model's ability to accurately interpret clinical notes while maintaining patient privacy.

Importance of Data Quality and Dataset Size

The quality and size of the training dataset significantly affect the model's performance. Poor-quality data or insufficiently diverse datasets can introduce biases, reduce diagnostic accuracy, or limit the model's ability to generalize. In clinical applications, the inclusion of high-quality, peer-reviewed literature, accurately labeled clinical notes, and validated patient data is crucial.

The Concept of Tokens and Tokenization

Models process text by breaking it down into smaller units known as tokens. Tokenization converts words, phrases, or characters into numerical representations the model can process. Effective tokenization is vital because it impacts comprehension, efficiency, and the coherence of generated outputs [13]. In clinical practice, accurate tokenization ensures that complex medical terminology, abbreviations, and numerical data (such as laboratory values) are appropriately understood and utilized by the model. For instance, if a model encounters the phrase "BP 120/80," improper tokenization could result in a failure to recognize this as a standard blood pressure measurement [14]. Fine-tuning helps ensure that medical terminology is accurately processed and interpreted [15].

Addressing Bias and Ensuring Reliability

Bias in AI models can arise when the data used during training are unbalanced, outdated, or reflect systemic inequities in healthcare delivery [16]. For example, if a model is trained primarily on patients from one demographic group, its predictions may be less accurate for individuals outside that group. This can lead to errors in diagnosis, treatment recommendations, or risk assessments, especially in populations already underserved by the healthcare system.

To minimize bias and enhance clinical reliability, developers employ several key strategies. First, they train models on large, diverse, and representative datasets that reflect the full spectrum of patient populations [17]. This helps ensure that the model performs consistently across age groups, ethnicities, and clinical conditions. Second, clinician input is incorporated during the fine-tuning phase, allowing experts to flag unsafe outputs and guide the model toward clinically sound reasoning [18]. Finally, models must be regularly updated to align with evolving medical standards, new guidelines, and changes in practice patterns. Without these safeguards, even a well-designed model can drift from clinical reality and become unreliable over time [19].

Integration with Clinical Workflows

To be truly useful in clinical practice, models must integrate seamlessly with existing systems like electronic health records (EHRs). Proper integration allows AI tools to provide decision support, generate clinical notes, and offer diagnostic insights directly within the physician's workflow [4].

Key Takeaways for Physicians Regarding Training:

- Training is a multiphase process involving pre-training on general text and fine-tuning with specialized clinical data.
- Fine-tuning enhances the model's relevance and accuracy for medical applications.
- Data privacy and regulatory compliance are essential when training models for clinical use.
- Biases must be addressed to ensure reliable and unbiased decision support.
- Effective tokenization is critical for accurate comprehension of medical terminology.

How Generative AI Produces Responses

Generative AI models produce responses through a systematic process involving probability calculations, prediction mechanisms, and sampling techniques. When presented with input data, such as a clinical question or a set of patient symptoms, the model processes the text by breaking it down into tokens and transforming these tokens into numerical representations. Using attention mechanisms, the model identifies the most relevant tokens and applies weights to prioritize significant information.

During response generation, the model relies on probability calculations to determine which words or phrases are most likely to follow based on the input provided. These predictions are derived from patterns the model has learned during training. Once the model generates probabilities for potential outputs, it employs sampling techniques to produce a coherent text. Standard sampling methods include greedy decoding, beam search, and temperature scaling.

Understanding this process helps you become a more effective and skeptical user of AI tools. You'll know that the model isn't pulling facts from a textbook; it's making predictions based on patterns. That means it can sometimes sound confident but be wrong. As a future physician, your job is to use AI as a support tool, not a final authority.

Step-by-Step Breakdown of How Prompts Are Processed:

1. **Input reception:** The model receives a prompt and converts it into tokens (numerical representations of words or phrases).
2. **Encoding:** The tokens are passed through the encoder, which applies self-attention mechanisms to identify relevant information and establish contextual relationships. The encoder evaluates each token by comparing it to every other token in the sequence, determining which pieces of information are most important.
3. **Contextual understanding:** The model interprets the tokens in relation to one another based on the attention scores assigned during encoding, prioritizing significant words or phrases while disregarding less relevant information.
4. **Prediction calculation:** The model calculates probabilities for all possible next tokens by analyzing learned patterns, predicting the most likely continuations.
5. **Sampling and output generation:** The model generates a response by selecting tokens according to these probabilities, using sampling methods.
6. **Common sampling methods:** When a large language model (LLM) generates text, it predicts the next token based on preceding context. This prediction comes in the form of a probability distribution across all possible tokens in its vocabulary. Several sampling methods then determine how the LLM selects the final token from this distribution, each impacting generated text's creativity, cohence and diversity. These sampling methods include: Greedy Decoding, Beam Search and Temperature Scaling.

   - **Greedy decoding:** Selects the highest probability token at each step. This produces predictable and structured outputs but can be overly rigid. Example application: generating a discharge summary from clinical notes where consistency is prioritized.
   - **Beam search:** Generates multiple potential sequences and evaluates them before selecting the most probable one. This improves coherence but can sometimes produce generic outputs that overlook specific details. Example application: generating a differential diagnosis list where completeness is important, but it may struggle to identify uncommon conditions.

- **Temperature scaling:** Adjusts the probability distribution to control creativity and variability:
  - **Lower temperature settings** produce more conservative and focused outputs, useful for generating diagnostic recommendations where accuracy is paramount.
  - **Higher temperatures** encourage diversity in the generated text, valuable for brainstorming treatment options or producing patient education materials that require a conversational tone.
  - The quality of the output depends on the quality of the training data, the sophistication of the attention mechanisms, and the appropriateness of the sampling techniques. Errors can occur when the model encounters scenarios for which it has insufficient training data or when it fails to correctly prioritize relevant information. Clinicians must be aware of these limitations and exercise caution when interpreting AI-generated outputs.

Limitations and Challenges of Generative AI

While generative AI offers significant potential, it is not without limitations. Understanding these is essential for clinicians.

Common Issues with Generative AI Outputs:

- **Hallucinations:** Producing plausible but factually incorrect or irrelevant information. This stems from relying on probability rather than genuine comprehension, incomplete/biased data, misinterpreting context, or overreliance on high-probability token generation. Hallucinations can lead to incorrect diagnoses, inappropriate treatment, flawed documentation, and misleading patient education. Clinicians must remain vigilant, critically assessing AI-generated outputs and validating them against clinical guidelines.
- **Bias:** Training data biases lead to skewed responses that may disproportionately affect minority or underrepresented groups, potentially resulting in suboptimal care. Addressing these biases requires using diverse and representative datasets, incorporating clinician feedback, and regularly updating models.
- **"Garbage In, Garbage Out":** The reliability of outputs is directly influenced by the quality of the training data. Poor-quality or incomplete datasets result in inaccurate, biased, or even harmful outputs.
- **Inadequate Contextual Understanding:** Difficulty integrating diverse information or recognizing subtleties, leading to potentially inappropriate or incomplete recommendations in complex cases. AI tools may overlook important subtleties in patient history or fail to recognize rare findings.

Ethical Considerations and the Importance of Human Oversight

As generative AI becomes more common in clinical settings, it brings not only powerful capabilities but also serious ethical responsibilities. One primary concern is patient privacy. AI models must be trained and utilized in a manner that complies with HIPAA and safeguards confidential health information. This is especially important when models are exposed to clinical notes, test results, or other sensitive data.

Bias is another concern. If the data used to train these systems reflects existing disparities in healthcare, such as unequal access to care or underrepresentation of certain groups, the AI may reinforce those inequities. That's why it's essential to use diverse, high-quality datasets and to involve clinicians in reviewing and fine-tuning these tools.

Transparency also matters. Clinicians need to understand how an AI system arrived at its suggestion, especially in high-stakes situations like diagnosis or treatment planning. Even without knowing all the technical details, physicians should be able to ask: "Why did the model say this?"

Accountability rests with the clinician, not the algorithm. AI tools can generate responses that sound fluent and confident, but that doesn't mean they're correct. These models don't truly understand medicine—they identify patterns in text. This can lead to what's called the "illusion of precision," where the language appears expert, even if the content is wrong or misleading.

This is why human oversight is essential. Before acting on an AI-generated recommendation, clinicians must ask whether it makes clinical sense. They should verify outputs against trusted guidelines, peer-reviewed literature, or their own judgment. AI can support clinical decisions—but it should never replace clinical reasoning. As future physicians, your responsibility is to lead with critical thinking, using AI as a tool, not a crutch.

How to Mitigate Limitations

As a future physician, you will likely rely on AI tools to assist with clinical documentation, decision support, and summarizing patient data. But these systems are not infallible. To use them responsibly, it's essential to understand how their limitations can be managed and what role you play in that process.

One strategy is *Reinforcement Learning with Human Feedback* (RLHF). In this method, AI systems are fine-tuned using input from clinicians who assess whether the model's outputs are accurate, clinically relevant, and aligned with medical standards. This approach has shown success in models like Med-PaLM, which was trained on medical datasets with physician input to improve its diagnostic accuracy and reduce hallucinations [20]. Commercial tools such as Nuance Dragon Medical One and Suki AI also incorporate real-time clinician feedback to continuously refine their outputs [21, 22].

Training data diversity is another key factor. When AI systems are developed using datasets that underrepresent certain populations, they risk amplifying existing health disparities. Research has shown that models trained predominantly on data from majority populations may underperform in racially and socioeconomically diverse groups [16]. Incorporating representative datasets improves generalizability and equity in care delivery.

Clinician feedback loops—built into some EHR-integrated AI systems—allow users to flag mistakes or suggest corrections. These mechanisms serve as continuous quality improvement tools, helping developers update and refine model behavior in real-world environments [17]. As a user, reporting model errors contributes directly to the safety and accuracy of future outputs.

Transparency is also critical. Although generative models can appear to "reason," they actually only simulate patterns based on statistical likelihood. Tools such as SHAP (SHapley Additive exPlanations) and LIME (Local Interpretable Model-agnostic Explanations) make AI outputs more interpretable by highlighting which features influenced a given prediction [23]. While you don't need to master these tools, you should feel empowered to ask, "Why did the model recommend this?"

Finally, *human oversight* remains paramount. AI should enhance—not replace—your clinical judgment. A 2024 position statement by the American Medical Association emphasized that clinicians bear ultimate responsibility for verifying AI-generated suggestions against established clinical guidelines and peer-reviewed evidence [24]. Even when an AI system sounds confident, its fluency does not necessarily equate to correctness.

Practical tips for physicians include cross-referencing AI outputs, using explainability tools (like IBM AI Explainability 360 and Google's What-If Tool), providing structured feedback through formal channels, ensuring ethical compliance (especially HIPAA), and monitoring AI performance over time.

Clinical Algorithms: A Foundational Precursor

AI is often layered on top of traditional *clinical algorithms,* decision trees, or flowcharts that guide diagnosis and treatment. While static algorithms follow rigid rules (e.g., if blood pressure > 180/110, give antihypertensives), AI systems can learn and adapt based on new data. Still, both aim to improve consistency, reduce error, and optimize care. Understanding this lineage helps clarify AI's role: not a radical departure, but an evolution of clinical decision tools.

Types of Clinical Algorithms

As AI evolves, it often builds upon or integrates with traditional clinical algorithms, structured processes used to guide decision-making. Understanding these categories can help you recognize where AI fits in:

- **Diagnostic algorithms** aim to identify disease (e.g., chest pain workups, rule-out MI pathways) [6].
- **Treatment algorithms** recommend interventions based on established criteria (e.g., hypertension guidelines) [25].
- **Predictive algorithms** estimate future outcomes (e.g., likelihood of readmission, ICU transfer) [26].
- **Prescriptive algorithms** take it a step further, recommending actions based on predicted outcomes (e.g., automatically adjusting insulin doses) [27].

AI-enhanced systems can perform all four functions, sometimes simultaneously (see Fig. 1.2) For instance, a sepsis prediction model may recognize clinical deterioration, suggest initiating antibiotics, and predict mortality risk, all based on continuously updated patient data [28].

Clinical Relevance

As a medical student, you're just starting to see how complex clinical decision-making can be—and how time-consuming documentation often is. You may not realize it yet, but artificial intelligence is already quietly working behind the scenes in many hospitals and clinics. While you won't need to program these tools, you *will* need to understand what they're doing and how to use them wisely.

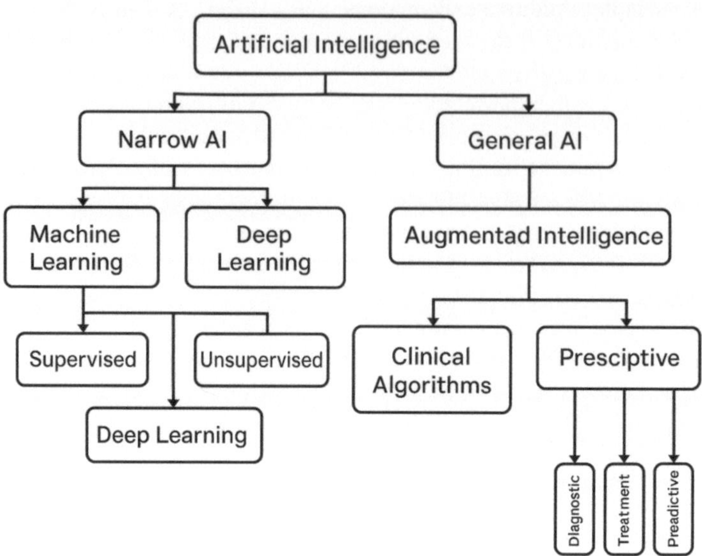

Fig. 1.2 Types of clinical algorithms and their relationship to AI

In practice, AI commonly shows up in three ways. First, there are *decision support* tools that work inside the electronic health record (EHR). These might flag abnormal lab values, suggest possible diagnoses, or prompt you to consider specific tests. Second, AI helps with *documentation*, using natural language models to draft or summarize clinical notes based on what you dictate or type. Third, *risk prediction* models review a patient's chart and calculate the likelihood of complications, such as sepsis, readmission, or in-hospital death.

These tools are designed to save time and reduce errors, but they aren't perfect. If used carelessly, they can lead to misdiagnosis or inappropriate treatment. Your role isn't to design these systems, but to engage with them critically. Ask yourself: Does this suggestion make clinical sense? Is there a better explanation? Can I back this up with evidence?

Using AI in medicine requires more than curiosity—it requires judgment. Your responsibility is to understand what these tools are good at, where they fall short, and how to integrate them into safe, evidence-based care.

Why It Matters

These distinctions are not just academic. Suppose you're using an AI system in the hospital, whether for documentation, diagnosis, or triage, you need to know how it was trained, what kind of data it uses, and what type of problem it's designed to solve. A deep learning model can excel at image recognition without needing to explain its reasoning. A machine learning model trained on outdated data may propagate past bias. Without conceptual fluency, you risk trusting a system you don't fully understand.

Real Tools Used Today

Artificial intelligence is no longer confined to academic research or speculative headlines. It is increasingly integrated into the daily tools used by physicians, residents, and medical students. From documentation aids to risk stratification models and adaptive learning platforms, AI systems are reshaping how clinicians interact with information, patients, and technology. Understanding these tools—and their limitations—is essential for any future practitioner.

One of the most prominent developments in medical AI is the emergence of large language models capable of clinical reasoning. Domain-tuned models such as Med-PaLM scored 67% on USMLE-style questions, clearing the usual 60% pass mark [29]. In comparison, GPT-4 reached 78% on full NBME practice forms [30], about 1.5 standard deviations above the average student score [31]. These numbers show that AI can match or exceed typical test performance, yet each model still commits errors that require clinician review.

OpenAI's GPT-4, a more general-purpose model, is now being incorporated into applications such as Microsoft Copilot, UpToDate AI, and Doximity DocsGPT. These tools summarize medical records, explain disease mechanisms, or generate clinical notes based on structured prompts. For students, these systems can support learning by helping synthesize complex material, but they still carry the risk of hallucinated or inaccurate outputs. Critical appraisal and human oversight remain essential.

AlphaFold, another major contribution from DeepMind, has advanced the field of molecular medicine by predicting three-dimensional protein structures from amino acid sequences [32, 33]. While this tool does not operate at the bedside, its influence on drug discovery and protein modeling is profound. Medical students are beginning to encounter its applications in pharmacology, oncology, and basic science modules focused on protein folding diseases and structure-guided therapy [34].

In clinical environments, several AI-powered tools are transforming the documentation process. Epic's NoteWriter is integrated into the electronic health record and assists with generating templated notes based on real-time inputs [35]. Abridge listens to clinician-patient conversations and drafts a structured SOAP note for review [36]. Nabla Copilot, designed for primary care and telehealth, uses AI to generate visit summaries, offer ICD-10 suggestions, and streamline follow-up instructions [37]. These systems can significantly reduce the cognitive and clerical burden of note-writing, particularly during busy rotations. However, students must learn to carefully verify and edit machine-generated content, as even minor errors in the medical record can lead to downstream consequences [38].

AI is also playing a growing role in clinical decision support. At institutions such as Duke University, tools like Sepsis Watch use real-time electronic health record data to predict the onset of sepsis several hours before traditional criteria are met [28]. Other models, including those integrated into Epic and Cerner platforms, forecast readmission risk, heart failure decompensation, or likelihood of ICU transfer. These predictions often appear as silent alerts or risk scores embedded within the workflow. For students, these tools are useful not only for anticipating deterioration but also for learning how algorithms interpret trends in lab values, vitals, and notes [39]. Yet these systems are not perfect; false positives, alert fatigue [40], and lack of transparency can undermine their effectiveness if not managed appropriately [41].

Sidebar: What Is Alert Fatigue?
Alert fatigue occurs when clinicians become desensitized to frequent notifications from clinical decision support systems, leading them to ignore or override both low-priority and high-urgency warnings. In AI-driven environments, this risk increases as predictive models generate more real-time alerts. When too many notifications compete for attention, it becomes harder to distinguish critical warnings from minor noise. The result is reduced trust in the system, slower clinical responses, and the potential for missed emergencies. Designing AI tools that balance sensitivity with clinical relevance is essential to reducing alert fatigue and preserving clinician attention.

AI in Medical Education: From Assessment to Adaptive Learning
Artificial intelligence is becoming increasingly embedded in medical education, not only in how students study but also in how they are assessed. One important example is the Objective Structured Clinical Examination, or OSCE. OSCEs are widely used in medical training to evaluate key clinical skills, such as communication, physical exam technique, diagnostic reasoning, and ethical judgment, under standardized conditions. Students rotate through a series of timed stations, each presenting a clinical scenario with a standardized patient or actor. Faculty assess the student's performance using structured rubrics, making OSCEs a cornerstone of competency-based education.

Today, AI is being used to both *generate* and *evaluate* OSCE stations. For instance, some platforms now use generative AI to design realistic clinical vignettes in ethics, communication, and reasoning. Others employ AI-driven avatars—simulated patients with verbal and emotional responses that adapt to the learner's tone, empathy, and word choice. This creates dynamic and individualized encounters that mimic real-world patient interactions [42]. These systems can also provide real-time feedback, helping students develop communication and empathy skills more effectively than static case materials.

Beyond simulation, AI is also being applied to assessment. Natural language processing models are now used at select institutions to evaluate students' written clinical rationales and open-ended exam responses. These tools can deliver structured feedback on reasoning, completeness, and clarity—offering formative input while reducing the burden on faculty graders [43]. While these technologies remain in early stages of deployment, there are ongoing concerns about fairness, transparency, and student trust. Ensuring these systems do not inadvertently penalize diverse communication styles or reasoning approaches is a critical area of ongoing research and oversight.

Meanwhile, adaptive learning platforms have become popular among students preparing for high-stakes exams or reviewing complex material. AI-powered tools like *Osmosis AI*, *Firecracker*, and *Jasper Health* analyze a student's learning behavior and quiz performance to identify knowledge gaps and generate targeted review materials. For example, a student struggling with cardiovascular physiology might receive a personalized learning plan that includes multiple-choice questions, animated explainer videos, and flashcards emphasizing high-yield cardiology content [44]. These platforms enable self-paced learning and reinforce mastery through repetition and spaced retrieval.

Interactive simulation platforms like *Body Interact* go even further, placing students in virtual clinical scenarios where they manage patient care. The patient's condition changes based on the learner's actions—mirroring the unpredictability of real clinical environments and offering immediate feedback [45].

Across all of these examples, the key takeaway is this: AI is no longer a distant future in medical education; it is already part of how students learn, communicate, and prepare for clinical care. Each tool adds new capabilities, but also new responsibilities. As a future clinician, it's not enough to ask whether an AI tool is helpful. You must ask how it works, what data it draws from, whether it has been validated, and how its suggestions should be interpreted. In the next chapter, we'll move from learning about AI tools to learning how to talk to them by crafting prompts that are clinically precise and context-aware.

Prompt Challenge

Why Prompting Matters

Prompt design is one of the most practical skills you can develop when working with large language models. This involves providing AI systems with clear, specific, and well-structured instructions. Prompting is not just for computer scientists. In the clinical setting, your ability to frame a question or summarize a case effectively can directly influence the quality and safety of AI-generated output.

Practice Exercise: Audience Adaptation

Begin with this exercise. Try asking a generative AI tool, "Describe artificial intelligence to a first-year medical student in 100 words." Then try adjusting your prompt for a different audience again: "Explain artificial intelligence to a patient with no medical background." Notice how the language, tone, and level of detail shift depending on the audience. This is more than a communication trick. It is a form of diagnostic reasoning. You are adapting how information is generated to meet the needs of a specific clinical or educational context.

Spot the Weak Prompt

Now examine a poorly constructed prompt such as: "Write me a good diagnosis for this patient." Why is this ineffective? The question is vague and underspecified and ignores context. A more effective prompt might read: "Given a 55-year-old male with chest pain, ST elevations in V2 through V4, and elevated troponin, what is the most likely diagnosis and what should be done next?"

Structuring Clinical Prompts

Think of writing a prompt as having a consultation with an AI colleague. The more structured and complete your request, the more clinically useful the output will be. Use the six-part Clinical LLM Prompt Template below to guide your thinking (see Table. 1.1).

This prompt template turns a vague question into a structured dialogue that large language models can follow reliably. Begin by filling in the Patient Snapshot and Clinical Task, so the model knows who the case involves and what you want. Add concrete vitals, labs, and imaging under Key Data to ground the response in objective facts. Specify the Audience and Tone to match the output to either professional colleagues or lay readers, and then set any Output Constraints such as word count or citation style to keep the answer concise and citable. Finally, include a Safety Check that instructs the model to flag missing information or potential contraindications. Completing all six fields produces a reproducible prompt that reduces hallucinations, makes the model's reasoning transparent, and speeds your review process when incorporating AI-generated content into patient notes or study materials.

By using this template to create prompts, you will build habits that mirror how you'll communicate with real-world AI tools, concise, complete, and clinically clear.

Table 1.1 Clinical prompt template

Clinical LLM prompt template	
1	**Patient snapshot** Start with a one-line summary that includes age, sex, and the reason for presentation. *Example:* "42-year-old woman with type 2 diabetes, hypertension, and 3-day history of pleuritic chest pain."
2	**Clinical task** Clearly state what you want the AI to do, generate a note, offer a differential, or explain a finding. *Example:* "Generate a focused SOAP note," or "list a three-item differential diagnosis."
3	**Key data** Include vitals, laboratory values, imaging findings, active medications, and any relevant past history. *Example:* "BP 138/82 mm hg, troponin I 0.03 ng/mL, CT angiogram negative for PE."
4	**Audience and tone** Indicate who the output is for and how it should sound, patient-friendly, or suitable for a resident or attending. *Example:* "Explain in patient-friendly language," or "write for a PGY-1 resident."
5	**Output constraints** Word limit, bullet versus prose, citation style, or formatting requests. *Example:* "No more than 150 words, use bullet points, cite sources in AMA style."
6	**Safety check** Instruct the model to flag missing data, contraindications, or uncertainty. *Example:* "If information is insufficient to form a safe plan, state 'additional data required'."

Clinical Reasoning in a Digital Age
As a clinician-in-training, learning to prompt effectively mirrors your broader diagnostic reasoning process. Whether drafting a note, summarizing a case, or requesting a consultation, the clarity of your thinking will shape the clarity of your communication—with patients, with colleagues, and increasingly, with machines.

Ethics and Equity Checkpoint

As artificial intelligence becomes more embedded in clinical workflows, it brings not only new opportunities but also serious ethical and equity challenges. These are not just theoretical concerns. They directly affect the safety, fairness, and trustworthiness of the care we deliver.

Algorithmic Opacity and Accountability
As a medical student, you're learning to justify clinical decisions based on evidence, guidelines, and patient context. But what happens when an AI system makes a recommendation, like flagging a patient as high risk for sepsis, and you can't explain why? This is the problem of *algorithmic opacity*. Many advanced AI systems, especially those built on deep learning architectures, are considered "black boxes" because their internal reasoning is difficult to interpret, even by their developers [46]. In medicine, this opacity complicates clinical accountability. If harm occurs due to an AI-generated suggestion, who bears responsibility: the physician who used it, the institution that approved it, or the company that built it? These questions remain unsettled in both clinical and legal settings [47].

Explainability and Clinical Trust
For AI to be useful in healthcare, it must be *explainable*. Explainability refers to the ability of a system to communicate the reasoning behind its output in a way that humans can understand and evaluate. Without it, AI can undermine rather than support clinical reasoning. Research shows that clinicians are less likely to trust and adopt AI tools when the decision-making process is unclear, even if the outputs are accurate [41]. Tools such as SHAP (SHapley Additive exPlanations) and LIME (Local Interpretable Model-agnostic Explanations) attempt to bridge this gap by showing which inputs most influenced a prediction [23]. These tools are still evolving, but they represent a critical step toward building systems that support, rather than replace, human judgment.

Bias and Health Equity
Bias in AI systems can worsen the very inequities that medicine seeks to address. AI models learn from existing healthcare data, and those data often reflect systemic disparities in access, treatment, and outcomes. For example, one study found that a widely used algorithm underestimated the health needs of Black patients compared to White patients with similar disease burdens because it relied on healthcare

spending as a proxy for illness severity [16]. If left uncorrected, such biases can lead to misdiagnosis or undertreatment of already marginalized groups.

In response to these concerns, the US Food and Drug Administration (FDA) issued its 2025 *Draft Guidance on Managing Bias in Device Learning Algorithms* [48]. The guidance encourages developers to evaluate performance across demographic subgroups and report the results transparently. It also emphasizes the need for representative training datasets and ongoing model evaluation after deployment. Without these safeguards, AI could entrench inequities rather than correct them.

Finally, the FDA calls attention to disparities in access to AI-enabled tools themselves. Suppose these technologies are only deployed in large academic centers or well-funded health systems. In that case, they may widen the gap between high- and low-resource settings, making the promise of AI one more factor in unequal care delivery. The 2025 FDA draft guidance on *Managing Bias in Device Learning Algorithms* directly addresses this concern. It urges developers to proactively identify and mitigate sources of bias at every stage of the model life cycle, from data curation and labeling to validation and deployment. The agency recommends stratified performance testing across demographic subgroups and emphasizes the importance of transparent reporting on model performance in diverse populations.

As a future clinician, your role will not be to build these models, but to understand their limitations, ask critical questions, and apply your judgment before acting on their suggestions.

Bias and Health Equity

Bias in AI models is not just a technical flaw; it's a clinical and ethical hazard. These models learn from historical data, which often reflects long-standing inequities in healthcare delivery. As a result, algorithms may inherit and even amplify disparities in diagnosis, treatment, and outcomes. For example, a risk prediction tool trained predominantly on White patients may misclassify disease severity in patients from underrepresented racial or ethnic groups.

Moreover, the guidance acknowledges disparities in access to AI-enabled devices and encourages equitable distribution in both high-resource and under-resourced settings. Without these safeguards, AI could entrench existing inequities rather than correct them.

Designing for Ethical Use

Ethical design means accounting for these risks from the beginning. Developers, institutions, and clinicians must ask: Does this model work equally well for all groups? What data were used to train it? Can it be audited or improved if it underperforms for a particular population?

The Role of the Medical Student

As a medical student, you are in a position to ask these questions early. You are not expected to solve them on your own. But your awareness of explainability, accountability, and fairness will shape how these tools are implemented in the years ahead.

AI in medicine is not just a technical evolution—it is an ethical one. The habits you build now in questioning, validating, and critiquing AI systems will help ensure they remain tools of equity rather than engines of harm.

Reflection Questions

These questions are designed to help you process and apply the material from this chapter. As generative AI becomes a routine part of clinical workflows, developing self-awareness, critical thinking, and ethical sensitivity will be essential. Use the prompts below to explore how you might integrate AI into your own clinical reasoning, responsibly, thoughtfully, and with a healthy balance of curiosity and skepticism.

Building Self-Awareness

- Where have you seen or used AI tools in your academic or clinical training so far? How did they affect your work or thinking?
- Reflect on the clinical vignette from the beginning of this chapter. If you were in Anna's position, how would you decide whether to accept, revise, or reject the AI-generated discharge summary?

Application and Skepticism

- What would you say to a colleague or attending who believes AI cannot be trusted in clinical care?
- Are there specific clinical tasks where you think AI tools are especially helpful or especially risky? Why?

Ethical Insight

- What is one ethical or equity concern about medical AI that stood out to you in this chapter? How might you bring that awareness into your future clinical practice?

Quick Recap Box

Artificial intelligence is already integrated into many aspects of modern clinical workflows, especially in documentation, risk prediction, and decision support. Most current tools rely on narrow AI models designed for specific tasks like image interpretation or discharge summary generation. These systems frequently use machine learning or deep learning methods to detect patterns, make predictions, or generate content.

Medical students do not need to become computer scientists, but they need to understand the tools they will likely encounter during training. This includes gaining fluency in the structure of prompts, awareness of how bias can affect AI performance, and the importance of maintaining clinical oversight even when technology appears helpful. As the field evolves, your ability to use AI wisely will become as essential as any physical exam skill.

What Would You Do?

Your attending has begun using an AI tool to auto-generate all discharge summaries for patients leaving the hospital. During your rotation, you notice that the tool consistently omits key psychosocial details, such as unstable housing, caregiver availability, or language barriers, that are essential for safe transitions of care. These details are clearly documented in the chart, but the AI does not incorporate them [49].

You feel uncomfortable signing off on the summaries without adding these important elements. At the same time, you worry about disrupting the workflow or appearing critical of the attending's enthusiasm for the new technology. As a third-year medical student, your authority is limited, but your responsibility to patient safety is not.

What should you do? Should you edit the summaries to include the omitted details? Should you raise the issue with the attending physician or bring it to the attention of the broader clinical team? Is there a professional and constructive way to raise questions about AI-generated documentation while maintaining collegiality?

This is more than a theoretical exercise. As a student, you may be one of the first people to notice when an AI tool produces outputs that are technically accurate but clinically incomplete. In this case, the AI-generated summary risks undermining the quality of the discharge plan by omitting critical social determinants of health. These oversights can lead to readmissions, medication errors, or unmet post-discharge needs.

Stepping in does not mean rejecting AI; it means ensuring that its outputs are interpreted and supplemented with human insight. Consider approaching the attending with curiosity rather than confrontation. For example: "I noticed the AI tool left out some of the social history. Do you think we should add that before finalizing the note?" This kind of question shows initiative and clinical judgment without undermining the attending's use of new technology.

In team-based care, even medical students can influence safety and quality. Learning when and how to speak up, particularly in response to technology-generated content, is a vital skill for the AI era. Discuss with your peers or instructors how you might handle this situation. What strategies promote both patient safety and respectful communication in environments shaped by rapidly evolving tools?

Use this scenario to reflect on how emerging technologies challenge traditional hierarchies of authority and how you, as a learner, can be an advocate for responsible innovation in clinical care.

Sidebar: AI in the News

In recent years, AI has captured national headlines with its performance on standardized exams and its rapid integration into hospital systems.

In 2023, researchers demonstrated that GPT-4, a large language model developed by OpenAI, could pass the USMLE Step 1 and Step 2 Clinical Knowledge exams with scores exceeding the median performance of medical students. This result sparked widespread discussion about whether AI could 1 day assist—or even replace—certain aspects of clinical reasoning and test preparation.

In 2024, Epic Systems began rolling out an AI-powered discharge summary tool integrated into its EHR. While early adopters praised the tool's efficiency, clinicians quickly identified critical flaws. These included incorrect medication dosages, omission of recent lab results, and inaccurate descriptions of clinical encounters. These early cases illustrate a key tension in AI integration: speed versus safety.

These developments raise important legal and ethical questions. Should AI-generated documentation be held to the same standards as human-authored notes? If an AI makes a mistake, who bears responsibility—the clinician who signed off, the vendor who built the system, or the institution that deployed it?

Discussion Prompt: If you were reviewing an AI-generated discharge note with factual errors, would you sign off on it? How would you explain your concerns to a supervising physician? Should AI-generated notes be legally treated like clinician-authored documentation?

Artificial intelligence is no longer a distant abstraction. It is embedded in the daily practice of modern medicine. From note generation to risk prediction, AI tools are reshaping how clinicians interact with information, make decisions, and deliver care. As this chapter has shown, using these tools responsibly requires more than technical awareness; it demands clinical judgment, ethical sensitivity, and a commitment to equity. You are not expected to master every algorithm's inner workings but to question outputs, identify risks, and maintain accountability. By building fluency in the language of AI and learning how to prompt these systems effectively, you position yourself as a user and a thoughtful steward of this evolving technology. In the next chapter, we turn from understanding AI to learning how to communicate with it, an essential step in shaping safe, efficient, patient-centered care.

Instructor Resource Appendix

Learning Objectives
After completing this chapter, students should be able to:

- Define artificial intelligence, machine learning, and deep learning in clinical context.
- Describe current AI tools used in clinical care and medical education.
- Demonstrate awareness of ethical challenges and health equity concerns related to AI.
- Construct effective prompts for clinical AI tools.
- Evaluate the limitations of AI-generated documentation and formulate appropriate responses.

Clinical Vignette: Teaching Notes

Scenario Summary
Anna, a third-year student, encounters an AI-assisted discharge summary generator. She hesitates to use it due to uncertainty about how the tool functions.

Instructional Goals
- Demonstrate AI integration in documentation.
- Discuss the limits of automation and human oversight.
- Explore the ethical implications of trust and responsibility.

Suggested Strategies
- Socratic Dialogue: Ask, "Who is ultimately responsible for errors in an AI-generated note?"
- Role-Play: Assign roles (Anna, resident, attending, patient) and simulate responses.
- Mini Variants: Introduce different AI errors (e.g., hallucinated medications) and assess risk.
- Writing Prompt: "Should hospitals require clinicians to sign off on all AI-generated notes?"

Prompt Challenge: Teaching Notes

Activity
Have students complete both exercises: explaining AI to a student and to a patient.

Discussion Questions
- How did tone, vocabulary, and assumptions change?
- What makes a prompt effective in clinical contexts?
- Can poor prompts lead to clinical harm?

Extension
Have students improve and compare outputs using structured and unstructured prompts.

Ethics and Equity Checkpoint: Facilitation Guide

Key Themes
Opacity, explainability, bias, fairness, and accountability.

Group Activity
Assign teams a dilemma (e.g., "Should a biased AI tool be deployed if it improves average outcomes?") and have them propose solutions.

Suggested Readings
- Obermeyer et al., 2019. Racial bias in clinical algorithms.
- AMA Policy on Augmented Intelligence.

Discussion Facilitation "What Would You Do?" Case.

Scenario Summary
A student sees omissions in AI-generated notes. Should they speak up?

Instructor Tips
- Emphasize psychological safety.
- Explore communication up the hierarchy.

Highlight Documentation of Concerns

Debrief Prompts
- When should students escalate an issue?
- What's the risk of remaining silent?
- How can AI safety culture be taught?

Quick Recap for Slides or Review

- AI is present in clinical environments today.
- Most tools are narrow and data-driven.
- Students must learn structured prompting, recognize AI bias, and maintain oversight.

Curricular Integration Suggestions

- Use this chapter in ethics, clinical reasoning, and EHR documentation workshops.
- Pair with flipped classroom models or case-based learning modules.
- Integrate animated explainers or OSCE simulation prompts.

For Faculty Use Only

References

1. Sezgin G, Maier C, Wertheimer J. Accuracy of AI-generated discharge summaries in a tertiary-care study. J Hosp Med. 2024;19(2):88–95.
2. U.S. Food and Drug Administration. Artificial Intelligence/Machine Learning (AI/ML)-Enabled Medical Devices List – Status Report April 2025. Silver Spring: FDA; 2025
3. Shortliffe EH, Buchanan BG. A model of inexact reasoning in medicine. Math Biosci. 1975;23:351–79. https://doi.org/10.1016/0025-5564(75)90047-4.
4. Jiang F, Jiang Y, Zhi H, Dong Y, Li H, Ma S, Wang Y, Dong Q, Shen H, Wang Y. Artificial intelligence in healthcare: past, present and future. Stroke and Vasc Neurol. 2017;2(4):230–43. https://doi.org/10.1136/svn-2017-000101.
5. Esteva A, Robicquet A, Ramsundar B, Kuleshov V, DePristo M, Chou K, Cui C, Corrado GS, Thrun S, Dean J. A guide to deep learning in healthcare. Nat Med. 2019;25(1):24–9. https://doi.org/10.1038/s41591-018-0316-z.
6. Topol EJ. High-performance medicine: the convergence of human and artificial intelligence. Nat Med. 2019;25(1):44–56. https://doi.org/10.1038/s41591-018-0300-7.
7. Yu KH, Beam AL, Kohane IS. Artificial intelligence in healthcare. Nat Biomed Eng. 2018;2(10):719–31. https://doi.org/10.1038/s41551-018-0305-z.
8. Vaswani A, Shazeer N, Parmar N, Uszkoreit J, Jones L, Gomez AN, … Polosukhin I. Attention is all you need. In Advances in neural information processing systems; 2017. p. 30
9. Radford A, Narasimhan K, Salimans T, Sutskever I. Improving language understanding by generative pre-training. OpenAI; 2018.
10. Devlin J, Chang MW, Lee K, Toutanova K. BERT: pre-training of deep bidirectional transformers for language understanding. In Proceedings of NAACL-HLT; 2019, pp. 4171–4186. https://doi.org/10.48550/arXiv.1810.04805.
11. Beam AL, Kohane IS. Big data and machine learning in health care. JAMA. 2018;319(13):1317–8.
12. Rajkomar A, Hardt M, Haraf D, Basu S, Huang J, Quinn J, et al. Ensuring fairness in machine learning to advance health equity. Ann Intern Med. 2018;169(12):866–72.
13. Névéol A, Dalianis H, Velupillai S, Savova G, Zweigenbaum P. Clinical natural language processing in languages other than English: opportunities and challenges. J Biomed Semant. 2018;9(1):12. https://doi.org/10.1186/s13326-018-0189-8.
14. Wang Y, Sohn S, Liu S, Shen F, Wang L, Atkinson EJ, Amin S, Liu H. A clinical text classification paradigm using weak supervision and deep representation. BMC Med Inform Decis Mak. 2018;18(Suppl 2):57. https://doi.org/10.1186/s12911-018-0623-5.

15. Alsentzer E, Murphy JR, Boag W, Weng WH, Jin D, Naumann T, McDermott M. Publicly available clinical BERT embeddings. In Proceedings of the 2nd clinical natural language processing workshop; 2019, pp. 72–78. https://aclanthology.org/W19-1909/
16. Obermeyer Z, Powers B, Vogeli C, Mullainathan S. Dissecting racial bias in an algorithm used to manage the health of populations. Science. 2019;366(6464):447–53. https://doi.org/10.1126/science.aax2342.
17. Rajkomar A, Hardt M, Howell MD, Corrado G, Chin MH. Ensuring fairness in machine learning to advance health equity. Ann Intern Med. 2018;169(12):866–72. https://doi.org/10.7326/M18-1990.
18. Finlayson SG, Bowers JD, Ito J, Zittrain JL, Beam AL, Kohane IS. The clinician and dataset shift in artificial intelligence. N Engl J Med. 2021;385(3):283–6. https://doi.org/10.1056/NEJMp2104626.
19. He J, Baxter SL, Xu J, Xu J, Zhou X, Zhang K. The practical implementation of artificial intelligence technologies in medicine. Nat Med. 2019;25(1):30–6. https://doi.org/10.1038/s41591-018-0307-0.
20. Singhal K, Azizi S, Tu T, et al. Large language models encode clinical knowledge. Nature. 2023;620(7972):172–80. https://doi.org/10.1038/s41586-023-05881-4.
21. Nuance Communications. Dragon Medical One: Cloud-based clinical speech recognition; 2023. https://www.nuance.com/healthcare/clinical-documentation/dragon-medical-one.html
22. Suki AI. Suki Assistant overview; 2023. https://www.suki.ai/.
23. Ribeiro MT, Singh S, Guestrin C.. Why should I trust you? Explaining the predictions of any classifier. In Proceedings of the 22nd ACM SIGKDD international conference on knowledge discovery and data mining; 2016, pp. 1135–1144. https://doi.org/10.1145/2939672.2939778.
24. American Medical Association. Augmented intelligence in health care: AMA policy and guidance; 2024. https://www.ama-assn.org/delivering-care/public-health/ama-principles-augmented-intelligence.
25. Sutton RT, Pincock D, Baumgart DC, Sadowski DC, Fedorak RN, Kroeker KI. An overview of clinical decision support systems: benefits, risks, and strategies for success. NPJ Digit Med. 2020;3(1):17. https://doi.org/10.1038/s41746-020-0221-y.
26. Rajkomar A, Dean J, Kohane I. Machine learning in medicine. N Engl J Med. 2019;380(14):1347–58. https://doi.org/10.1056/NEJMra1814259.
27. Sendak MP, D'Arcy J, Kashyap S, Gao M, Nichols M, Corey K, Ratliff W, Balu S. A path for translation of machine learning products into healthcare delivery. EMJ Innovations. 2020;4(1):70–5. https://doi.org/10.33590/emjinnov/20-00021.
28. Henry KE, Hager DN, Pronovost PJ, Saria S. A targeted real-time early warning score (TREWScore) for septic shock. Sci Transl Med. 2015;7(299):299ra122. https://doi.org/10.1126/scitranslmed.aab3719.
29. Nori H, King N, McKinney SM, Carignan D, Horvitz E. Evaluating GPT-4 and large language models on medical licensing examinations. NPJ Digit Med. 2023;6:106. https://doi.org/10.1038/s41746-023-00936-9.
30. Singhal K, Azizi S, Tu T, Mahdavi SS, Wei J, Chung H-W, et al. Large language models encode clinical knowledge. Nature. 2023;622:572–7. https://doi.org/10.1038/s41586-023-06422-2.
31. National Board of Medical Examiners. Step 2 CK score interpretation guidelines. Philadelphia: NBME; 2024.
32. Jumper J, Evans R, Pritzel A, Green T, Figurnov M, Ronneberger O, et al. Highly accurate protein structure prediction with AlphaFold. Nature. 2021;596(7873):583–9. https://doi.org/10.1038/s41586-021-03819-2.
33. Callaway E. What AlphaFold means for biologists. Nature. 2022;604(7906):201–4. https://doi.org/10.1038/d41586-022-00997-5.
34. Senior AW, Evans R, Jumper J, Kirkpatrick J, Sifre L, Green T, et al. Improved protein structure prediction using potentials from deep learning. Nature. 2020;577(7792):706–10. https://doi.org/10.1038/s41586-019-1923-7.

35. Patel BN, Rosenberg L, Willcox G, Baltaxe E, Lyons M, Irvin J, Rajpurkar P. Ambient clinical intelligence in healthcare: early experiences with automated documentation and hands-free order entry. NPJ Digit Med. 2023;6(1):89. https://doi.org/10.1038/s41746-023-00889-4.
36. Abridge. Abridge and Epic partner to bring generative AI to clinical documentation. Business Wire; 2023. https://www.businesswire.com/news/home/20230912524323/en/Abridge-and-Epic-Partner-to-Bring-Generative-AI-to-Clinical-Documentation
37. Nabla. Nabla Copilot: AI medical scribe for clinicians; 2024. https://www.nabla.com/copilot
38. Liu V, Lin S, Tseng E, et al. Quality assurance informs large-scale use of ambient AI clinical documentation. NEJM AI. 2025;1(2)
39. Ghassemi M, Naumann T, Schulam P, Beam AL, Chen IY, Ranganath R.A review of challenges and opportunities in machine learning for health. IN AMIA joint summits on translational science proceedings; 2021, pp. 191–200. https://www.ncbi.nlm.nih.gov/pmc/articles/PMC8130462/
40. Ancker JS, Edwards A, Nosal S, Hauser D, Mauer E, Kaushal R. Effects of workload, work complexity, and repeated alerts on alert fatigue in a clinical decision support system. BMC Med Inform Decis Mak. 2017;17(1):36. https://doi.org/10.1186/s12911-017-0430-8.
41. Tonekaboni S, Joshi S, McCradden MD, Goldenberg A. What clinicians want: contextualizing explainable machine learning for clinical end use. In Machine learning for healthcare conference; 2019, pp. 359–380. https://proceedings.mlr.press/v106/tonekaboni19a.html
42. Huang W, Chen T, Davis D. Simulated patients and AI avatars in clinical communication training: opportunities and challenges. Med Teach. 2023;45(2):123–30. https://doi.org/10.1080/0142159X.2022.2146821.
43. Chowdhury N, Adhikari A, Chen H. Use of natural language processing in evaluating medical students' written assessments: a pilot study. J Med Educat Curri Develop. 2022;9:23821205221124857. https://doi.org/10.1177/23821205221124857.
44. Osmosis. Personalized learning with AI-driven adaptive review tools; 2024. Retrieved from https://www.osmosis.org
45. González-González CS, Infante Moro JC, Infante Moro A. Implementation of virtual simulation tools in clinical education: the body interact experience. BMC Med Educ. 2021;21(1):202. https://doi.org/10.1186/s12909-021-02647-3.
46. Doshi-Velez F, Kim B. Towards a rigorous science of interpretable machine learning. arXiv preprint, arXiv:1702.08608; 2017. https://arxiv.org/abs/1702.08608
47. Price WN. Black-box medicine. Harv J Law Technol. 2017;28(2):419–67.
48. U.S. Food and Drug Administration. Draft guidance: managing bias in device learning algorithms. Silver Spring: Center for Devices and Radiological Health; 2025.
49. Jones M, Patel L, Chen DL. Social determinants under-documented by automated discharge tools: a cross-sectional audit. BMJ Qual Safety. 2024;33(4):255–62. https://doi.org/10.1136/bmjqs-2023-016789.

Chapter 2
Data and Algorithms

Learning Objectives

By the end of this chapter, students will be able to:

- **Differentiate** among structured, semi-structured, and unstructured data in clinical contexts
- **Explain** the processes of data preprocessing and feature engineering in healthcare datasets
- **Identify** various types of algorithms used in medical AI, including rule-based systems, machine learning, and deep learning
- **Evaluate** the ethical implications of data bias, algorithmic transparency, and accountability in AI applications
- **Apply** knowledge through interactive case studies and simulations to reinforce understanding

Section 1: The Role of Data in Medical AI

Clinical Relevance

In modern healthcare, data forms the foundation of decision-making, diagnostics, and treatment planning. The integration of artificial intelligence (AI) into clinical workflows has only magnified the value of data, enabling more precise, timely, and personalized care. AI systems are designed to analyze large, complex datasets to identify patterns, forecast outcomes, and support clinicians in making informed decisions.

Visualizations of research data or results in this manuscript were generated, refined, corrected, edited, or formatted with the assistance of artificial intelligence (AI) tools, specifically OpenAI's ChatGPT 4.0, 2024. All content has been thoroughly reviewed, revised, and approved by the author(s) to ensure scientific accuracy and preserve the integrity of the original material.

© The Author(s), under exclusive license to Springer Nature Switzerland AG 2025

C. Quinn, *Generative AI for the Medical Student*,
https://doi.org/10.1007/978-3-032-01613-3_2

For example, AI algorithms can assist with early disease detection by analyzing imaging data, monitor patient vitals in real time to predict complications, and even recommend treatment plans based on historical cases. The success of these systems, however, depends on the quality, structure, and completeness of the data they use [1].

Data Sources in Healthcare

To understand how AI generates insights, it is essential to examine the different types of clinical data it relies on. These data originate from a wide range of healthcare processes and settings, each contributing unique and complementary information about patient health.

- **Electronic Health Records (EHRs):**
  EHRs are digital versions of patients' charts. They capture medical history, diagnoses, medications, allergies, immunizations, vital signs, and lab results. Because they span time and settings, EHRs offer a longitudinal view of patient care, making them essential for training AI systems that require temporal context.
- **Medical Imaging:**
  Imaging modalities such as X-rays, MRIs, CT scans, and ultrasounds produce visual data crucial for diagnosis. Deep learning algorithms are particularly adept at identifying abnormalities in these images, sometimes flagging subtle patterns missed by the human eye.
- **Wearable Devices and Remote Monitoring:**
  Devices like smartwatches, glucose monitors, and home pulse oximeters continuously record physiological data. These real-time streams are valuable for monitoring chronic conditions and predicting acute events, offering a richer dataset than episodic clinical visits alone.
- **Laboratory and Pathology Reports:**
  Laboratory values and pathology findings provide quantitative measures of disease. AI can uncover trends or correlations in this structured data, improving diagnostic accuracy and enabling predictive models.
- **Genomic and Molecular Data:**
  Advances in precision medicine have generated large volumes of data on genetic sequences and molecular markers. AI tools are increasingly used to identify genetic risk factors and suggest tailored treatments based on individual genomic profiles.
- **Patient-Generated Health Data (PGHD):**
  Patients now contribute data through apps, symptom trackers, surveys, and home logs. These insights, which include pain scores, mood tracking, or medication adherence, are particularly helpful in chronic disease management and behavioral health.
- **Administrative and Claims Data:**
  Although less clinically focused, billing and claims data reveal patterns in healthcare utilization, disparities, and resource allocation. When integrated, these datasets help inform health system performance and care delivery models.

Importance of Data Quality and Integration

The performance and safety of AI models in medicine depend directly on the quality of the data they analyze. Incomplete, inaccurate, or biased data can mislead algorithms and compromise patient safety. As a result, ensuring high standards for data accuracy, consistency, and representativeness is essential [2].

Another challenge lies in integrating diverse data types from multiple systems. Different hospitals may use different formats, terminologies, or units of measurement. Achieving interoperability—so that systems can talk to each other and interpret the same data correctly—requires standardization efforts such as the adoption of common vocabularies (e.g., SNOMED CT, LOINC) and data exchange protocols (e.g., HL7, FHIR) [3].

In short, without high-quality, integrated data, even the most sophisticated AI model will struggle to deliver clinically meaningful results.

Section 2: Types of Data in Healthcare

To understand how artificial intelligence functions in medicine, it's essential to first examine the raw materials it works with—clinical data. Every day, healthcare generates vast amounts of information, from vital signs and imaging to dictated notes and genomic sequences. But not all data are equally usable by AI. The structure and format of data influence how easily it can be processed, interpreted, and acted upon.

Broadly, healthcare data fall into three categories: structured, semi-structured, and unstructured. Understanding the differences among them helps explain both the promise and limitations of AI in medicine.

Structured Data

Structured data are highly organized and easily digestible by machines. These data are stored in fixed fields within tables, often appearing as numbers or coded categories in the electronic health record (EHR). They are standardized, labeled, and predictable.

Examples Include

- Vital signs: temperature, blood pressure, respiratory rate
- Laboratory results: serum creatinine and white blood cell count
- Medication lists: drug name, dose, and frequency
- ICD-10 codes: standardized diagnostic labels, such as "E11.9" for type 2 diabetes without complications

Why It Matters
Structured data are the easiest for algorithms to process. They are frequently used in calculating risk scores (e.g., CHA_2DS_2-VASc for stroke) or detecting trends over time (e.g., serial creatinine elevations in acute kidney injury) [4].

Semi-structured Data

Semi-structured data have some internal organization, but they don't conform to rigid tables or schemas. They include tags or labels that allow partial automation and interpretation by machines. This middle-ground format often serves as a bridge between structured and unstructured sources.

Examples Include
- **XML files:** Clinical documents wrapped in tags such as `<patient>`, `<diagnosis>`, or `<medication>`
- **JSON records:** Short for *JavaScript Object Notation*, JSON is a compact, human-readable format used to exchange data between systems. It is widely used in mobile health applications and EHR integrations. For example:

```
json
CopyEdit
{
  "name": "John Doe",
  "age": 42,
  "diagnosis": "Pneumonia"
}
```

Why It Matters
Semi-structured data allow for easier data exchange between systems. They are particularly useful for AI tools that ingest information from mobile apps, wearable devices, or external healthcare institutions. These formats support data interoperability and serve as stepping stones to structured storage [5].

Unstructured Data

Unstructured data make up the bulk of clinical documentation. They include text, images, audio, and other formats that lack a predefined organizational schema. These data require advanced tools, such as natural language processing (NLP) or image recognition, to be understood by AI.

Examples Include

- Free-text clinical notes: "Patient is a 64-year-old male with worsening dyspnea and orthopnea."
- Radiology images: DICOM-formatted CT scans, X-rays, and MRIs
- Audio recordings: Dictated notes or patient interviews
- Scanned documents: PDFs of outside records or lab reports

Why It Matters

Unstructured data hold much of the clinical insight used in decision-making. AI systems that can extract key phrases from narrative notes or detect pathology in medical images are particularly valuable. However, these systems are also more complex, and their accuracy depends heavily on the quality of training data [6].

Try It Yourself: Interactive Classification

To build intuition, examine a sample electronic health record (EHR) or simulated patient chart. For each element, ask the following:

- Is it structured, like a lab result or ICD code?
- Is it semi-structured, like a JSON file from a wearable app?
- Is it unstructured, like a narrative progress note or radiology scan?

You can use the interactive worksheet below (Fig. 2.1) to parse the elements of the EHR.

Reflection Questions

1. Which types of data are easiest for AI systems to analyze? Why?
2. Which types of data are most likely to contain valuable but hard-to-extract insights?
3. How might data format affect the design, function, or reliability of an AI system?

Understanding the structure of healthcare data is only the beginning. Before AI systems can use these data to make predictions or offer clinical support, the data must be cleaned, standardized, and refined, a process known as data preprocessing. In the next section, we'll explore how this critical step transforms raw clinical inputs into trustworthy signals that AI can act on.

Data Item	Example	Your Classification
Blood pressure reading	142/90 mmHg	
Radiology image	CT scan of the chest (DICOM format)	
Progress note	"Patient reports chest pain worsening overnight."	
Lab report in XML	<lab><test>WBC</test><value>11.2</value></lab>	
Medication list	Lisinopril 10 mg daily	
Dictated audio note	MP3 recording of physicianpatient encounter -	
JSON from health app	{"steps": 8200, "heart_rate": 76}	
Diagnosis code	I10 – Essential hypertension	

Fig. 2.1 Interactive worksheet: categorizing healthcare data

Section 3: Data Preprocessing and Feature Engineering

Before artificial intelligence (AI) can analyze healthcare data, that data must be prepared in ways that make it clean, complete, and consistent. This stage of preparation is called data preprocessing, and it is one of the most important steps in developing safe and reliable AI tools. Once the data is cleaned, the next step is called feature engineering. This involves choosing which parts of the data the AI model will focus on when learning how to make predictions.

Even the most brilliant physician cannot make a good diagnosis if a patient's chart is missing lab results, includes medication errors, or contains conflicting information. The same applies to AI systems. They can only be as useful as the data they are given.

What Is Data Preprocessing?

Data preprocessing encompasses all the steps taken to prepare raw clinical data so that AI models can effectively understand and utilize it (see Fig. 2.2). Most healthcare data, when first collected, is messy. There may be missing lab values, conflicting documentation, or measurements recorded in different units (such as weight in kilograms vs. pounds). Preprocessing addresses these issues, ensuring the AI model doesn't learn from flawed information.

Here are four common preprocessing tasks:

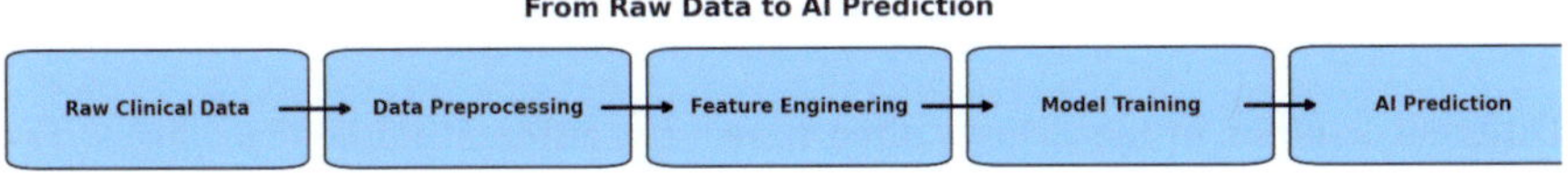

Fig. 2.2 Data preprocessing

Handling Missing Data

In real-world practice, patient records are often incomplete. A potassium level may not have been drawn, or a vital sign might not have been recorded. If an AI system tries to learn from data that includes too many gaps, it can make incorrect assumptions.

There are a few ways to manage missing data:

- **Omit** the record entirely (which may reduce the sample size).
- **Impute** or estimate the missing value using information from similar patients.
- **Flag** the data as missing so the model can treat it cautiously.

Clinical Example A model predicting hypokalemia might encounter a record with no potassium value. Rather than guess blindly, preprocessing could estimate a likely range based on the patient's medications and renal function [7].

Correcting Errors and Inconsistencies

Sometimes, data entries contain mistakes. A blood pressure reading of "900/40" is likely a data entry error. A medication might be listed twice or spelled incorrectly. These inconsistencies must be corrected before training a model.

Why This Matters Just like a resident reviewing a chart for errors before rounds, an AI system needs clean data to form valid clinical conclusions.

Standardizing Units and Terminology

Medical data come from many different hospitals, clinics, and devices. Each may use its own formats and language. One chart might list weight in pounds, another in kilograms. One note might say "heart attack," while another says "myocardial infarction."

To address this, data preprocessing converts all units to a common system and utilizes standardized clinical terms. These are often drawn from vocabularies like **SNOMED CT** (a system for clinical terms) or **LOINC** (used for lab tests) [8, 9].

Why This Matters Standardization ensures that data from different sources can be meaningfully combined. Without it, models trained at one hospital might fail at another.

Normalization

Different features in the dataset often have very different numerical ranges. For example, systolic blood pressure might range from 90 to 200, while troponin values might go from 0.01 to 5. If an AI model sees only the raw numbers, it may think blood pressure is more important simply because the values are bigger.

Normalization means putting all data on the same scale, such as from 0 to 1. This ensures that each variable contributes equally to the model's learning process, not just the ones with large numbers [10].

Clinical Analogy You wouldn't conclude that a weight of 200 pounds is more clinically important than an oxygen saturation of 95% just because the number is larger. Normalization prevents AI from making that mistake.

What Is Feature Engineering?

Once the data is cleaned and standardized, the next task is to decide what parts of the data the AI model will actually use to make decisions. This process is called feature engineering.

In AI, a feature is just a single variable or data point that may be helpful in predicting an outcome. This could be age, heart rate, sodium level, or something more complex, such as the rate of change in creatinine over time [11].

There are two main parts to feature engineering:

Feature Selection

This means choosing the most important data elements for the task at hand. Not every data point in a chart is helpful for every prediction.

Example If we want to predict whether a patient will be readmitted after surgery, we might select:

- Age
- Type of surgery
- Length of hospital stay
- Comorbidities
- Discharge medications

Removing irrelevant features (like hair color or height) reduces noise and improves model accuracy [12].

Feature Creation (or Transformation)

This involves building new features from existing data. Sometimes, a combination of variables tells a better story than a single one.

Example Instead of using raw glucose values, a model might look at whether the patient's glucose is rising or falling. Or instead of using systolic and diastolic pressures separately, it might combine them into pulse pressure.

Why This Matters Good features make AI smarter. They allow it to think more like a clinician by focusing on clinically meaningful patterns.

Why This Matters for Medical Students

As a future physician, you may not be building AI models, but you will certainly use them. When you encounter an AI-generated risk score or diagnostic suggestion, your ability to interpret that output depends on knowing how the model was trained.

If the model was trained using incomplete data, uncorrected errors, or irrelevant features, it could offer unsafe recommendations. Just as you learn to question a lab result based on how the sample was collected, you should learn to question AI output based on how the data was prepared.

Preprocessing and feature engineering may seem like technical topics, but they form the foundation of every clinical AI tool. A trustworthy tool begins with trustworthy data.

What Is Data Preprocessing?

Data preprocessing refers to all the steps taken to clean, organize, and standardize data before it is used to train or operate an AI system. Most raw data—especially in healthcare—is messy, inconsistent, and incomplete. Preprocessing helps transform that messy data into a usable format.

Common Preprocessing Tasks in Medicine

1. **Handling Missing Data**

   In the real world, patient charts are often incomplete. A lab test may not have been ordered, or a vital sign wasn't recorded. An AI system needs a strategy for dealing with these missing values. Options include ignoring those records, estimating the missing data based on similar patients, or using clinical reasoning to fill in gaps.

Example A patient's potassium level is missing from their chart. Should the AI assume it's normal? Should it skip the patient altogether? Or should it make a conservative estimate based on the patient's clinical profile?

2. **Correcting Errors and Inconsistencies**
   Sometimes, the data contains mistakes. A temperature recorded as 400 degrees is clearly an error. A medication name may be misspelled or entered twice. AI systems need clean, accurate data to avoid making dangerous conclusions.
3. **Standardizing Units and Terminology**
   Healthcare data comes from many sources, such as different hospitals, devices, or systems. One system may record weight in pounds, another in kilograms. One chart may use the term "myocardial infarction," and another may write "heart attack." AI tools must be trained using consistent formats and terminology.

Example If one data source lists a heart rate as "HR = 88 bpm" and another says "88 beats/min," both must be recognized as the same thing.

4. **De-identifying Patient Information**
   Before patient data is used to train AI systems, especially in research or commercial settings, personal identifiers (like names, dates of birth, or addresses) must be removed to protect privacy. This is a crucial preprocessing step for regulatory and ethical compliance.

What Is Feature Engineering?

Once the data is clean and consistent, the next step is to decide what parts of the data will actually be used by the AI system to make decisions. This is known as feature engineering (see Fig. 2.3.)

In this context, a "feature" is simply an individual data point or variable that might help predict an outcome.

Think of Features as Clinical Clues

Imagine you're seeing a patient with chest pain. You mentally consider the person's age, history of hypertension, ECG findings, troponin level, and smoking history. These are all **features**—important clues that help you assess risk.

In the same way, when an AI system is trained to predict whether a patient will go into shock, the system needs to decide which features to consider. Should it include heart rate? Blood pressure? Recent hemoglobin drop? Number of medications?

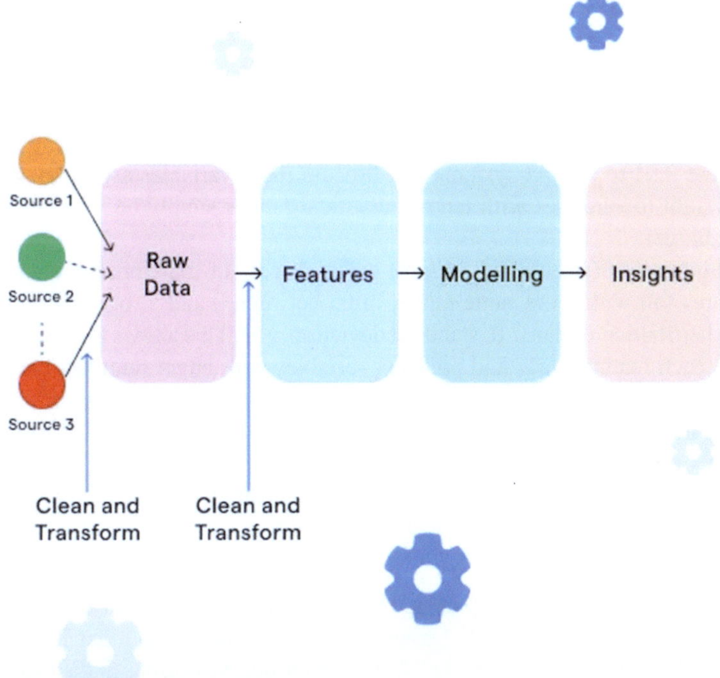

Fig. 2.3 Process of feature engineering

Feature Selection and Engineering

- **Feature selection** involves choosing the most relevant variables for the task at hand.
- **Feature engineering** involves creating new, more useful variables from the existing data.

Example 1: Feature Selection
For predicting readmission after surgery, features might include age, type of surgery, length of stay, discharge medications, and comorbidities.

Example 2: Feature Engineering
Rather than using raw blood glucose levels, a model might use the trend in glucose over time (e.g., "rising," "falling," or "stable") as a feature. Or instead of using each individual vital sign, it might combine them into an early warning score.

These engineered features often make models more accurate and more reflective of real clinical reasoning.

Normalization: Putting Data on the Same Scale

Even when units are consistent, the range of values across different variables can vary significantly. For example, systolic blood pressure might range from 90 to 180, while age might range from 0 to 100, and troponin levels could span tiny decimal values like 0.01 to 5.0. AI systems that process these variables as-is may give too much weight to variables with larger numerical ranges simply because their numbers are bigger.

Normalization (also called *scaling*) is the process of transforming data so that all features fall within the same range, often between 0 and 1, or with a standard normal distribution (mean = 0, standard deviation = 1). This allows the AI system to evaluate each feature fairly and prevents variables with larger numbers from overshadowing others.

Without normalization, an AI model might give undue importance to features with larger numeric ranges (like blood pressure) and overlook others (like troponin), even if they are clinically critical. Normalization ensures that each feature contributes proportionally to the model's learning process.

Clinical Analogy
Think of this like comparing a patient's weight in pounds with their oxygen saturation in percentages. You wouldn't assume weight is more important just because "200" is a bigger number than "95." Yet without normalization, that's exactly the kind of assumption an AI model might make. Normalization ensures the algorithm interprets values on different scales fairly, without favoring one variable simply due to its numeric range.

Example: Min-Max Normalization in a Clinical Dataset
To see how this works, let's apply min-max normalization to a small dataset used to predict 30-day hospital readmission. The dataset includes three features:

Patient	Age (years)	Systolic BP (mmHg)	Troponin (ng/mL)
A	75	160	0.5
B	45	120	0.2
C	60	140	0.9

As you can see, the raw values are on very different scales. Age ranges from 45 to 75, systolic blood pressure from 120 to 160, and troponin from 0.2 to 0.9. If we fed these raw values into a machine learning model, it might mistakenly treat systolic blood pressure as more important simply because the numbers are larger.

Step 1: Apply Min-Max Normalization
To level the playing field, we use the following formula:

$$\mathbf{X\_normalized} = \left(\mathbf{x} - \min\left(\mathbf{x}\right)\right) / \left(\max\left(\mathbf{x}\right) - \min\left(\mathbf{x}\right)\right)$$

Let's apply this step-by-step to each feature:

Age (Min = 45, Max = 75):

- Patient A: (75–45)/(75–45) = 1.0
- Patient B: (45–45)/(75–45) = 0.0
- Patient C: (60–45)/(75–45) = 0.5

Systolic BP (Min = 120, Max = 160):

- Patient A: (160–120)/(160–120) = 1.0
- Patient B: (120–120)/(160–120) = 0.0
- Patient C: (140–120)/(160–120) = 0.5

Troponin (Min = 0.2, Max = 0.9):

- Patient A: (0.5–0.2)/(0.9–0.2) ≈ 0.43
- Patient B: (0.2–0.2)/(0.9–0.2) = 0.0
- Patient C: (0.9–0.2)/(0.9–0.2) = 1.0

Normalized Table:

Patient	Age (normalized)	BP (normalized)	Troponin (normalized)
A	1.0	1.0	0.43
B	0.0	0.0	0.0
C	0.5	0.5	1.0

Interpretation

Now, each feature is scaled from 0 to 1. This allows the model to compare clinical variables more objectively, without bias toward the measurement scale. In other words, it will weigh each input based on relevance to the prediction task, not just its raw size. For students, this example underscores the critical role of preprocessing in developing safe, equitable AI tools that reflect clinical priorities, not just mathematical ones.

Why It Matters for Medical Students

You don't need to build AI systems yourself, but you should understand how the data was prepared before trusting an algorithm's output. If the system learned from incomplete, incorrect, or biased data, or if key features were excluded, it might deliver unsafe or misleading recommendations.

Just like interpreting a lab result requires understanding how the test was collected and processed, interpreting AI output requires understanding where the data came from and how it was handled.

Case Study Preprocess a dataset to prepare it for input into a machine learning model.

Interactive Worksheet: Data Normalization in Clinical AI

In this activity, you will practice applying min-max normalization to clinical data. This technique rescales values so they fall between 0 and 1, allowing algorithms to fairly compare features that originally use different units or ranges.

Step 1: Original Clinical Data

Use the data below to calculate normalized values using the formula:

$$x\_\text{normalized} = \left(x - \min(x)\right) / \left(\max(x) - \min(x)\right)$$

Patient	Age (years)	Systolic BP (mmHg)	Troponin (ng/mL)
A	75	160	0.5
B	45	120	0.2
C	60	140	0.9

Step 2: Your Normalized Values

Now calculate and enter the normalized values for each variable below. Hint: first find the minimum and maximum for each column.

Patient	Normalized age	Normalized BP	Normalized troponin
A			
B			
C			

Step 3: Reflection

1. Which feature had the largest original range? How did that affect normalization?
2. Why might an AI model perform better using normalized inputs instead of raw values?
3. Can you think of clinical variables that should not be normalized? Why?

Section 4: From Data to Decisions—How AI Learns in Medicine

Once healthcare data has been cleaned and prepared, the next step is teaching the AI system how to make sense of it. This process is called training a model, and while the technical details can be complex, the basic concept is easy to understand.

At its core, an AI model learns from examples. Just as medical students learn clinical reasoning by reviewing cases and seeing patterns, AI systems do something similar: they look at thousands, or even millions, of examples to find relationships between data inputs and clinical outcomes.

What Is a Model?

An AI model is a mathematical tool that takes data (the inputs) and produces a prediction, classification, or recommendation (the output) [13, 14]. For example:

- Input: age, symptoms, and lab results
- Output: risk of sepsis within 12 h

The model learns to connect the dots between inputs and outcomes based on prior examples. This process is called **training**, and the examples it learns from are called training data.

A Clinical Analogy: Think Like a Clinician

Imagine a new resident sees a patient with shortness of breath. Based on years of exposure to teaching cases, they know that when shortness of breath occurs with leg swelling, orthopnea, and an S3 gallop, a diagnosis of heart failure is likely. This isn't because they memorized a rulebook; it's because they've seen enough patterns to recognize the diagnosis.

AI works the same way. It does not understand medicine the way humans do. But it learns associations by detecting statistical patterns in large datasets.

Supervised Learning: The Most Common Approach in Medicine

Most clinical AI tools use a method called supervised learning [15]. In this approach, the model is given examples where both the inputs and the correct answers are already known. The goal is for the model to learn how to make the right prediction when it sees similar data in the future.

Example

- Input: Patient is 73 years old, sodium = 128, systolic BP = 92, creatinine = 2.1.
- Known Outcome: The patient was transferred to the ICU within 24 h.
- After seeing thousands of such examples, the model begins to learn which combinations of features are associated with deterioration, and it can predict the likelihood of ICU transfer for new patients.

Training and Testing

To make sure the model doesn't just memorize the examples, data scientists divide the dataset into two parts:

- **Training data:** Used to teach the model
- **Testing data:** Used to check whether the model can generalize to new, unseen cases

This process is like preparing for Step 1: studying with practice questions (training), and then taking a mock exam (testing) to see if you can apply the knowledge to new problems.

Evaluating Model Performance

To ensure AI models are reliable and safe for clinical use, their performance must be rigorously evaluated using several metrics [16]:

- **Accuracy:** The proportion of correct predictions made by the model.
- **Sensitivity (Recall):** The model's ability to correctly identify patients with a condition.
- **Specificity:** The model's ability to correctly identify patients without the condition.
- **Precision:** The proportion of positive identifications that were actually correct.
- **Area Under the Receiver Operating Characteristic Curve (AUC-ROC):** This is a metric used to evaluate how well a model separates two groups, such as patients with a disease versus those without it. The ROC curve is a graph that shows how a model's sensitivity (true positive rate) and 1-specificity (false-positive rate) change at different thresholds [17].

Clinical Analogy Evaluating an AI model is akin to assessing a new diagnostic test. Just as you would consider a test's sensitivity and specificity before using it in practice, AI models must demonstrate high-performance metrics to be trusted in clinical settings.

Clinical Decision Support Systems (CDSS)

Clinical decision support systems (CDSS) are tools that integrate AI models into clinical workflows, providing healthcare professionals with patient-specific assessments or recommendations to aid decision-making [18].

Example in Practice A CDSS might alert a clinician to a potential drug interaction based on a patient's current medications or suggest additional tests when certain risk factors are present.

Why This Matters CDSS can enhance diagnostic accuracy, reduce errors, and improve patient outcomes by providing timely, evidence-based information at the point of care.

Accuracy Isn't Everything

A model's accuracy tells us how often it makes the correct prediction. But that's not the only metric that matters. In medicine, we also need to know the following:

- **Sensitivity:** How well does the model identify true positives? (e.g., detecting all real cases of sepsis)
- **Specificity:** How well does the model avoid false alarms?
- **Calibration:** Does the predicted risk match the actual risk?

Imagine a model that predicts sepsis risk with 95% accuracy. It identifies the majority of patients on a ward as being at risk for sepsis. Since sepsis is rare, very few of those patients develop sepsis. However, the constant sepsis alarms the model sends out annoy the clinicians on the ward, and they begin to ignore the model entirely. This is not a helpful tool. Evaluation metrics must be chosen based on clinical context, not just statistical performance.

Limitations and Considerations

While AI holds great promise in healthcare, it's essential to recognize its limitations:

- **Data Quality:** AI models are only as good as the data they're trained on. Inaccurate or biased data can lead to unreliable predictions.
- **Interpretability:** Some AI models operate as "black boxes," making it difficult to understand how they arrive at specific conclusions. This lack of transparency can hinder clinical trust and adoption.
- **Ethical and Legal Concerns:** Issues such as patient privacy, data security, and accountability for AI-driven decisions must be carefully managed.

Clinical Analogy Using an AI model without understanding its limitations is akin to relying on a diagnostic test without knowing its false-positive or false-negative rates. Clinicians must critically appraise AI tools, just as they do with any medical test or intervention.

Why This Matters for Medical Students

You may never build an AI model, but you will be asked to interpret one. You might be shown a risk score in the EHR or an AI-generated suggestion in a patient's chart. To use that information wisely, you need to know:

- What kind of data did the model learned from
- Whether the model has been tested on patients like yours

- How to weigh the model's output against your clinical judgment

Remember: AI is a tool, not a decision-maker. And like any tool, its value depends on how well it is understood and used by skilled professionals.

Section 5: Overview of Algorithms in Medical AI

In clinical medicine, artificial intelligence can take many forms. Some systems follow simple sets of instructions. Others learn patterns from vast amounts of data (see Table 2.1), Understanding the differences between these approaches is essential for interpreting how AI tools work and how much trust to place in their outputs.

Not all AI is created equally. Rule-based systems are straightforward and predictable. Machine learning models are flexible and adaptive. Deep learning networks are powerful but often opaque. Each has a different role to play in healthcare, and knowing their strengths and limitations can help you evaluate when and how to use them.

Rule-Based Systems: The Earliest Form of Medical AI

Rule-based systems are the simplest kind of AI. They rely on fixed logic, sets of "if this, then that" statements, to make decisions. These systems do not learn from experience. Instead, they apply predefined clinical rules every time they are used.

For example, imagine a clinical decision support tool in the emergency department that flags a possible diagnosis of appendicitis when a patient has right lower quadrant pain, a fever over 100.4 degrees, and an elevated white blood cell count. That system is not "thinking" in any meaningful sense. It is executing a programmed checklist.

Table 2.1 Algorithm type comparisons

Algorithm type	How it works	Example use	Strengths	Limitations
Rule-based systems	Follows fixed "if-then" logic written by humans	EHR alerts for vaccinations or drug interactions	Simple, transparent, and easy to audit	Rigid and cannot adapt to new information
Machine learning	Learns from labeled examples in structured data	Predicting 30-day readmission risk or sepsis scores	Flexible and accurate for structured data tasks	May lack transparency; performance depends on data
Deep learning	Learns complex patterns from images, text, or audio	Classifying chest X-rays or reading pathology slides	Excels at interpreting complex, unstructured data	Opaque decision-making; requires large datasets

Chapter 1 introduced a historical example of this type of system, MYCIN. Although it never reached clinical deployment, it was a proof of concept that expert medical logic could be encoded into a machine. These early efforts laid the groundwork for more advanced AI applications in use today.

Rule-based systems are still widely used today. You've likely seen them embedded in electronic health records as best practice alerts, age-based vaccination reminders, or order sets triggered by lab values. These tools are valuable because they are easy to understand and easy to audit. However, they are also limited. They cannot handle unexpected cases, learn from new data, or adjust to subtle patterns that fall outside of their programming [19].

Machine Learning: Learning from Patterns in Data

Machine learning represents a more flexible form of AI (see Fig. 2.4). Instead of following rules created by humans, machine learning systems learn how to make decisions by examining large sets of labeled data. These systems are trained to find patterns that predict clinical outcomes [20].

Consider a hospital that wants to reduce 30-day readmission rates after surgery. A machine learning model could be trained on thousands of past patient records, each labeled to indicate whether the patient was readmitted. The model would learn how different factors, such as age, type of surgery, length of stay, discharge medications, and lab values, relate to the likelihood of readmission. After training, it could predict the readmission risk for a new patient based on those same features.

Several types of machine learning models are commonly used in clinical care. Logistic regression models are frequently used to predict binary outcomes, such as

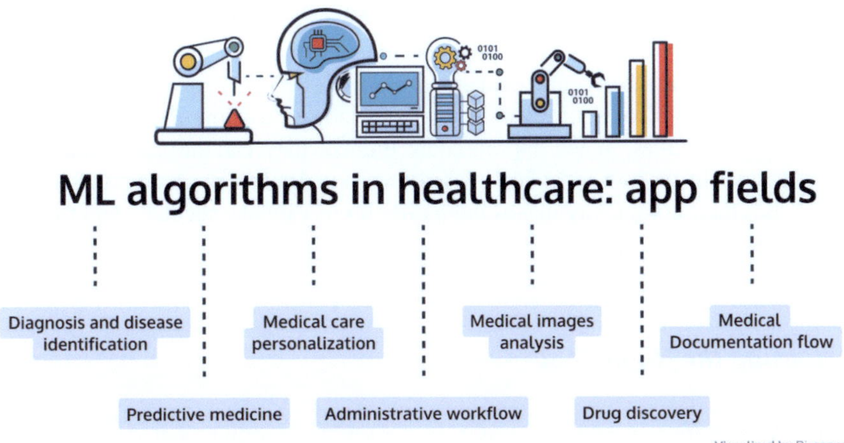

Fig. 2.4 Machine learning uses in healthcare

mortality or readmission. Decision trees and random forests divide data into branching paths, mimicking diagnostic reasoning. Other models, like support vector machines and gradient boosting, are used in more complex classification tasks, including imaging interpretation or genomic analysis [21].

Machine learning models can handle noisy or incomplete data and often outperform rule-based systems in accuracy. However, they require very large, high-quality datasets to be reliable. While they are more adaptable than rule-based systems, they can still be difficult to explain clearly to clinicians or patients.

Deep Learning: A Powerful and Complex Tool

Deep learning is a specialized type of machine learning. These systems are based on artificial neural networks, which are loosely inspired by the human brain's information processing. Deep learning models are especially useful when the input data is complex and unstructured, such as medical images, audio recordings, or free-text clinical notes.

For instance, a deep learning model trained on thousands of chest X-rays can learn to recognize signs of pneumonia, pleural effusion, or lung nodules. Unlike traditional machine learning models that require humans to define specific features, like heart size or lung opacity, deep learning systems learn those patterns on their own [22].

Deep learning is also used in natural language processing, where models extract clinical concepts from physician notes or summarize conversations between doctors and patients. In pathology, deep learning models can accurately identify cancer cells in digitized biopsy slides [23].

Despite their power, deep learning models are often criticized for being "black boxes." That means they produce outputs without offering clear explanations for how they reached their conclusions. In high-stakes clinical environments, this lack of transparency can be problematic. If a deep learning model suggests a diagnosis or recommends a treatment, clinicians need to understand whether the suggestion is reasonable and based on sound evidence.

These models also require vast amounts of labeled training data and powerful computing resources. When appropriately trained, they can surpass human-level performance in narrow tasks like classifying skin lesions or interpreting retinal scans. But their complexity makes them difficult to validate, regulate, and troubleshoot [23].

Choosing the Right Tool

The choice between rule-based systems, machine learning, and deep learning depends on the clinical problem at hand (see Fig. 2.5). Rule-based tools are ideal for predictable, standardized workflows where transparency is important. Machine learning is well-suited for risk prediction and triage systems that rely on patterns in

Scenario	Rule-Based	Machine Learning	Deep Learning
Triage of ED Chest Pain	If age > 50 and chest pain and troponin > 0.04, trigger cardiac workup	Uses EHR data to estimate probability of ACS based on prior cases	Not commonly applied due to limited image involvement
30-Day Readmission Risk	Fixed thresholds for length of stay, comorbidities flag risk	Predicts risk from patterns in historical patient data	Rare use; requires large unstructured datasets
Radiology Image Analysis	Not used; requires structured rules not suited to images	Can predict radiology turnaround delays based on workload and case type	Analyzes CT/X-ray to detect pneumonia, masses, or fractures

Fig. 2.5 Choosing the right clinical tools

structured data. Deep learning excels when the task involves interpreting complex visual or linguistic inputs, such as X-rays or progress notes.

No one model type is perfect. Each carries trade-offs between explainability, flexibility, and performance. As a medical student, your goal is not to build these systems, but to understand their foundations well enough to evaluate their outputs critically. You must ask not only what the model predicts but also how it was trained, what kind of data it uses, and whether its recommendations make clinical sense.

In a world where algorithms are becoming part of the care team, this kind of reasoning is a core competency for modern medical practice.

With a foundational understanding of the various AI algorithms utilized in medical practice, we now turn our attention to the practical aspects of integrating these technologies into clinical workflows. The next section will explore the challenges and strategies associated with implementing AI tools in healthcare settings, ensuring they augment clinical decision-making effectively and ethically.

Section 6: Emerging Technologies in Medical AI

Artificial intelligence is not a single technology but a collection of evolving approaches. As foundational systems like rule-based tools and machine learning models continue to mature, several newer methods are beginning to influence the practice of medicine. These emerging technologies are not yet universally adopted, but they hold great promise and pose new challenges for the future physician.

This section introduces three areas where AI innovation is rapidly accelerating: natural language processing, computer vision, and reinforcement learning. Each offers unique capabilities that may soon reshape how we deliver and document care.

Natural Language Processing: Making Sense of Clinical Text

Much of healthcare runs on free text. Progress notes, discharge summaries, operative reports, pathology comments, and patient histories all contain valuable information that lives outside of structured data fields. Traditional algorithms struggle to utilize this type of unstructured information, but natural language processing (NLP) is specifically designed to do exactly that.

NLP systems are trained to read and interpret language. In medicine, this allows AI tools to extract diagnoses, medications, procedures, or symptoms from clinician-authored notes. For example, an NLP tool might scan an emergency department note and identify that the patient has a documented penicillin allergy, even if it is not listed in the allergy field.

Some systems go further. Generative language models can now summarize entire patient encounters, extract billing codes, or convert dictated narratives into structured SOAP notes. Others help with chart review by flagging mentions of missed follow-ups, abnormal findings, or changes in treatment plans buried in long progress notes.

Many modern NLP tools, including those used in medical chart summarization, rely on transformer-based models like BERT or GPT-4, which are trained to understand clinical context at scale. For instance, Nuance's DAX Copilot uses GPT-4 to generate clinical notes from doctor-patient conversations [24] automatically.

Despite these advances, NLP in medicine remains a challenging field. Clinical language is dense, full of abbreviations, and often inconsistent. One provider might write "HTN," another "hypertension," and a third "elevated BP." The system must learn to recognize that all of these refer to the same concept. Furthermore, understanding negation, knowing the difference between "no chest pain" and "chest pain," requires sophisticated processing.

Even when the technology works, human oversight is essential. NLP tools can misunderstand sarcasm, mislabel symptoms, or overlook context. They are powerful assistants but not replacements for clinical reasoning.

Computer Vision: Teaching AI to See Like a Clinician

Computer vision allows machines to interpret visual data. In medicine, this usually means analyzing images like chest X-rays, CT scans, pathology slides, or retinal photographs. Rather than looking at numbers or words, these systems learn from pixels.

Deep learning models trained on tens of thousands of medical images can learn to identify subtle features that might be missed by the human eye. For example, AI systems have been shown to detect lung nodules, diabetic retinopathy, or melanoma with accuracy that rivals or even exceeds that of trained specialists.

Computer vision is most widely utilized in radiology, dermatology, pathology, and ophthalmology, specialties that rely heavily on visual interpretation. Several tools have received FDA clearance for specific clinical applications. For instance, IDx-DR (now marketed as LumineticsCore) is approved to autonomously detect diabetic retinopathy from retinal images without requiring clinician input [25]. Similarly, Aidoc offers FDA-cleared solutions that assist radiologists by flagging potential findings such as pulmonary embolisms or intracranial hemorrhages on CT scans [26]. In pathology, AI-powered tools such as Paige Prostate and Ibex Prostate Detect have received FDA clearance to aid in the identification of prostate cancer in digital pathology slides [27, 28].

These tools are categorized into two regulatory classes: assistive AI, which supports but does not replace human interpretation, and autonomous AI, which can render clinical judgments independently. The FDA has established guidelines for both categories, emphasizing transparency, explainability, and real-world validation to ensure that AI performance remains safe and effective across diverse clinical settings [29].

These tools are not perfect. They can be fooled by poor image quality, unusual anatomy, or unexpected artifacts. Just as a tired clinician can misread an X-ray, an AI model trained on ideal cases may struggle with real-world variation. That is why most AI vision systems are used for triage or second opinions, not as final diagnostic authorities.

The key for students is to understand what these systems can and cannot do. If an AI flags a suspicious mass on a chest X-ray, it is still your responsibility to interpret that alert in the full clinical context.

Reinforcement Learning: AI That Learns by Doing

Most clinical AI today is based on supervised learning, where the system learns from labeled examples. Reinforcement learning, by contrast, is based on trial and error. The model interacts with an environment, receives feedback based on its actions, and gradually learns to make better decisions to achieve a goal.

This approach is inspired by how humans learn from experience. A child learns to ride a bike not by reading a manual, but by trying, falling, adjusting, and trying again. In medicine, reinforcement learning models are being explored for tasks that require sequential decision-making, such as adjusting ventilator settings in the ICU or personalizing chemotherapy regimens based on patient response.

For example, a reinforcement learning model might simulate hundreds of treatment pathways for a patient with sepsis and identify a strategy that optimizes fluid management and vasopressor use. These systems can evaluate long-term consequences, not just immediate outcomes, which makes them particularly promising for chronic disease management or dynamic care environments.

However, this technology is still largely experimental in healthcare. Training reinforcement learning systems safely requires accurate simulations or enormous historical datasets. In high-stakes clinical settings, trial and error carries obvious risks. That is why these models are currently used more in research than in practice. For instance, recent studies have explored reinforcement learning to optimize mechanical ventilation settings in intensive care units, showing potential improvements in patient outcomes [30].

Even so, reinforcement learning reflects the next frontier in clinical AI: systems that not only recognize patterns but also learn to act and adapt in complex environments.

Discussion Prompt

Debate with your classmates or reflect in writing: What are the greatest opportunities and most pressing concerns related to these emerging AI technologies?

Consider questions like the following:

- Can NLP be trusted to capture key clinical nuances?
- Should computer vision systems be used in place of radiologist reads?
- How do we test reinforcement learning models ethically in human care?

Each of these technologies carries promise. But the path from innovation to safe implementation is long, and future physicians will play a key role in navigating that transition.

Sidebar: Real-World Examples of Emerging AI Technologies

Natural Language Processing (NLP)

Clinical Use: An NLP tool integrated into the EHR scans physician notes for unlisted symptoms and automatically suggests ICD-10 codes.

Example: A system detects "worsening fatigue" and "recent weight loss" in a free-text progress note and flags the chart for possible cancer workup.

Benefit: Saves time on coding and improves documentation completeness.

Challenge: Misinterprets statements like "no weight loss" as a positive finding unless properly trained.

Computer Vision

Clinical Use: AI software analyzes retinal photographs to screen for diabetic retinopathy during a primary care visit.

Example: The system identifies early retinal microaneurysms before the patient experiences symptoms, allowing earlier referral to ophthalmology.

Benefit: Increases screening access, especially in underserved areas.

Challenge: Accuracy drops with poor image quality or variations in retinal pigmentation.

(continued)

Reinforcement Learning

Clinical Use: In a simulation-based ICU environment, a reinforcement learning agent learns optimal fluid resuscitation strategies for septic shock.

Example: After evaluating thousands of ICU cases, the system proposes stepwise vasopressor adjustments that reduce mortality in test environments.

Benefit: Optimizes care decisions over time, especially in dynamic conditions.

Challenge: Still experimental and not yet validated for live patient care.

Section 7: Ethical Considerations

As artificial intelligence becomes a more routine part of clinical care, physicians must confront not only technical and diagnostic challenges but also ethical ones. These issues are not abstract; they affect real patients and real decisions. Understanding how AI systems can go wrong, and who is responsible when they do, is part of being a safe and thoughtful clinician in the digital age.

This section explores four major areas of ethical concern: data bias, algorithmic transparency, informed consent, and accountability.

Data Bias: When the Model Learns the Wrong Lessons

AI systems learn from data. If the data are flawed, the system may make flawed decisions. This is known as data bias. In healthcare, bias can arise from many sources. For instance, if a dataset contains mostly White, urban, insured patients, then the AI trained on that data may perform poorly when used on patients who are Black, rural, or uninsured [31].

A notable example involves a commercial risk prediction tool used in the United States, which was found to underestimate the health needs of Black patients. The model used healthcare spending as a proxy for health status. Because Black patients historically received less care, even when equally sick, the model assumed they were healthier than they really were. This led to fewer referrals and less care for those who needed it most [32].

Bias does not always come from bad intentions. Often, it stems from historical inequalities built into the healthcare system. But when an AI model reflects or amplifies those inequalities, the consequences are real. Clinicians must be alert to the possibility that "objective" outputs may be skewed by unfair inputs.

Algorithmic Transparency: Understanding How the Model Thinks

Another ethical challenge is transparency. Many modern AI tools, especially those that rely on deep learning, do not explain their decisions in ways that are easy to understand. These models process massive amounts of data and return a result, such as a diagnosis or a risk score, without showing how they got there.

In medicine, that can be dangerous. Imagine an AI tool that recommends discharging a patient with chest pain. If the physician cannot understand how the model reached that conclusion, it becomes difficult to judge whether the recommendation is safe. Trust in medicine depends on reasoning that can be explained and defended.

Lack of transparency also makes it harder to catch errors. A clinician reviewing a medication list can often spot a mistake quickly. But when an AI system outputs a risk score of 0.17 for sepsis, there is no obvious way to check its logic. This puts the physician in a difficult position. They must act on a number without knowing how it was calculated.

To address this, tools like SHAP (SHapley Additive exPlanations) and LIME (Local Interpretable Model-agnostic Explanations) have been developed to provide insights into model predictions. SHAP assigns each feature an importance value for a particular prediction, while LIME approximates the model locally to explain individual predictions [33]. These tools enhance interpretability and allow clinicians to better understand and trust AI outputs.

Informed Consent: Disclosing AI's Role in Care

Informed consent is a cornerstone of ethical medical practice. As AI becomes more integrated into clinical decision-making, questions arise about whether patients should be informed when AI tools are involved in their care. Some ethicists argue that patients should be made aware of AI's role, especially if it significantly influences diagnoses or treatment plans.

A recent study of patient perspectives found that many individuals prefer transparency when AI is involved in their healthcare. They expressed a desire to be told when an AI tool contributes to decision-making, especially in serious or complex cases [34]. Including a brief disclosure during the informed consent process may help preserve patient autonomy and reinforce trust.

Accountability: Who Is Responsible When AI Goes Wrong?

Finally, there is the question of responsibility. If an AI tool makes a recommendation that leads to harm, who is accountable?

Consider a case where an AI system suggests an incorrect antibiotic. The physician follows the recommendation, and the patient develops complications. Is the physician at fault for trusting the tool? Is the hospital liable for deploying it? Should the software company be held responsible for its design?

These questions are still being debated in law and policy. However, in clinical training, the answer is clear. Until professional guidelines say otherwise, physicians remain responsible for the decisions they make, even if AI influences those decisions. This means that using AI does not replace clinical judgment; it must enhance it.

Accountability also extends to institutions. Hospitals must monitor the performance of AI systems, track errors, and adjust policies accordingly. If a tool underperforms in certain populations or settings, it should be revised or removed. Developers, too, must be held to ethical design standards. A model that performs well on paper but fails in practice is not safe.

For students, the key lesson is this: AI is not a shield from responsibility. If you use a model's output, you own the outcome. That makes it all the more important to understand how these tools work and where their limits lie.

Group Activity: An Ethical Dilemma in Practice

Case Scenario

At a large academic hospital, an AI tool is deployed to identify patients eligible for early palliative care referral. The tool performs well during internal validation and is rolled out across the system. Six months later, staff notice a pattern: patients who do not speak English are being referred much less often, even when they meet the clinical criteria.

A review finds that the training data mainly came from English-speaking patients. As a result, the model struggles to interpret documentation from encounters conducted through interpreters. Key terms like "prognosis," "pain control," and "goals of care" are inconsistently recognized.

Discussion Questions

1. What kind of bias occurred in this scenario?
2. What were the unintended consequences for patients?
3. Who should be held accountable for addressing the issue?
4. How would you raise your concerns if you were a student on that service?
5. How could this model be improved or replaced?

This case challenges you to think critically about fairness, transparency, and responsibility. In the age of AI-assisted care, ethical practice includes not only knowing what the model says but also asking why and for whom it may be wrong.

Sidebar: The Learned Intermediary Doctrine in the Age of Medical AI

The learned intermediary doctrine has long shielded pharmaceutical manufacturers from direct liability to patients. Rooted in traditional tort law, it assumes that prescribing physicians, acting as "learned intermediaries," are best positioned to evaluate drug risks and benefits and communicate those risks to patients. This doctrine provides manufacturers with a legal safe harbor: as long as they adequately warn the physician, their duty to the patient is fulfilled.

But what happens when artificial intelligence (AI) disrupts this triangular relationship?

Modern AI tools, especially those incorporating black-box algorithms, are increasingly capable of evaluating patient data, suggesting treatments, and even warning about contraindications. In some direct-to-consumer digital health applications, AI may recommend medications without any physician input. As such tools grow more autonomous and their role in clinical care expands, and questions emerge about whether AI can or should be viewed as a "learned intermediary."

Legally, AI is not a licensed medical professional. It cannot testify, hold malpractice insurance, or exercise clinical judgment in the legal sense. Yet it may substantially influence, or even make, medical decisions. This challenges the foundations of the learned intermediary doctrine, especially when AI replaces or circumvents human physicians in the decision-making process.

In cases where AI acts independently or offers recommendations directly to patients, plaintiffs may argue that the doctrine should not apply since the physician is no longer the sole gatekeeper of risk communication. On the other hand, if physicians use AI merely as a tool, validating its suggestions within a traditional patient encounter, the doctrine remains intact.

Furthermore, AI's opacity complicates attribution of responsibility. When physicians cannot explain how an AI system reached its conclusion, and manufacturers claim no control over its outputs, courts face difficulty in assigning fault. In such cases, traditional legal shields may erode, prompting calls for reform.

Some legal scholars have proposed adapting the doctrine to reflect these new realities better. One suggestion is formally recognizing hybrid decision-making models, where a human physician and an AI system contribute to medical decisions. In this scenario, the physician remains the responsible party but must understand and critically evaluate the AI's input. Another proposal is to require developers to ensure that AI-generated outputs are explainable and traceable, so physicians and courts can review how recommendations were formed. Additionally, manufacturers may be expected to provide drug safety information in formats optimized for human and machine consumption, allowing AI tools to process the most current warnings and clinical guidance accurately.

In short, the learned intermediary doctrine stands at a crossroads. While it has long served as a bulwark in products liability, its applicability in AI-mediated care will depend on how courts view the evolving roles of physicians, patients, and algorithms in the therapeutic decision chain.

Section 8: Interdisciplinary Collaboration

Artificial intelligence (AI) in healthcare is not developed in isolation. It emerges from the concerted efforts of clinicians, engineers, data scientists, designers, and ethicists. To create AI tools that are safe, effective, and clinically relevant, these diverse groups must collaborate effectively. For medical students, understanding how to contribute meaningfully to this collaboration is as crucial as understanding how to use AI in practice.

Why Medicine Needs Team Science

AI tools are the result of extensive processes involving design, training, testing, and validation. Clinicians provide essential context to ensure these tools address real-world clinical needs. For instance, an algorithm predicting postoperative complications might be technically accurate but clinically unhelpful if it generates alerts too late, requires unnecessary data entry, or overlooks patient-specific factors.

While medical insight grounds the development process, it is not sufficient alone. Engineers bring expertise in constructing models, managing large datasets, and solving optimization problems. Ethicists ensure that tools promote fairness, protect privacy, and respect patient autonomy. Effective collaboration requires clear communication among all team members.

The Clinician's Role in AI Development

As a future physician, even if you do not write code or build machine learning models, your role is pivotal. You are responsible for defining clinical problems: identifying pain points in current workflows, common errors, or decisions that could benefit from data-driven support (see Fig. 2.6).

Testing tools in realistic settings is also part of your role. This involves assessing when AI outputs are useful, confusing, or misleading. For example, when a predictive model flags a patient as high risk, can you understand why? Does the recommendation align with your clinical judgment? Your feedback is crucial for refining these tools.

Advocating for patients is another key responsibility. You understand their needs, values, and concerns. If an AI model fails to account for language barriers, social

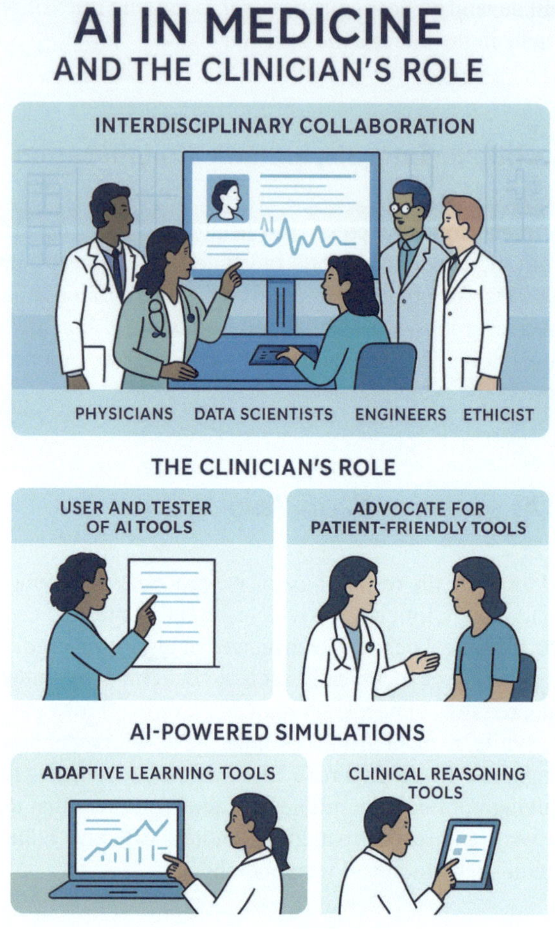

Fig. 2.6 AI requires interdisciplinary collaboration

determinants of health, or population diversity, it is incumbent upon you to raise these issues. Your voice ensures that technology serves people, not just systems.

Communication Across Disciplines

One of the greatest challenges in interdisciplinary work is language. Data scientists and software engineers may use terms like "features," "model accuracy," or "training sets," while clinicians discuss diagnoses, differential reasoning, or patient safety. Miscommunication can derail a project before it begins.

To bridge this gap, consider the following strategies:

- **Translate clinical problems into technical terms**: Instead of saying "patients are getting missed," explain that delayed lab reviews or inconsistent triage criteria may lead to late interventions.
- **Ask clarifying questions**: If a developer mentions a model's "precision" or "recall," inquire about what that means for clinical safety or patient outcomes.
- **Use case-based examples**: A real patient story is often more effective than a theoretical description, grounding the conversation in shared understanding.

Challenges to Interdisciplinary Collaboration

Despite the benefits, interdisciplinary collaboration faces challenges such as misaligned incentives, communication breakdowns, and differences in workflow expectations between developers and clinicians. Addressing these barriers requires institutional support, shared goals, and ongoing dialogue among team members.

How Medical Students Learn with AI

Medical students increasingly interact with AI tools not only in patient care but also in their own training. These tools are used to simulate clinical scenarios, generate personalized learning plans, and provide feedback on diagnostic reasoning.

AI-Driven Simulations in Education

During Objective Structured Clinical Examinations (OSCEs) or virtual clinical scenarios, AI may simulate patient responses or evaluate communication skills. These simulations allow students to experience how AI functions in diagnostic triage or symptom assessment. For instance, an AI-driven case might dynamically adjust a patient's condition based on the student's questions or physical exam findings.

Personalized Learning with Adaptive Platforms

AI-powered systems like intelligent tutoring platforms can analyze a student's strengths and weaknesses, offering targeted content. If a student repeatedly struggles with interpreting arterial blood gases (ABGs) or electrocardiograms (ECGs), the platform may automatically prioritize these topics in future sessions. This kind of adaptive learning is increasingly common in preparation for licensing examinations.

Feedback on Clinical Reasoning

Some medical schools use AI tools to evaluate written clinical reasoning exercises or SOAP notes. These systems may highlight missing elements, suggest evidence-based differential diagnoses, or prompt the student to clarify vague language. Importantly, students must still review and verify these suggestions, ensuring human oversight remains central.

Notably, institutions like the University of California, San Diego (UCSD), have successfully implemented AI tools such as COMPOSER, a deep learning model that predicts sepsis risk in emergency department patients. COMPOSER continuously monitors over 150 patient variables and alerts clinicians to high-risk cases, leading to a 17% reduction in sepsis-related mortality [35]. This example underscores the importance of interdisciplinary collaboration in developing and deploying effective AI solutions in healthcare.

Summary

This chapter provides a comprehensive overview of the types of data and algorithms integral to medical AI. Through interactive activities and discussions, students will gain practical insights into how AI technologies are developed and applied in healthcare settings. Emphasis on ethical considerations and interdisciplinary collaboration prepares students to navigate the complexities of AI integration in medicine.

Instructor's Guide: Chapter—Data and Algorithms

Learning Objectives

After completing this chapter, students should be able to:

- Distinguish between structured, semi-structured, and unstructured clinical data
- Describe how data preprocessing, including normalization and feature engineering, prepares data for AI models
- Explain key performance metrics such as accuracy, sensitivity, specificity, and AUC in clinical AI evaluation
- Compare rule-based systems, machine learning, and deep learning using real-world examples
- Recognize ethical challenges in AI use, such as bias and algorithmic opacity
- Understand how medical students interact with AI tools in education and practice

Section-by-Section Instructional Strategies

Section 1: Types of Data in Healthcare

- Use real EHR screenshots (de-identified) to highlight examples of each data type.
- Prompt students to categorize types of data from short clinical notes or lab panels.

Section 2: Data Preprocessing and Feature Engineering

- Work through a lab test example (e.g., HbA1c) showing how missing values are imputed and normalized.
- Introduce feature engineering by asking students to brainstorm new variables (e.g., pulse pressure).

Section 3: Model Evaluation Metrics

- Present confusion matrices for binary classification tasks.
- Discuss trade-offs using different clinical scenarios (e.g., cancer screening vs. ICU alerts).

Section 4: Overview of Algorithms in Medical AI

- Use patient case vignettes to show how different algorithm types handle the same task.
- Prompt discussion: "Why might a deep learning system outperform a rule-based one in radiology?"

Section 5: Emerging Technologies

- Assign groups to research and present one emerging AI technology (e.g., NLP or reinforcement learning).
- Discuss examples of AI hallucinations or failures in image interpretation.

Section 6: Ethical Considerations

- Case-based ethics discussion: present a real-world incident of bias in a predictive model.
- Debate prompt: Should AI outputs be legally considered clinical recommendations?

Section 7: Interdisciplinary Collaboration

- Use the provided role-playing exercise to simulate a meeting between AI developers and clinicians.
- Encourage students to reflect on communication gaps between technical and clinical experts.

Section 8: How Medical Students Learn with AI

- Have students log and reflect on their encounters with AI tools in clinical skills or documentation.
- Facilitate a discussion on how AI might alter the student-patient relationship.

Quick Recap Points for Lecture Slides

- Clinical data varies in structure and influences model design.
- Preprocessing and feature selection determine model performance.
- Evaluation metrics must match the clinical goal.
- Rule-based, ML, and DL models serve different needs.
- AI can amplify bias if not monitored.
- Students will encounter AI in both clinical training and educational tools.

To consider adding if we decide to provide the students with a course portal

Interdisciplinary Collaboration in Action

In real-world clinical AI development, teams often include physicians, data scientists, software engineers, UX designers, and clinical ethicists. Each member brings a distinct perspective. To help you experience this kind of collaboration, we've created a role-based simulation where students work together to design an AI tool for early cancer detection.

You can access the full activity—including role briefs and discussion questions—in Appendix B or through the course portal.

As you participate, consider the following:

- What clinical information do developers need that they might not realize?
- How should an ethicist respond if a model works better in one population than another?
- What does a successful partnership between clinicians and engineers look like?

Worksheet: Interdisciplinary Collaboration in Medical AI

This worksheet is designed to help you explore your role in interdisciplinary AI development. In this exercise, you will simulate a collaborative meeting between clinicians and technical team members to design a new AI-based diagnostic tool.

Role-Playing Scenario

You are participating in a simulated planning meeting to design an AI tool that helps emergency physicians triage patients presenting with chest pain. The AI should identify patients at high risk for a cardiac event within 72 h.

Each student will take on a role in the interdisciplinary development team. Some of these roles fall outside traditional clinical training. To support your participation, use the accompanying one-page role briefs that explain each team member's responsibilities and priorities.

Assigned Roles and Guidance

Assign one role per student. Use the role brief sheets for background context, suggested discussion points, and guiding questions. Roles include:

- Medical student (clinical perspective)
- Emergency medicine attending (clinical leadership)
- Data scientist (model development and data design)
- UX designer (interface and usability design)
- Clinical ethicist (safety, bias, and fairness oversight)

Discussion Tasks

- Identify the clinical problem to solve and translate it into a technical goal.
- Discuss the types of data the model should use and potential challenges in accessing or interpreting it.
- Decide how the model should present risk scores to physicians.
- Anticipate challenges related to safety, patient consent, and equity.
- Design a user interface layout or describe how the alert should appear within the clinical workflow.

Post-exercise Reflection Questions

1. How did your assigned role shape your perspective in the discussion?
2. What challenges did your group encounter when trying to balance clinical needs and technical feasibility?
3. What strategies helped you communicate effectively across disciplines?
4. How can you apply these insights in your future clinical or academic work?

Role Briefs: Interdisciplinary Collaboration in AI

Medical Student

You represent the voice of learners and junior clinicians.

Your role is to:

- Share how clinical tasks are experienced by students
- Identify areas where AI might support learning or reduce clerical burden
- Flag concerns where overreliance on automation might hinder training
- Ask clarifying questions when technical terms are unclear

Emergency Medicine Attending

You are the clinical lead with deep experience in frontline decision-making.

Your role is to:

- Define the real-world clinical workflow in the ED
- Explain what information physicians need to make quick and accurate decisions
- Identify risks of over-alerting or alert fatigue
- Prioritize features that improve patient safety and reduce decision-making time

Data Scientist

You specialize in building models that identify patterns in data.

Your role is to:

- Ask what the model should predict (e.g., cardiac event in 72 h)
- Decide which inputs to include (e.g., ECG, vitals, troponins)
- Explain how accuracy, bias, and missing data could affect performance
- Make trade-offs between complexity and interpretability

UX Designer

You are responsible for how users interact with the tool.

Your role is to:

- Ensure the AI tool fits seamlessly into the clinician's workflow
- Design alerts that are clear, concise, and nonintrusive
- Ask: Where should this alert appear? What should it look like?
- Consider accessibility, mobile compatibility, and colorblind safety

Clinical Ethicist

You focus on fairness, transparency, and accountability.

Your role is to:

- Ask whether the model works equally well for all patient populations
- Identify ways to make the tool explainable
- Raise concerns about consent, privacy, and unintended harm
- Suggest how equity concerns can be addressed

References

1. Ranjbar A, Ravn J. Data quality in healthcare for the purpose of artificial intelligence: a case study on ECG digitalization. Stud Health Technol Inform. 2023;305:471–4. https://doi.org/10.3233/SHTI230534.
2. Schwabe D, Becker K, Seyferth M, Klaß A, Schäffter T. The METRIC-framework for assessing data quality for trustworthy AI in medicine: a systematic review. npj Digital Med. 2024;7:45. https://doi.org/10.1038/s41746-024-01196-4.
3. Luo Y, et al. Novel AI model may enhance health data interoperability. northwestern medicine news center. 2024. Retrieved from https://news.feinberg.northwestern.edu/2024/08/07/novel-ai-model-may-enhance-health-data-interoperability/
4. HealthTech Magazine. Structured vs. unstructured data in healthcare. 2023, May. Retrieved from https://healthtechmagazine.net/article/2023/05/structured-vs-unstructured-data-healthcare-perfcon
5. CrowdStrike. What is semi-structured data? 2024. Retrieved from https://www.crowdstrike.com/en-us/cybersecurity-101/cloud-security/semi-structured-data/
6. Sciforce. Turning chaos into clarity: mastering unstructured healthcare data with AI. 2024, July 17. Retrieved from https://medium.com/sciforce/turning-chaos-into-clarity-mastering-unstructured-healthcare-data-with-ai-a105406e89d8
7. Bess L. Enhancing healthcare with data preprocessing: a real-world AI application. 2024. Retrieved from https://www.linkedin.com/pulse/enhancing-healthcare-data-preprocessing-real-world-ai-lee-bess-1ou9c
8. Netguru. Data preprocessing: artificial intelligence explained. n.d. Retrieved from https://www.netguru.com/glossary/data-preprocessing

9. Astera Software. Data preprocessing: concepts, importance, & tools. 2025. Retrieved from https://www.astera.com/type/blog/data-preprocessing/
10. IBM. What is feature engineering? n.d. Retrieved from https://www.ibm.com/think/topics/feature-engineering
11. IBM. What is feature engineering? n.d. Retrieved from https://www.ibm.com/think/topics/feature-engineering accessed 5/19/25.
12. Soni S, Roberts K. Feature engineering with clinical expert knowledge: a case study assessment of machine learning model complexity and performance. J Biomed Inform. 2020;108:103514. https://doi.org/10.1016/j.jbi.2020.103514
13. Briganti G, Le Moine O. Artificial intelligence in medicine: today and tomorrow. Front Med. 2020;7:27. https://doi.org/10.3389/fmed.2020.00027.
14. Harrer S, Shah P, Antony B, Hu J. Artificial intelligence for clinical trial design. Trends in Pharmacol Sci. 2019;40(8):577–91. https://doi.org/10.1016/j.tips.2019.06.004.
15. Owkin. What is unsupervised vs supervised learning? | A-Z of AI for healthcare. n.d. Retrieved May 19, 2025, from https://www.owkin.com/a-z-of-ai-for-healthcare/unsupervised-vs-supervised-learning
16. Park SH, Han K. Methodologic guide for evaluating clinical performance and effect of artificial intelligence technology for medical diagnosis and prediction. Radiology. 2018;286(3):800–9. https://doi.org/10.1148/radiol.2017171920.
17. Mandrekar JN. Receiver operating characteristic curve in diagnostic test assessment. J Thorac Oncol. 2010;5(9):1315–6. https://doi.org/10.1097/JTO.0b013e3181ec173d.
18. Shortliffe EH, Sepúlveda MJ. Clinical decision support in the era of artificial intelligence. JAMA. 2018;320(21):2199–200. https://doi.org/10.1001/jama.2018.17163.
19. Malik S, Bansal M, Meena D, Gupta S. Rule-based system for effective clinical decision support. Procedia Comput Sci. 2023;218:1645–52. https://doi.org/10.1016/j.procs.2023.10.030.
20. Pfob A, Lu S-C, Sidey-Gibbons C. Machine learning in medicine: a practical introduction to techniques for data pre-processing, hyperparameter tuning, and model comparison. BMC Med Res Methodol. 2022;22:282. https://doi.org/10.1186/s12874-022-01758-8BioMedCentral.
21. Ma Y, Wang Y, Li L, Wang Y. Effective hospital readmission prediction models using machine learning: a systematic review. BMC Health Serv Res. 2022;22:1085. https://doi.org/10.1186/s12913-022-08748-y.
22. Khobahi S, Agarwal C, Ghaffari M. Deep learning for chest X-ray analysis: a survey. Med Image Anal. 2021;73:102193. https://doi.org/10.1016/j.media.2021.102193.
23. Ahmed MU, Saeed S, Abid A. A review of recent advances in deep learning models for chest diseases detection using chest X-ray images. J Healthcare Eng. 2022;2022:7802035. https://doi.org/10.1155/2022/7802035.
24. Nuance Communications. Nuance and Microsoft announce the first fully AI-automated clinical documentation application for healthcare. 2023, March 20. Retrieved from https://news.nuance.com/2023-03-20-Nuance-and-Microsoft-Announce-the-First-Fully-AI-Automated-Clinical-Documentation-Application-for-Healthcare
25. U.S. Food and Drug Administration. FDA permits marketing of artificial intelligence-based device to detect certain diabetes-related eye problems. 2018, April 11. Retrieved from https://www.fda.gov/news-events/press-announcements/fda-permits-marketing-artificial-intelligence-based-device-detect-certain-diabetes-related-eye
26. Aidoc. Aidoc granted AI industry-first FDA clearance for triage of incidental pulmonary embolism. 2020, August 26. Retrieved from https://www.aidoc.com/about/news/fda-incidental-pulmonary-embolism/
27. U.S. Food and Drug Administration. FDA authorizes software that can help identify prostate cancer. 2021, September 21. Retrieved from https://www.fda.gov/news-events/press-announcements/fda-authorizes-software-can-help-identify-prostate-cancer
28. Ibex Medical Analytics. Ibex medical analytics receives first FDA 510(k) clearance. 2025, January 24. Retrieved from https://ibex-ai.com/fda-510k-clearance/

29. U.S. Food and Drug Administration. Artificial intelligence and machine learning in software as a medical device. 2021. Retrieved from https://www.fda.gov/medical-devices/software-medical-device-samd/artificial-intelligence-and-machine-learning-software-medical-device
30. Liu S, Xu Q, Xu Z, Liu Z, Sun X, Xie G, Feng M, See KC. Reinforcement learning to optimize ventilator settings for patients on invasive mechanical ventilation: retrospective study. J Med Internet Res. 2024;26:e44494. https://doi.org/10.2196/44494.
31. Chen F, Wang L, Hong J, Jiang J, Zhou L. Unmasking bias in AI: a systematic review of bias detection and mitigation strategies in electronic health record-based models. 2023. arXiv preprint arXiv:2310.19917. https://arxiv.org/abs/2310.19917arXiv.
32. Obermeyer Z, Powers B, Vogeli C, Mullainathan S. Dissecting racial bias in an algorithm used to manage the health of populations. Science. 2019;366(6464):447–53. https://doi.org/10.1126/science.aax2342.
33. DataCamp. Explainable AI: understanding and trusting machine learning models. n.d. Retrieved from https://www.datacamp.com/tutorial/explainable-ai-understanding-and-trusting-machine-learning-models
34. McCradden MD, Baba A, Saha A, Ahmad T. Patient perspectives on informed consent for medical AI. Digital Health. 2024;10:20552076241247938. https://doi.org/10.1177/20552076241247938.
35. Boussina A, Shashikumar SP, Malhotra A, Owens RL, El-Kareh R, Longhurst CA, et al. Impact of a deep learning sepsis prediction model on quality of care and survival. npj Digital Med. 2024;7(1):14. https://doi.org/10.1038/s41746-023-00986-6.

Chapter 3
The AI Toolkit

Learning Objectives

By the end of this chapter, students will be able to:

1. **Define natural language processing (NLP)** and explain its role in analyzing clinical documentation, decision-making, and patient communication
2. **Describe the architecture and function of large language models (LLMs)** and how they differ from earlier rule-based or keyword-matching systems
3. **Identify common use cases of NLP in healthcare**, such as clinical summarization, decision support, ambient documentation, and patient education
4. **Explain how LLMs generate humanlike language** and the clinical implications of their capacity to synthesize, summarize, and translate information
5. **Critically evaluate the benefits and risks of using generative AI in clinical settings**, including hallucinations, bias, overreliance, and misinformation
6. **Describe key components of prompt engineering** and how well-structured prompts can improve the reliability of AI outputs in a clinical context
7. **Compare the performance of NLP-based tools** to traditional clinical documentation and decision-support systems
8. **Discuss the ethical, legal, and regulatory considerations** surrounding the use of LLMs in healthcare documentation and communication
9. **Apply NLP tools to practical exercises** involving chart summarization, simulated patient communication, and clinical question answering
10. **Reflect on their role as future clinicians** in responsibly guiding the use of generative AI tools to enhance, not replace, clinical reasoning and patient care

---

Visualizations of research data or results in this manuscript were generated, refined, corrected, edited, or formatted with the assistance of artificial intelligence (AI) tools, specifically OpenAI's ChatGPT 4.0, 2024. All content has been thoroughly reviewed, revised, and approved by the author(s) to ensure scientific accuracy and preserve the integrity of the original material.

© The Author(s), under exclusive license to Springer Nature Switzerland AG 2025

C. Quinn, *Generative AI for the Medical Student*,
https://doi.org/10.1007/978-3-032-01613-3_3

Clinical Vignette: "The Prompt That Backfired"

It was supposed to be a quick task. Marianna, a fourth-year medical student finishing her sub-internship, had been asked to draft simple discharge instructions for a patient newly diagnosed with type 2 diabetes. Short on time and eager to be efficient, she turned to her favorite AI assistant and typed, "Write a simple explanation of diabetes for a patient." Within seconds, the AI generated a polished summary that was clear, friendly, and easy to read.

But when Marianna reviewed the instructions with her attending, she was met with concern.

"This tells the patient to cut out all carbohydrates," the attending said. "That's not part of our dietary plan."

"And there's no mention of how to store insulin or manage hypoglycemia," added the pharmacist during rounds. "This isn't safe to send home."

Marianna realized the AI had done precisely what she asked. The problem wasn't the tool; it was the prompt. She hadn't included details about the patient's medications, dietary goals, or discharge plan. The AI produced a general answer, but one that wasn't tailored to the clinical context.

That night, Marianna revisited the case and rewrote her prompt: "Write discharge instructions for a newly diagnosed type 2 diabetic patient on insulin. The patient has only moderate health literacy. Emphasize diet, exercise, glucose monitoring, and follow-up appointments." The response was markedly better, safer, more specific, and clinically appropriate.

A good AI output starts with a good prompt.

This experience sparked a team-wide discussion:

- What makes a good prompt?
- How do you instruct AI tools responsibly?
- And how do you ensure the technology supports care without compromising it?

Before exploring specific AI models, let's start by remembering that ***primary care's "Four Cs,"*** *First Contact, Comprehensiveness, Coordination, and Continuity, set a unique stage for any AI system aiming to support frontline clinicians* [1].

Why Primary Care Demands a Different Kind of AI

Before diving into specific AI tools, it's essential to understand what makes primary care fundamentally different from other medical settings and why that difference matters. The field is built around four foundational principles, often referred to as the "Four Cs" of primary care: First Contact, Comprehensiveness, Coordination, and Continuity [1].

The Four Cs of Primary Care

1. **First Contact**: Primary care is usually the patient's entry point into the health system. Clinicians encounter vague, undifferentiated symptoms, such as fatigue or cough, that require broad, hypothesis-free evaluation.
2. **Comprehensiveness**: One clinician manages acute issues, chronic diseases, preventive screenings, and behavioral health, all in the same setting.
3. **Coordination**: Primary care is a central hub that connects patients to specialists, imaging, community services, and follow-up care.
4. **Continuity**: Long-term relationships over months or years allow clinicians to monitor subtle changes, track social context, and build trust.

Each principle places unique demands on any AI system operating in this environment. For example, an AI assistant designed for primary care must make sense of a wide range of clinical scenarios, adjust across multiple visits, and handle incomplete or loosely structured input. It can't rely on clean datasets or narrow diagnoses like an AI model built for radiology might.

As you'll see in the next section, **natural language processing (NLP)** is particularly well-suited for this kind of setting. Primary care records are full of unstructured text, progress notes, referral letters, and patient-reported symptoms. These messy data sources hold enormous clinical value. NLP tools are designed to extract meaning from them and turn narrative into insight.

Natural Language Processing (NLP) in Medicine

To build effective models for those "Four Cs," we first need to understand how primary-care EMR data differ from specialty-care records.

To appreciate NLP's challenges and opportunities, note that **primary-care EMRs** differ from specialty or inpatient systems in four key ways: risk profile, visit frequency, multimorbidity complexity, and data span, requiring tailored preprocessing steps.

EMR Data in Primary Care Versus Specialty Care

Primary-care EMR data contrast with hospital or specialty systems across four dimensions:

- **Baseline Risk Profile**: Lower acuity and rarer events than inpatient populations.
- **Visit Granularity**: Frequent, shorter visits capture incremental changes over time.
- **Complexity Type**: Multimorbidity and social-determinant notes dominate over single-disease focus.
- **Time Course**: Data may span years or decades rather than acute episodes.

Recognizing these differences is critical when preparing and normalizing data for ML in primary-care contexts.

Natural language processing, or NLP, is the branch of artificial intelligence that helps machines understand and generate human language. This is especially useful in clinical environments where much of the documentation exists in free-text form (see Fig. 3.1). NLP summarizes physician notes, extracts information from radiology reports, and interprets patient instructions [2]. These tasks all depend on accurately understanding complex language in real-world clinical settings.

NLP systems such as GPT-4 and Med-PaLM are designed to handle unstructured text by analyzing and generating human language in formats commonly found in clinical settings. These systems can interpret clinical notes, summarize radiology findings, and respond to patient inquiries.

A key innovation underlying these systems is a model architecture known as the transformer. More on this topic later.

In clinical practice, NLP appears in tools like Epic's NoteWriter (which drafts templated notes) [3] (which listens to conversations and creates SOAP notes), and DocsGPT [4] (which drafts responses to patient messages). These tools help clinicians reduce clerical burden, automate documentation, and communicate more clearly.

Beyond documentation, NLP can be used to:

- Extract structured data from unstructured clinical notes
- Flag potential drug interactions by parsing prior prescriptions
- Identify high-risk patients from written histories
- Predict mortality or hospitalization risks in critical care settings

Some advanced NLP systems even support decision-making by generating differential diagnoses based on a patient's narrative history. Powered by NLP, chatbots are increasingly used for pre-visit screening, post-visit education, and triage support, offering responses in natural-sounding language.

Despite its promise, NLP has limitations that are especially relevant in clinical settings (see Fig. 3.2). Clinical notes often contain jargon, abbreviations, and ambiguous phrases that even the most advanced systems can misinterpret. For example, one hospital tested an NLP model for emergency triage. It consistently

Documentation Automation
Tools like Epic NoteWriter help draft notes using voice input or templates.

Patient Communication
Chatbots explain conditions and provide follow-up education in plain language

Clinical Prediction
NLP helps flag high-risk patients by analyzing clinical notes and patterns

Fig. 3.1 How physicians use NLP **tools**

Risk Category	Clinical Example	Potential Harm	Mitigation Strategy
Misinterpretation	NLP misreads "cold" as a viral illness instead of "cold extremities," missing signs of early circulatory shock.	Delayed recognition and treatment of shock.	Manually review outputs for ambiguous terms; use structured input fields when possible.
Bias in Training Data	An NLP model trained on urban hospital data fails to recognize rural health patterns.	Inaccurate assessments, misdiagnosis, or poor triage in underrepresented populations.	Train on diverse, representative datasets; conduct external validation across care settings.
Hallucination	AI-generated discharge note includes medication instructions not found in the patient chart.	Patient harm due to inappropriate treatment or instructions.	Require human review of generated text; limit use of generative tools for high-risk outputs.
Lack of Explainability	AI suggests a diagnosis but the logic behind it is opaque to clinicians and developers.	Reduced clinician trust and inability to validate AI recommendations.	Use models with explainability tools such as saliency maps or rationales;
			educate users on limitations.

Fig. 3.2 Clinical NLP risk matrix

interpreted the word "cold" as a viral illness, even when the physician's note clearly referred to "cold extremities," a possible shock indicator. This misreading demonstrates the risk of relying on models that do not fully grasp clinical nuance.

Bias in training data also presents serious challenges. If a model is trained mostly on data from urban hospitals, it may perform poorly in rural clinics where demographics and health conditions differ. A more specific risk, known as **training-set mismatch**, arises when hospital-trained models stumble in community practices. Even a well-performing AI model can fail spectacularly if it has never seen data like yours. Hospital datasets often exhibit varying disease rates, coding styles, and patient demographics compared to those in neighborhood practices. Without sampling from a range of primary-care sites—urban, rural, and high- and low-resource—models may misinterpret routine findings or miss critical signals, undermining their reliability in front-line clinics. Clinical consequences of biased training data can include missed diagnoses, inappropriate triage recommendations, or misleading health education materials.

Another concern is hallucination. NLP models sometimes generate fabricated details, offering confident but incorrect statements. This makes human oversight indispensable. Clinicians must know these risks and when to verify or challenge a system's conclusions.

As the field evolves, transparency and explainability are essential. Clinicians must understand what the system is doing, what data it was trained on, and how to assess its reliability. NLP is not a replacement for clinical judgment but a tool that works best when paired with it.

While NLP helps clinicians make sense of unstructured text, many diagnostic decisions hinge on interpreting visual data, from X-rays to histopathology slides. For that, we turn to a different class of models designed to process images: convolutional neural networks.

Sidebar: Tech Spotlight: CNNs and RAG
Convolutional neural networks (CNNs) excel at extracting spatial patterns from images—think CT scans and histopathology slides. CNNs apply filters across pixels, highlighting edges, textures, or lesions. While Chap. 4 goes deeper into imaging applications, here we note that CNN representations can feed into text analyses (e.g., image-captioning prompts).

Retrieval-augmented generation (RAG) combines a retrieval system (like a clinical database) with a generative model. RAG first fetches relevant documents and then prompts the model to synthesize grounded summaries. This hybrid approach reduces hallucinations by anchoring outputs in real data. You'll see full case studies of RAG in Chap. 7's "Patient Education" section.

Convolutional Neural Networks (CNNs) in Clinical Practice

What Are CNNs and How Do They Work?

Convolutional neural networks, or CNNs, are a specialized type of deep learning algorithm designed to interpret visual data. In healthcare, they are especially useful for analyzing medical images, such as chest X-rays, MRI scans, and CT images. Unlike traditional image processing methods that rely on hand-crafted features, CNNs learn directly from raw image data. They automatically detect patterns by passing images through a series of computational layers that mimic how a human might study an image, from simple shapes to complex patterns.

At their core, CNNs include multiple layers. The initial layers recognize basic features like edges or color gradients. Deeper layers combine these features to detect more complex structures, such as lesions, tumors, or anatomical boundaries. This layered architecture makes CNNs highly effective for tasks such as classification (e.g., pneumonia vs. no pneumonia), detection (e.g., spotting a small lung nodule), and segmentation (e.g., outlining the borders of a tumor). Think of it like a radiologist scanning a CT scan in increasing detail, the CNN does the same, but computationally.

How CNNs Differ from Other AI Models

Compared to traditional rule-based systems or even standard machine learning algorithms, CNNs offer a critical advantage in handling image data. Rule-based systems follow predefined logic and struggle with variability in images. Standard machine learning often requires extensive feature engineering. CNNs, by contrast, excel at identifying features automatically, making them ideal for the complex, high-dimensional data found in medical imaging.

Clinical Applications of CNNs

CNNs have found real-world use in a variety of diagnostic and therapeutic scenarios:

In **disease classification**, CNNs help distinguish between conditions based on image features. For instance, they have been trained to identify diabetic retinopathy in retinal fundus photographs and classify breast masses as benign or malignant on mammograms.

For **tumor segmentation**, CNNs can outline the boundaries of brain tumors on MRI scans, guiding both surgical planning and radiation therapy.

In **lesion detection**, CNNs support radiologists by flagging abnormalities in large image volumes that may be overlooked during routine reads, such as detecting small liver metastases or identifying pulmonary embolisms on CT angiography [6].

CNNs are also employed in **anatomical structure identification**, helping to delineate organs and vessels in complex regions like the abdomen or pelvis. This is essential for robotic surgery planning or augmented reality visualization.

During the **COVID-19 pandemic**, CNNs were adapted to identify characteristic findings in chest X-rays and CTs to help triage patients, especially in settings where PCR testing was not readily available [7].

Outside of traditional imaging, CNNs are used to interpret **echocardiograms** [8] to assess heart wall motion and analyze **electrocardiograms (ECGs)** [9, 10] to detect arrhythmias like atrial fibrillation with high sensitivity.

Benefits of CNNs in Clinical Workflows

The integration of CNNs into clinical workflows offers several advantages. They enhance diagnostic speed, enabling faster clinical decisions. They reduce human error by acting as a second reader, highlighting areas of concern. CNNs also promote standardization by offering consistent interpretations, regardless of time of day or clinician fatigue. In busy practices, CNNs can prioritize abnormal scans for immediate review, improving triage and workflow efficiency.

Challenges and Limitations

CNNs require large, well-annotated datasets for training, which is often a barrier in healthcare due to data privacy regulations and limited availability of expert-labeled data. A model trained on data from one hospital may not perform well in another, a problem known as poor generalizability. CNNs are also criticized for their opacity: they can generate accurate predictions without being able to explain their reasoning, creating a trust gap for clinicians.

Bias is another concern. The CNN may not perform equally across all demographic groups if the training data underrepresents specific populations. For example, a model trained predominantly on images from lighter-skinned patients might underperform when interpreting dermatologic images from patients with darker skin.

Improving Trust and Transparency
Researchers are developing methods to explain CNN decisions, aiming to build trust in clinical settings. Visualization tools like heatmaps and saliency maps highlight areas of the image that influenced the model's decision, making it easier for clinicians to understand and validate the output.

The Future of CNNs in Medicine
CNNs are increasingly integrated into multimodal systems that combine image analysis with electronic health record data, lab results, and natural language processing of clinical notes. This fusion enables a more holistic view of the patient, supporting decision-making across specialties. With proper validation, CNNs will likely become essential tools that complement, not replace, clinical expertise. They will help physicians provide faster, safer, and more precise care.

As we shift to retrieval-augmented methods, remember that primary care demands cohorts defined by **whole-person complexity**, not narrow disease labels. In primary care, patients rarely present with a single issue. Effective cohorts, therefore, include multiple chronic disease codes, indicators of social determinants such as housing stability, and observation windows that extend over years. This whole-person approach ensures that AI outputs truly reflect the interwoven health and life factors central to family medicine practice.

Just as different clinical tools serve different diagnostic tasks, different model architectures are optimized for various data types. CNNs are best suited for spatial data. But what about information that's embedded in time or text? To process those, we need models designed for sequences, such as transformers.

Transformer Architectures in Clinical AI

Transformers revolutionized how AI models handle sequential data by introducing a **self-attention** mechanism that lets the model simultaneously weigh the importance of every word, or data point, against every other [11]. Rather than processing one token at a time (as RNNs do), transformers create a web of connections that capture local detail and global context in a single pass. For a refresher on tokens and tokenization, see Chap. 2.

Transformers revolutionize how models process language by letting every token "look at" every other token. First, the text undergoes tokenization, breaking a sentence into discrete units (words or subwords). Then the model computes three vectors for each token: a Query, a Key, and a Value. Self-attention multiplies Queries by Keys (dot products) to assign scores that reflect contextual relevance. Finally, it weights each token's Value by these scores and sums them to produce a context-rich representation. In practice, this means the word "bark" in "the dog's bark" pays more attention to "dog" than to "tree," resolving ambiguity on the fly. You can explore the mathematical details of this process in Chap. 2a, Sect. 2a.3. By explicitly linking tokens across the entire sequence, self-attention empowers transformers to capture long-range dependencies, key for interpreting complex clinical narratives.

For you as a medical student, this means transformer-based models such as Clinical BERT, which is tuned on electronic health record notes, can quickly summarize long progress notes, highlight key findings, and even suggest relevant guidelines without losing sight of the overall narrative [12]. In practical terms, a transformer-powered assistant might read a multipage admission note and pull out exactly the lab trends, medication changes, and social history details you need to formulate a care plan, all in seconds.

Key advantages for clinical use include the following:

- **Speed and Scalability:** Parallel processing enables the swift analysis of large batches of notes or imaging reports.
- **Context-Rich Understanding:** Self-attention ensures that distant mentions—like a past surgery noted months ago—still inform today's summary.
- **Flexibility Across Modalities:** Transformers can be extended to handle text, imaging features, and even structured data in a unified framework.

By mastering the basics of transformers, you'll better appreciate why downstream methods, like retrieval-augmented generation, build on their ability to "understand" and index vast amounts of clinical information before retrieving the most pertinent knowledge.

Introducing RAG: Retrieval-Augmented Generation

Retrieval-augmented generation, or RAG, represents an evolution in how AI models access and use information. Rather than relying solely on pre-trained knowledge, RAG models can retrieve relevant, up-to-date data from trusted sources, such as electronic health records or medical literature, and use it to ground their generated outputs. *(For hands-on clinical use of RAG tools, see Section "Feedback loops & continuous learning".)*

How RAG Works in Clinical Contexts

RAG systems function in three stages. First, the system retrieves relevant information from a structured or semi-structured database. Then, this data is integrated into the prompt for the AI model. Finally, the model generates a response that incorporates both the query and the retrieved knowledge, improving the factual grounding of the output.

How RAG Differs from Other AI Approaches
Common LLMs, such as pure generative models or rule-based systems, often lack the context specificity required in complex fields like healthcare.

RAG Versus Pure Generative Models: These large language models generate outputs based on patterns learned from training data. While they can produce coherent responses, they might not always be accurate or relevant, especially in a dynamic field like healthcare, where new research and clinical guidelines are constantly emerging.

RAG Versus Rule-Based Systems: These rely on pre-defined rules and are limited by the knowledge encoded within them. They struggle to adapt to new data or unexpected scenarios and are often rigid and unable to handle the nuanced decision-making required in healthcare.

Benefits of RAG in Healthcare
RAG enhances accuracy in clinical decision support by enabling real-time access to recent clinical guidelines, case studies, and patient data. It reduces hallucinations. It can personalize responses to specific patient populations using proprietary datasets. RAG ensures data security by retrieving information from compliant, secure databases, keeping sensitive patient data protected. It also provides traceability; clinicians can examine the sources that inform the AI's output, which is a critical feature for maintaining trust and meeting regulatory expectations.

Clinical Applications of RAG
In practice, RAG is being used for automated chart review, clinical triage, and generation of patient-specific education materials. For example, a RAG system might generate a differential diagnosis by combining patient symptoms from an EHR with recent literature on rare diseases. Using authoritative databases like UpToDate or PubMed, RAG also helps power tools that answer clinicians' questions in real time [13].

Defining targets and metrics must also match primary-care priorities of prevention and continuity. Instead of predicting immediate events, primary-care models often benefit from **longer horizons,** for example, forecasting fall risk 6–12 months ahead.

Challenges and Future Directions
While RAG systems improve transparency and adaptability, they rely heavily on the quality and structure of their source data. Inconsistent formats or outdated content can lead to misleading outputs. To address this, efforts are underway to standardize medical databases and improve interoperability. RAG will likely become foundational in AI-supported medical practice as these systems mature, offering clinicians fast, context-aware, and verifiable insights.

Finally, because no two clinics are identical, robust deployment requires **local validation** and ongoing monitoring for data-drift and model-drift. Before rolling out any AI tool, test it on your own clinic's patient data to confirm it works in your setting. After deployment, set up systems to detect when incoming data patterns shift (data-drift) or when performance degrades (model-drift), and involve frontline staff in periodic reviews. This combination of local validation and staff-driven governance is key to keeping AI accurate, fair, and trustworthy over time.

Even the most advanced AI systems depend on how clinicians interact with them. The next section explores how to craft prompts that guide models toward safe, accurate, and clinically useful outputs.

Sidebar: Understanding Data-Drift

What Is Data-Drift?

Data-drift occurs when the statistical properties of incoming real-world data change over time compared with the data on which an AI model was trained. In clinical practice, this might mean shifts in patient demographics (age, comorbidities), new coding conventions, changes in documentation workflows, or evolving disease patterns (e.g., the rise of a novel infectious agent).

Why It Matters

- **Degraded Performance:** A model that once accurately predicted a 90% risk of hospitalization may become less reliable if patients' characteristics or record-keeping styles change.
- **Unintended Bias:** When data drift disproportionately affects records, groups underrepresented in the original training set may suffer more.

Detection Strategies

1. **Statistical Monitoring:** Regularly compare feature distributions (e.g., age, lab values) in new data against the training baseline using techniques like population-stability index (PSI).
2. **Performance Tracking:** Continuously track key model metrics (accuracy, sensitivity, specificity). Sudden drops can signal drift.

Mitigation Approaches

- **Retraining/Updating:** Periodically retrain the model on a mixed dataset that includes recent records.
- **Adaptive Algorithms:** Use online learning techniques that adjust model parameters as new data arrive.
- **Governance Oversight:** Involve clinicians in reviewing drift alerts and deciding when to deploy updated models.

Keeping an eye on data-drift ensures that AI tools remain accurate, fair, and safe as clinical environments evolve.

Prompt Engineering: Guiding AI with Clinical Precision

Prompt engineering is the art of writing clear, structured inputs that help AI systems, especially large language models (LLMs), produce useful and safe clinical responses. Just like a poorly phrased consult request can confuse a specialist, a vague AI prompt can lead to inaccurate or irrelevant answers. This isn't just inconvenient in clinical settings; it can affect safety, efficiency, and trust.

An effective prompt starts with a **clinical context**: include the patient's age, sex, and presenting symptoms. Then, add **relevant findings**, such as lab values, medications, and key history. Finally, finish with a **specific request**: What exactly do you want the AI to do? Summarize findings? Propose a differential? Draft a note?

Compare the following examples:

- *"What's wrong with this patient?"*
  This vague prompt provides no anchor and invites speculative output.
- *"A 68-year-old woman with atrial fibrillation presents with shortness of breath. BNP is elevated, and chest X-ray shows pulmonary edema. What are the likely causes and next steps?"*
  This version mirrors a real clinical handoff. It provides structured data and a clear question, making the AI more likely to return a focused and medically appropriate response.

Back in Chap. 1 (Section "Prompt challenge"), you explored how subtle changes in prompt wording can lead to dramatically different outputs. That "Prompt Challenge" showed how precision and context guide AI behavior. This section builds on that foundation by exploring structured prompting strategies that mirror clinical reasoning.

As you continue through this chapter, you'll have a chance to practice crafting your own prompts and evaluating how prompt structure affects output quality. Think of prompt engineering not just as a technical skill, but as a new kind of clinical communication, where clarity and specificity shape safety, just as they do in real-world medicine. Please review the checklist below when writing your clinical prompts.

Prompt Engineering Checklist for Medical Students

☐ Start with clear patient context (age, sex, chief complaint).
☐ Include relevant clinical data (labs, meds, vitals, imaging).
☐ Use specific language, and avoid vague or broad questions.
☐ Frame the task explicitly (e.g., "Summarize findings", "List possible diagnoses").
☐ Follow clinical logic, for example, mimic case presentations or SOAP format.
☐ Ask for step-by-step reasoning if appropriate (chain-of-thought (CoT)).
☐ Break complex tasks into smaller parts (ReAct prompting).
☐ Avoid ambiguous language or incomplete prompts.
☐ Review and revise the prompt if the output is incorrect or confusing.
☐ Match prompt format to clinical use case (e.g., triage, note drafting).

Advanced Prompting Techniques in Healthcare AI
As large language models (LLMs) become increasingly integral to healthcare, refining prompt engineering strategies is essential for maximizing their utility. Here are several advanced techniques tailored for clinical applications:

1. **Chain-of-Thought Prompting**

Encourage the AI to reason through problems step-by-step by including prompts like "Let's analyze this step by step." This approach enhances the model's ability to handle complex clinical reasoning tasks.

Chain-of-Thought (CoT) Prompting for Clinical Reasoning
Chain-of-thought prompting is a technique that encourages AI models to break down complex problems into a series of intermediate reasoning steps before arriving at a final answer. By explicitly prompting the AI to "think step-by-step" or "analyze this systematically," you can dramatically improve performance on tasks requiring multistep reasoning.

How Chain-of-Thought Works
CoT prompting works by:

- Signaling to the AI that a step-by-step approach is needed
- Creating space for intermediate reasoning to be articulated
- Allowing verification of each logical step in the reasoning process
- Reducing errors by catching flawed reasoning earlier in the process

Clinical Applications for Physicians in Training

Example 1: Diagnostic Reasoning for Acute Abdominal Pain
Standard Prompt:

What's the diagnosis for a 45-year-old male with right lower quadrant (RLQ) pain, fever, and leukocytosis?

Chain-of-Thought Prompt:

A 45-year-old male presents with right lower quadrant pain, fever, and leukocytosis. Let's analyze this step-by-step to determine the most likely diagnosis.

CoT Response:

Let me think through this systematically:

Step 1: Identify the key clinical features

- Middle-aged male (45 years)
- Right lower quadrant (RLQ) pain
- Fever
- Leukocytosis (elevated white blood cell count)

Step 2: Consider anatomic structures in the RLQ

– Appendix
– Terminal ileum
– Cecum
– Right ovary/fallopian tube (not applicable in male)
– Ureter
– Psoas muscle

Step 3: Match symptoms to potential conditions

– Acute appendicitis: RLQ pain, fever, leukocytosis—*STRONG MATCH*
– Ileocecal Crohn's disease: Can present with RLQ pain and fever, but typically has chronic symptoms
– Cecal diverticulitis: Possible but less common than left-sided diverticulitis
– Kidney stone/pyelonephritis: Typically flank pain rather than RLQ
– Psoas abscess: Uncommon, typically secondary to another process

Step 4: Evaluate probability based on epidemiology

– Acute appendicitis is the most common surgical emergency of the abdomen.
– Peak incidence includes middle-aged adults.
– Classic triad includes pain, fever, and leukocytosis.

Step 5: Consider additional information needed

– Migration of pain from periumbilical to RLQ (McBurney's point)
– Presence of rebound tenderness and guarding
– Anorexia or nausea/vomiting
– Urinalysis to rule out urinary causes
– Imaging (CT or ultrasound) findings

Given the information provided, acute appendicitis is the most likely diagnosis, though further history, physical examination findings, and imaging would be helpful to confirm.

Example 2: Management of Diabetic Ketoacidosis (DKA)
Standard Prompt:

How do you manage diabetic ketoacidosis?

Chain-of-Thought Prompt:

Let's work through managing diabetic ketoacidosis step-by-step, considering the priorities and potential complications at each stage.

CoT Response:

Let me approach DKA management systematically:

Step 1: Initial assessment and stabilization

– Assess ABCs (airway, breathing, circulation).
– Obtain IV access (preferably two large-bore IVs).
– Start cardiac monitoring and continuous pulse oximetry.
– Check vital signs including temperature.
– Order immediate labs: glucose, electrolytes, blood gas, ketones, CBC, and urinalysis

- Calculate anion gap: Na - (Cl + HCO_3).

Step 2: Fluid resuscitation

- Initial fluid: 0.9% NaCl (normal saline).
- Rate: 15–20 mL/kg/hr for the first hour (typically 1–1.5L for adults)
- Reassess volume status after initial bolus.
- Continue fluid replacement, typically 250–500 mL/h based on hemodynamics.
- Monitor for fluid overload in elderly or those with cardiac/renal disease.
- Goal: restore intravascular volume and improve tissue perfusion.

Step 3: Insulin therapy

- Start IV regular insulin after fluid initiation.
- Bolus: 0.1 units/kg (optional, often skipped in moderate cases).
- Continuous infusion: 0.1 units/kg/hr.
- Goal: reduce serum glucose by 50–75 mg/dL/hr.
- Do not lower glucose too rapidly (risk of cerebral edema).
- Continue until anion gap closes and ketoacidosis resolves.

Step 4: Electrolyte management

- Potassium: Most patients have total body potassium deficit despite normal/high initial levels.

  *If K+ <3.3 mEq/L: Hold insulin, and give potassium until >3.3.
  *If K+ 3.3–5.3 mEq/L: Add 20–30 mEq KCl to each liter of IV fluid.
  *If K+ >5.3 mEq/L: Hold potassium, and check frequently.

- Bicarbonate: Generally not recommended unless pH <6.9 or severe hyperkalemia.
- Phosphate: Replace if <1.0 mg/dL or symptomatic.

Step 5: Transitioning care

- When glucose reaches ~200 mg/dL: Switch to D5W or D5 1/2NS with continued insulin.
- When patient can eat: Start subcutaneous insulin.
- Overlap IV and subcutaneous insulin for 1–2 hours before discontinuing IV insulin.
- Address underlying precipitating cause (infection, noncompliance, new onset).

Step 6: Monitoring and complication prevention

- Hourly glucose checks.
- Electrolytes every 2–4 h until stable.
- Watch for cerebral edema (headache, altered mental status, hypertension, bradycardia).
- Monitor for hypoglycemia during treatment.
- Assess for resolution: glucose <200 mg/dL, bicarbonate ≥15 mEq/L, pH >7.3, anion gap normalized.

Step 7: Patient education before discharge

- Review sick day management.
- Ensure proper insulin administration technique.
- Discuss precipitating factors and prevention.
- Arrange appropriate follow-up.

This step-by-step approach ensures systematic management addressing all critical aspects of DKA care.

Example 3: Interpreting Arterial Blood Gas Results
Standard Prompt:

Interpret this ABG: pH 7.28, $PaCO_2$ 60 mmHg, PaO_2 85 mmHg, and HCO_3- 28 mEq/L

Chain-of-Thought Prompt:

Let's systematically interpret this arterial blood gas (pH 7.28, $PaCO_2$ 60 mmHg, PaO_2 85 mmHg, HCO_3- 28 mEq/L) by working through each component step-by-step.

CoT Response:

I'll interpret this ABG systematically:

Step 1: Assess the pH

- Normal pH range: 7.35–7.45.
- Patient's pH: 7.28.
- Interpretation: pH is below normal range → acidemia is present.

Step 2: Determine if the primary disorder is respiratory or metabolic

- Look at $PaCO_2$ (respiratory component):

Normal $PaCO_2$: 35–45 mmHg.
Patient's $PaCO_2$: 60 mmHg.
Interpretation: $PaCO_2$ is elevated → respiratory acidosis component.

- Look at HCO_3- (metabolic component):

*Normal HCO3-: 22–26 mEq/L.
*Patient's HCO3-: 28 mEq/L.
*Interpretation: HCO_3- is elevated → metabolic alkalosis component.

Step 3: Identify the primary disorder

- We have acidemia (low pH).
- With both respiratory acidosis (high $PaCO_2$) and metabolic alkalosis (high HCO_3-).
- Since the pH is acidemic, the respiratory acidosis must be the dominant disorder.
- The elevated HCO_3- represents either compensation or a mixed disorder.

Step 4: Determine if compensation is appropriate

- For acute respiratory acidosis:

*Expected HCO_3- increase: 1 mEq/L for every 10 mmHg increase in $PaCO_2$.

*$PaCO_2$ is elevated by ~15–20 mmHg → expected HCO_3- increase of ~1.5-2 mEq/L.
*Expected HCO_3- would be ~23.5–24 mEq/L.

- For chronic respiratory acidosis:

  * Expected HCO_3- increase: 3.5 mEq/L for every 10 mmHg increase in $PaCO_2$
  * $PaCO_2$ is elevated by ~15–20 mmHg → expected HCO_3- increase of ~5.25–7 mEq/L
  * Expected HCO_3- would be ~27.25–29 mEq/L

- Patient's actual HCO_3-: 28 mEq/L.
- This is consistent with chronic compensation or possibly a mixed disorder.

Step 5: Assess oxygenation

- PaO_2: 85 mmHg.
- This is within normal limits (80–100 mmHg).
- No hypoxemia is present.

Step 6: Form final interpretation

- Primary disorder: Chronic respiratory acidosis (elevated $PaCO_2$ with appropriate metabolic compensation via increased HCO_3-)
- Alternatively: Mixed respiratory acidosis and metabolic alkalosis with respiratory acidosis dominating
- Oxygenation: Normal

Step 7: Consider clinical context

- Chronic respiratory acidosis is commonly seen in:

  • COPD
  • Obesity hypoventilation syndrome
  • Neuromuscular disorders
  • Severe kyphoscoliosis

- If the patient also has a reason for metabolic alkalosis (diuretic use, vomiting, nasogastric suction), a true mixed disorder may be present.

Final interpretation: Chronic respiratory acidosis with appropriate metabolic compensation. Normal oxygenation.

Benefits for Physicians in Training

Chain-of-thought prompting offers several advantages for medical trainees:

1. Mirrors clinical reasoning processes: Aligns with the systematic approach taught in medical education
2. Educational tool: Demonstrates expert-level reasoning that trainees can learn from and emulate
3. Prevents diagnostic errors: Reduces cognitive biases by forcing consideration of each step

4. Improves documentation: Provides a framework for clearly documenting clinical reasoning in notes
5. Preparation for case presentations: Helps organize thoughts for structured case presentations to attendings
6. Exam preparation: Trains the reasoning process needed for board exams and clinical scenarios
7. Feedback tool: Allows preceptors to identify specific gaps in a trainee's reasoning process

By incorporating phrases like "Let's analyze this step-by-step," "Let me think through this systematically," or "Let's work through this methodically" into your prompts, you can leverage chain-of-thought prompting to enhance clinical reasoning and decision-making throughout your medical training.

2. **Role-Based Prompting**

Role-based prompting is a technique where you instruct the AI to adopt a specific role, perspective, or expertise when generating responses. By defining a particular role, you provide the AI with context about the expected knowledge base, communication style, and approach to problem-solving that should be reflected in its response.

How Role-Based Prompting Works

When using role-based prompting, you typically:

- Specify the role the AI should adopt (e.g., "Act as an experienced cardiologist")
- Provide context about the situation or problem
- Describe the task or question to be addressed
- Optionally, specify the intended audience or outcome

This technique leverages the AI's ability to adapt its knowledge representation and communication style to match different professional perspectives.

Benefits in Medical Education

For medical students, role-based prompting offers several advantages:

- Exposes students to different clinical reasoning patterns across specialties
- Helps prepare for different rotations by modeling specialty-specific thinking
- Demonstrates how different healthcare professionals might approach the same case
- Provides practice in communicating with different audiences (patients, colleagues, specialists)

Example: Role-Based Prompting for a Medical Student

Example Prompt:

Act as an experienced emergency medicine attending physician supervising a third-year medical student. The student has just evaluated their first patient with suspected acute coronary syndrome: a 62-year-old male with 40 minutes of substernal chest pressure, diaphoresis, and shortness of breath. The student seems uncertain about next steps in management.

Provide guidance to this medical student, including:

- Your immediate clinical concerns and priorities
- Which diagnostic tests should be ordered immediately
- Initial management steps while awaiting results
- Key risk stratification factors to consider
- How to present this case efficiently to the team

Remember that your goal is both patient care and learning appropriate clinical reasoning for emergency medicine.

Example Response
Alright, let's pause here and work through this case together. Good job completing the initial assessment of this patient.

First, I want to acknowledge that this presentation is concerning for ACS until proven otherwise, and we need to move efficiently while remaining thorough.

1. Immediate Clinical Concerns and Priorities:

    - This is a high-risk presentation with classic ACS symptoms.
    - Our priority is rapid assessment, stabilization, and initiation of appropriate therapy.
    - We need to determine: Is this STEMI, NSTEMI, unstable angina, or another cause of chest pain?
    - Remember our "door-to-balloon" time goal of <90 minutes if this is a STEMI.

2. Immediate Diagnostic Tests:

    - 12-lead ECG—this should be done within 10 minutes of arrival.
    - Cardiac biomarkers (troponin)—order now and plan for serial measurements.
    - Basic labs: CBC, CMP, and coagulation studies.
    - Portable chest X-ray.
    - Consider point-of-care ultrasound to assess for obvious wall motion abnormalities or alternative diagnoses.

3. Initial Management (Before Results Return):

    - Establish IV access with two large-bore IVs.
    - Supplemental oxygen only if hypoxemic (SpO2 <90%).
    - Cardiac monitoring.
    - "MONA" approach with modifications:

        – Morphine: We're using this less frequently now due to potential masking of symptoms and outcomes concerns.
        – Oxygen: As mentioned, only if hypoxemic.
        – Nitroglycerine: 0.4 mg SL if SBP >90mmHg and no contraindications.
        – Aspirin: 325 mg chewed immediately unless true allergy.

    - Additional medications to consider:

- P2Y12 inhibitor (e.g., ticagrelor, clopidogrel)
- Anticoagulation (e.g., heparin)
- Beta-blocker if no contraindications and after ruling out STEMI with right ventricular involvement

4. Risk Stratification Factors:

    - Demographic factors: Age >65, male sex
    - Medical history: Prior MI/CAD, diabetes, kidney disease, PVD
    - Presentation: Duration of symptoms, response to nitrates, hemodynamic stability
    - ECG changes: ST elevation/depression, T-wave inversions, new LBBB
    - Troponin elevation
    - HEART, TIMI, or GRACE score calculation
    - Killip classification if ACS confirmed

5. Efficient Case Presentation:

    - Start with one-liner: "Mr. X is a 62-year-old male with hypertension and hyperlipidemia presenting with 40 min of substernal chest pressure, diaphoresis, and shortness of breath concerning for ACS."
    - Relevant history and exam findings focusing on cardiac and pulmonary systems.
    - Key vitals and abnormal findings.
    - Initial ECG interpretation.
    - Differential diagnosis with ACS at the top.
    - Initial management already started.
    - Specific questions or concerns.

Remember, in emergency medicine, we often must act before we have all the information. With chest pain patients, we work to rule in/out life-threatening diagnoses first while keeping a broad differential. After you see the ECG, let's review it together and adjust our management plan accordingly.

Any questions about our approach so far?

Variations of Role-Based Prompting for Medical Students

You can use role-based prompting to practice different clinical scenarios:

- *Specialty-Specific Guidance:* Act as a [pediatric neurologist/infectious disease specialist/etc.] consulting on a case of [clinical scenario].
- *Different Communication Contexts:* Act as an internal medicine resident explaining a new diabetes diagnosis to a patient with limited health literacy.
- *Interprofessional Collaboration:* Act as a physical therapist providing recommendations for postoperative mobility for a patient who has undergone total knee replacement.
- *Different Training Levels:* Act as a PGY-3 resident providing feedback to a medical student on their first lumbar puncture procedure.

- *Patient Education:* Act as a family physician, explaining the importance of vaccination to a hesitant parent.

By experimenting with different roles, medical students can gain exposure to diverse perspectives and approaches to clinical problems, enhancing their preparation for various clinical rotations and interdisciplinary collaboration.

3. **Iterative Refinement in Clinical Contexts**

What Is Iterative Refinement and Why It Matters to You

As a medical student, you're developing a core professional habit: refining your thinking as new information becomes available. This is exactly what iterative refinement means in the context of AI prompting. You begin with a broad query and progressively narrow the focus, adding details just as you would when working through a differential diagnosis or developing a care plan. This approach aligns closely with clinical reasoning and allows AI to respond in ways that are more accurate, relevant, and patient-specific.

Mastering iterative prompting now will equip you to use AI tools more effectively throughout your training and career, whether you're working through complex cases, conducting evidence-based research, or preparing personalized patient education materials.

Clinical Example 1: Building a Differential Diagnosis
This example shows how successive details help an AI tool deliver more clinically useful responses.

- **Initial Prompt (General):** "What are the possible causes of chest pain?"
- **Refinement 1 (Add Demographics):** "What are the most likely causes of chest pain in a 42-year-old male?"
- **Refinement 2 (Add Risk Factors):** "…with obesity, hypertension, and family history of heart disease?"
- **Refinement 3 (Add Symptoms):** "…described as 'pressure' radiating to the left arm?"
- **Refinement 4 (Add Physical Findings):** "…with tachycardia (HR 110), elevated BP (162/95), and diaphoresis, no murmurs?"
- **Refinement 5 (Add Diagnostic Data):** "…ECG shows ST-segment elevation in V2–V4; troponin is 0.8 ng/mL?"

Clinical Example 2: Developing a Treatment Plan
Here, the model is guided step-by-step toward individualized care:

- **Initial Prompt (General):** "What are standard treatment approaches for community-acquired pneumonia?"
- **Refinement 1 (Add Age):** "…for a 68-year-old female?"
- **Refinement 2 (Add Comorbidities):** "…with type 2 diabetes and CKD (eGFR 40)?"
- **Refinement 3 (Add Clinical Status):** "…hemodynamically stable, hypoxic on 2L O_2?"

- **Refinement 4 (Add Allergies):** "…with severe penicillin allergy, anaphylaxis?"
- **Refinement 5 (Add Microbiology):** "…*Klebsiella pneumoniae* sensitive to fluoroquinolones, resistant to macrolides?"

Clinical Example 3: Tailoring Patient Education
This scenario shows how social and cultural factors shape communication strategies:

- **Initial Prompt (General):** "How should I explain diabetes management to a patient?"
- **Refinement 1 (Add Demographics):** "…to a newly diagnosed 54-year-old?"
- **Refinement 2 (Add Health Literacy):** "…with limited health literacy?"
- **Refinement 3 (Add Patient Concerns):** "…who is anxious about insulin injections?"
- **Refinement 4 (Add Social Context):** "…who lives alone with limited social support?"
- **Refinement 5 (Add Cultural Considerations):** "…Spanish-speaking, with cultural misconceptions about insulin?"

Takeaway for Medical Students
These examples show that refining prompts in stages allows AI to deliver responses that mirror the granularity and nuance of good clinical thinking. Like clinical problem-solving, prompting is a process, not a one-shot question. This habit reinforces your diagnostic discipline, strengthens your communication with AI, and helps you extract reliable, patient-centered insights.

Benefits of Iterative Refinement in Your Clinical Practice
As a medical student, you're building habits that will shape how you think, document, and make decisions for the rest of your career. Iterative refinement is not just a prompting technique; it's a cognitive tool that mirrors how clinicians naturally work through uncertainty and evolving patient data. Integrating this approach into your workflow can help you interact more effectively with patients and AI systems:

- **Mirrors your clinical reasoning process:** This method aligns with how you'll naturally approach cases—starting with broad possibilities and refining your assessment as more data becomes available. It reinforces the diagnostic habits you're already learning in rounds and preceptorships.
- **Helps you avoid information overload:** By isolating one detail at a time, iterative refinement trains you to evaluate each new piece of data in context, rather than becoming overwhelmed by the full complexity of a case all at once.
- **Adapts to evolving clinical scenarios:** When new lab results arrive or a patient's symptoms change, you can update your prompts in real time. This flexibility mirrors how working diagnoses are updated as clinical conditions evolve.
- **Enhances your learning:** Seeing how AI narrows its responses with each added input helps you visualize how a differential diagnosis changes with accumulating data—an invaluable exercise for strengthening clinical judgment.

- **Improves your documentation:** The stepwise logic used in refined prompting parallels the structure of a well-written clinical note. It helps you document not just your conclusions, but how you arrived at them.
- **Makes efficient use of AI assistance:** Rather than repeating a full case history in every prompt, you can build on previous inputs. This saves time and encourages more precise and clinically relevant output from the model.

When to Be Cautious

While iterative refinement is powerful, be mindful of these potential pitfalls:

- **Confirmation bias:** As you refine your prompts, stay open to alternative diagnoses that may not fit your initial hypothesis
- **Emergency situations:** In time-critical scenarios, you may need to act on limited information rather than waiting for complete data
- **Overreliance on technology:** Remember that AI tools complement, but don't replace, your clinical judgment and expertise

Your Turn: Practice Exercise

Scenario A 76-year-old female presents to the emergency department with acute confusion.

Try crafting a series of increasingly refined prompts as you would receive the following information:

1. Start with just the chief complaint.
2. Add that she has a history of hypertension and atrial fibrillation.
3. Add that her temperature is 38.9°C (102°F).
4. Add that urinalysis shows bacteria and WBCs.
5. Add that she's on warfarin with an INR of 4.7.

Applying This to Your Current Clinical Rotations

Here are three ways you can begin practicing iterative refinement during your training:

1. **Case presentations:** Before presenting to your attending, try using iterative refinement with an AI tool to develop your differential diagnosis and management plan

2. **Unfamiliar conditions:** When encountering a condition you haven't seen before, use this technique to guide your learning about diagnosis and management
3. **Preparation for rounds:** Practice crafting refined prompts based on your patients' evolving clinical pictures

Remember, iterative refinement in AI prompting closely parallels the SOAP note process and case presentations you're already learning. Both involve systematically incorporating new information to refine your understanding of the patient's condition and determine the most appropriate next steps in care.

4. **Few-Shot Prompting: Teaching by Example**

Few-shot prompting guides an AI model by showing it a few examples of what you want, before asking it to generate new content on its own. The term "few-shot" comes from machine learning and refers to the model learning from just a few reference cases instead of thousands (as in traditional training). In practical terms, this means you can "teach" an AI assistant how to respond simply by showing it two or three well-crafted examples within your prompt.

In clinical settings, few-shot prompting is particularly useful for generating structured, medically appropriate responses. It helps ensure that the AI mirrors your tone, logic, and reasoning style—especially when drafting differential diagnoses, discharge summaries, or patient instructions.

Few-Shot Prompting for Clinical Applications
Here's how a physician might use this technique to support diagnostic reasoning:

Prompt to the AI:

"I need help creating differential diagnoses for patient cases. I'll provide several examples of patient presentations. For each case, generate a prioritized list of possible diagnoses, along with one-sentence justifications for each."

Examples Included in the Prompt
Example 1

Patient Presentation: 68-year-old male with sudden onset of right-sided weakness and slurred speech.

Differential Diagnosis:

1. Ischemic stroke—sudden focal neurologic deficit in an elderly patient.
2. Intracerebral hemorrhage—acute symptoms could also result from a hemorrhage.
3. Brain tumor—less likely given acuity, but possible in the setting of new focal signs.

Example 2

Patient Presentation: 25-year-old female with fever, sore throat, and tender cervical lymph nodes.

Differential Diagnosis:

1. Streptococcal pharyngitis is a common bacterial cause in young adults with these symptoms.

2. Infectious mononucleosis often presents similarly with lymphadenopathy and fatigue.
3. Viral pharyngitis is most likely if symptoms are mild and self-limited.

Your Turn
Patient Presentation: 54-year-old male with epigastric pain after meals, unintentional weight loss, and fatigue.

[AI generates similar structure with justifications.]

This few-shot approach provides the AI with the following:

1. **Clear structure**: The example shows the expected format (prioritized list with justifications).
2. **Clinical reasoning patterns**: Demonstrates how physicians prioritize diagnoses based on clinical presentation.
3. **Appropriate medical terminology**: Sets the expected level of medical language.
4. **Reasoning transparency**: Shows how to justify each diagnosis consideration.

When the physician inputs the final case (35-year-old with severe headache), the AI can follow the established pattern to produce a clinically appropriate differential diagnosis that might include subarachnoid hemorrhage, meningitis, migraine, and other relevant conditions.

By giving the AI these examples first, you prime it to match your reasoning style and expectations. If you want to teach the AI what *not* to do, you can also include negative examples illustrating poor or irrelevant responses.

Benefits in Clinical Practice
Few-shot prompting is particularly valuable in medicine because:

- It helps align AI outputs with standard clinical reasoning processes
- It reduces the need for extensive prompt engineering for each new clinical question
- It can be customized to individual practice styles or specialty-specific approaches
- It creates more predictable and reliable outputs for clinical decision support

Physicians can create libraries of few-shot examples for common clinical tasks like generating differential diagnoses, interpreting lab results, creating patient education materials, or drafting clinical notes with consistent structure and content.

Why This Matters for Medical Students
Few-shot prompting gives you precise control over how the AI responds. It helps you practice the structure and logic of clinical reasoning while improving the usefulness of the AI's output. Think of it like teaching a medical student: show them a couple of ideal responses, and then ask them to try one themselves. It's a simple but powerful way to shape AI assistance to match professional standards.

5. **Politeness and Encouragement: Shaping How AI Responds**

When interacting with large language models, the tone of your prompt matters. Using polite, collaborative, or encouraging language can improve the AI's response's quality, completeness, and tone. For example, a prompt like "Please walk me through this step-by-step" is more likely to produce structured, helpful output than a blunt command like "Explain this."

Surprisingly, this effect is not just anecdotal; it reflects how these models are trained. Most modern language models, including those used in medicine, are fine-tuned on datasets that include human dialogues where cooperative and respectful language signals a shared goal. The model responds in kind. Encouraging phrases such as "Take a deep breath and work through this carefully" or "Let's approach this together step-by-step" can activate the model's internal templates for coaching, empathy, or instruction.

This is particularly useful when using AI to simulate teaching scenarios, role-play patient education, or generate motivational scripts. It also reduces the chance of receiving terse, vague, or overly technical replies, especially in high-stakes or emotionally sensitive prompts.

For medical students, this is a reminder that how you ask affects what you get. Practicing respectful, specific, and collaborative prompting prepares you not only to work with AI more effectively but also to communicate more thoughtfully with patients and colleagues.

6. **ReAct (Reasoning + Acting) Prompting**

ReAct prompting is a technique that combines reasoning (thinking step by step) with acting (taking specific actions based on that reasoning) in an iterative cycle. This approach helps AI models perform better on complex tasks by:

1. Breaking down problems into manageable steps
2. Explicitly reasoning through each step
3. Taking appropriate actions based on this reasoning
4. Observing the results of those actions
5. Using these observations to inform the next cycle of reasoning

ReAct is particularly effective for tasks requiring both critical thinking and information gathering or decision-making.

How ReAct Works

In a ReAct framework, the AI alternates between:

- **Thought:** Explicit step-by-step reasoning about the current situation
- **Action:** A specific action to take based on the reasoning
- **Observation:** The result of the action, which informs the next thought

Example: A Physician Using ReAct for Patient Care

Here's how a physician might use ReAct prompting for a complex patient case:

Patient: 67-year-old male presenting with unexplained weight loss, fatigue, and intermittent abdominal pain for the past 3 months.

Thought: The patient has concerning symptoms that could indicate several conditions, including cancer, chronic infection, or metabolic disorders. I need to gather more information systematically to narrow down the possibilities.

Action: Review patient history for risk factors and previous conditions.

Observation: Patient has history of smoking (40-pack years), type 2 diabetes (well-controlled), and family history of colorectal cancer in father.

Thought: The smoking history increases risk for several malignancies, and the family history of colorectal cancer is particularly relevant given the abdominal symptoms. I should focus my physical examination and initial diagnostic plan.

Action: Perform targeted physical examination focusing on abdominal assessment, lymph nodes, and general condition.

Observation: Patient has mild tenderness in the left lower quadrant, no palpable masses. Appears pale with minimal peripheral lymphadenopathy.

Thought: The physical findings are nonspecific but concerning. Given the constellation of symptoms, age, risk factors, and family history, I need to rule out colorectal cancer and other GI malignancies as a priority while also considering other possibilities.

Action: Order initial diagnostic tests: CBC, comprehensive metabolic panel, fecal occult blood test, and abdominal CT scan.

Observation: Lab results show mild anemia (Hgb 11.2), elevated inflammatory markers. Fecal occult blood test positive. CT scan shows irregular wall thickening in the sigmoid colon with regional lymphadenopathy.

Thought: These findings are highly suggestive of colorectal cancer. I need to confirm the diagnosis with direct visualization and biopsy, stage the disease, and prepare to discuss treatment options with the patient.

Action: Refer for urgent colonoscopy with biopsy of the suspicious area.

This ReAct approach helps the physician:

- Systematically work through differential diagnoses
- Document their reasoning process clearly
- Ensure each diagnostic step builds logically on previous findings
- Avoid premature conclusion-jumping
- Create a clear record of their clinical reasoning and decision-making

ReAct prompting is particularly valuable in medicine, where complex decisions benefit from structured thinking, careful documentation, and evidence-based action. It can help physicians avoid cognitive biases and ensure thorough consideration of all relevant information before arriving at a diagnosis or treatment plan.

For medical students, the skills involved in writing an effective prompt parallel those used in preparing a focused case presentation. It sharpens clinical reasoning, encourages precision, and reinforces thoughtful communication, skills essential in both human and AI-assisted care.

7. **Prompt** Crafting **Workshop (Interactive Section)**

In this section, students will:

- Compare vague and structured prompts to observe quality differences in AI output
- Rewrite flawed prompts to make them more precise and more clinically useful
- Create prompts for three audiences: a patient, a nurse, and an attending physician

Practice and Application

Prompt Crafting Workshop: Practice and Application

One of the most effective ways to build your confidence with AI tools is through active experimentation. This interactive section offers you a hands-on opportunity to practice and refine the skill of prompt engineering. Much like learning to write a clinical note or present a case, crafting prompts becomes more intuitive through repetition, feedback, and peer learning.

Why Practice Matters

Effective prompting is a skill that develops over time. Just as vague questions in rounds can confuse a consultant, vague prompts to an AI system often yield vague, unhelpful answers. This workshop bridges that gap by allowing you to directly compare the quality of AI output across different styles of input.

Workshop Activities

You'll begin by examining real examples of vague prompts such as "Explain heart failure" and comparing them to structured, audience-specific alternatives like "Explain systolic heart failure to a 65-year-old patient with low health literacy who is concerned about fluid retention." The difference in the relevance and tone of the AI's response will be immediately clear.

Next, you'll engage in guided rewriting exercises. You'll be given a flawed prompt and asked to improve it using the principles of prompt clarity, context, specificity, and role awareness. For instance, a poor prompt like "What's the treatment for pneumonia?" might be refined to "For a 72-year-old female with community-acquired pneumonia, type 2 diabetes, and penicillin allergy, what are recommended inpatient antibiotic regimens?" (see Fig. 3.3 for a refresher on how to structure prompts).

In small groups, you'll practice creating prompts for three different healthcare audiences:

- A patient (prioritizing clarity and compassion)
- A nurse (emphasizing logistics and handoff communication)
- An attending physician (focusing on differential diagnosis and clinical reasoning)

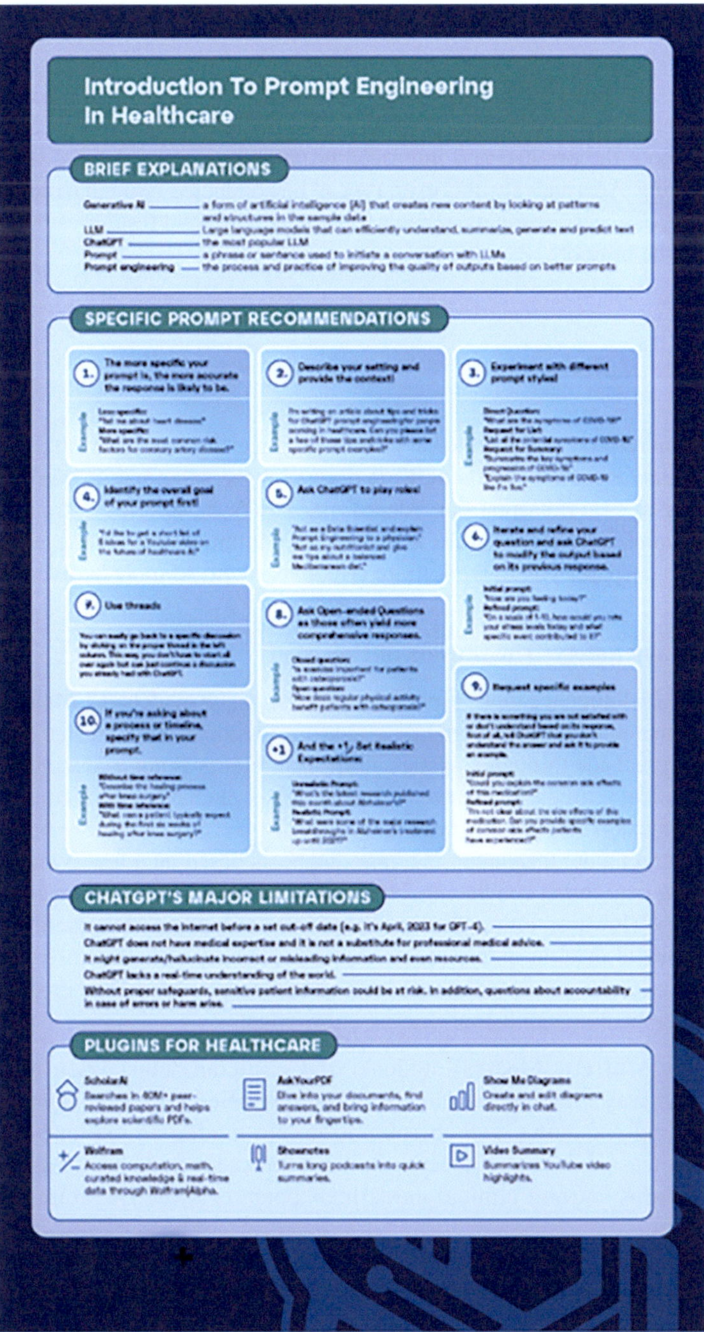

Fig. 3.3 Guide to prompt engineering

Optional Tools and Formats

Your instructor may choose to integrate AI tools directly by using a sandboxed version of a large language model (such as GPT-4 or Claude) during the session. You can enter both the original and improved prompts and evaluate the differences in output quality. Alternatively, this exercise can be conducted through structured role-play, with your peers acting as AI tools to simulate different responses based on the quality of the prompt.

Educational Takeaway

This section reinforces the idea that prompt engineering is not just a digital skill—it is a clinical communication skill. It draws on the same habits you're already developing in case presentations: identifying key facts, filtering extraneous data, framing a question appropriately, and tailoring communication to the audience. In doing so, it prepares you to work more effectively with AI tools in diverse clinical contexts.

8. **Ethics and Safety: The Illusion of Precision**

Artificial intelligence tools, especially large language models (LLMs), often produce text that sounds fluent, confident, and professional. This creates a powerful illusion of precision through language alone. But fluency is not a guarantee of accuracy. In clinical settings, where even small mistakes can have serious consequences, this illusion can be dangerous (see Fig. 3.4).

Consider a model that suggests a rare diagnosis based on a few symptoms. The explanation may sound convincing, complete with plausible reasoning and medical terminology. However, unless the model has been trained on high-quality, domain-specific clinical data, or unless the prompt is extremely well-structured, there is a high risk that the response will be misleading or outright wrong. The model is simulating understanding, not demonstrating knowledge.

Why This Matters Medical students and clinicians must learn to treat AI outputs the way they treat advice from an unverified colleague—with skepticism, critical reasoning, and corroboration. No model, no matter how fluent, should be trusted without review. Students must always check AI-generated content against current clinical guidelines, peer-reviewed literature, or expert supervision.

Protecting Patient Privacy Another ethical issue arises when students or clinicians include patient-specific data in AI prompts. Entering protected health information (PHI)—like names, medical record numbers, or detailed health histories—into online tools may violate HIPAA and institutional policies, even if the tool appears secure. Students must be trained to recognize and exclude identifying details from

Fig. 3.4 A review of ethics and safety

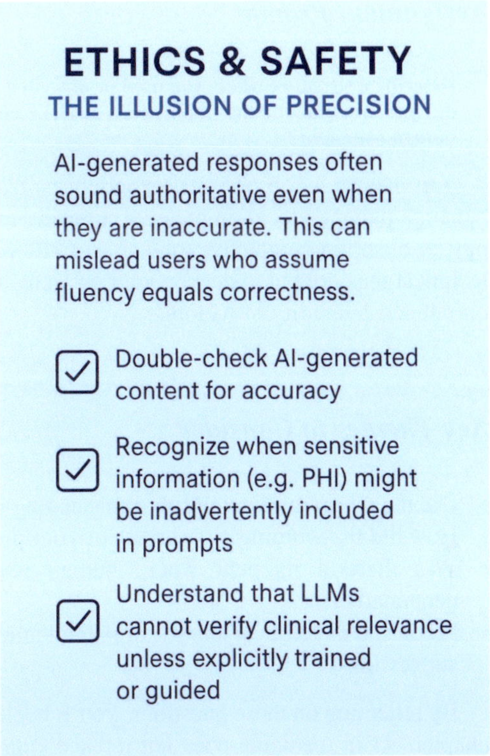

ETHICS & SAFETY

THE ILLUSION OF PRECISION

AI-generated responses often sound authoritative even when they are inaccurate. This can mislead users who assume fluency equals correctness.

- Double-check AI-generated content for accuracy
- Recognize when sensitive information (e.g. PHI) might be inadvertently included in prompts
- Understand that LLMs cannot verify clinical relevance unless explicitly trained or guided

any prompt unless they are using a locally compliant AI system authorized by their institution.

Understanding Model Limitations LLMs cannot independently assess clinical relevance. They lack a model of real-world consequences and cannot distinguish between medically urgent and trivial outputs unless explicitly designed and trained to do so. They are not search engines or databases; they generate plausible-sounding completions based on statistical patterns in the data they were trained on.

Clinical Takeaway Always validate AI output. Use AI to augment, not replace, clinical judgment. Understand when and where it is appropriate to use these tools, and always ensure patient privacy is protected.

9. **Reflection Assignment: Guiding the Tools We Use**

Artificial intelligence is rapidly becoming a fixture in medical education and clinical environments. Yet its effectiveness hinges not on the technology alone but on your skill, judgment, and responsibility as you operate it. This final section encourages you to step back from the technical details and reflect on your own evolving role as a future physician-AI collaborator.

Assignment Prompt

Describe a situation where you used or observed an AI tool in medical training. What did you learn about the importance of clear communication, prompt structure, or human oversight?

You may draw on personal experiences, from experimenting with ChatGPT to generate patient education material, to using image recognition software in radiology, or observing predictive tools in an EHR system. The goal is not to assess your technical mastery but to deepen your awareness of how you as a clinician shape the output and reliability of AI tools.

Key Themes to Consider

- Did the AI produce a helpful or misleading result?
- How did the wording or structure of your prompt affect the output?
- Was there a moment where human review caught or corrected an AI-generated error?
- What role did clinical context or patient nuance play in making sense of the AI's suggestions?

By reflecting on these questions, you'll begin to internalize a central tenet of this chapter: AI in medicine does not replace your judgment. Rather, it magnifies the quality of that judgment, for better or worse, depending on how well you guide it. This assignment closes the chapter with a forward-looking mindset: empowering you to not only use AI, but to use it wisely.

This exercise reinforces the chapter's key theme: that AI is only as useful and safe as you, the clinician who guides it.

Let's consolidate what you've learned with a quick reference guide to the key AI tools introduced in this chapter.

10. **Recap Box: What You Should Now Understand**

This chapter has introduced several foundational tools in generative AI and their direct applications in clinical practice (see Fig. 3.5). As future physicians, your ability to collaborate with these tools will shape how effectively and safely they are used to enhance patient care. Here are the key takeaways:

Natural Language Processing (NLP)
NLP enables computers to interpret, extract, and generate human language. In medicine, it powers clinical documentation systems that turn spoken notes into structured text, supports automated summarization of complex patient histories, and fuels chatbots that provide patients with follow-up instructions in plain language. It also underlies search tools that help clinicians retrieve guidelines and literature from unstructured notes.

Fig. 3.5 AI tools for clinical care

Natural Language Processing Processes and understands text and speech

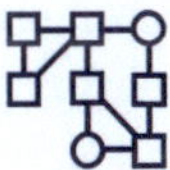

Retrieval-Augmented Generation Combines generating text with information retrieval

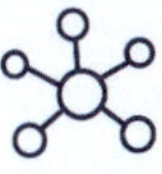

Transformer Processes sequential and contextual data

Prompt Engineering Crafts effective inputs for AI systems

Oversight Ensures ethical and safe AI deployment

Convolutional Neural Networks (CNNs)

CNNs are the workhorses of modern medical image analysis. They excel in identifying tumors on CT scans, segmenting organs in MRIs, and classifying dermatologic or retinal findings. These deep learning models learn spatial patterns in images and are being used to improve speed and accuracy in radiology, oncology, and even robotic surgery planning.

Retrieval-Augmented Generation (RAG)

RAG models blend large language models with structured clinical databases, ensuring that AI-generated answers are not just fluent but also grounded in authoritative information. In contrast to models that hallucinate or omit key facts, RAG enables physicians to query AI systems that cite recent guidelines, literature, or EHR entries—making it a powerful tool for decision support and evidence-based practice.

Transformer Models

Transformers harness self-attention to process entire sequences of clinical text in parallel, allowing each word or token to "attend" dynamically to every other token when building its context-aware representation. This architecture replaces the step-by-step recurrence of older models, dramatically speeding up training and improving the capture of long-range dependencies, essential for interpreting complex patient narratives and linking symptoms appearing far apart in a medical history. By computing Query, Key, and Value vectors and using their dot-product scores to weight information flow, transformers excel at disambiguating terminology (e.g., distinguishing "lead" as an ECG component vs. a chemical element) and at generating coherent, contextually grounded summaries of patient data. Described initially by Vaswani et al. in 2017, this paradigm underpins virtually all state-of-the-art clinical language models today

Prompt Engineering
The ability to write clear, focused prompts is now a core digital literacy skill for clinicians. Whether generating a discharge summary, simulating a patient conversation, or reviewing differential diagnoses, how you ask is just as important as what you ask. Prompt engineering requires clinical clarity, structured information, and awareness of audience, mirroring skills already familiar to students from rounds, consults, and patient interviews.

Human Oversight
No AI tool, regardless of power or design, can substitute for clinical judgment. Medical AI may produce authoritative-sounding answers that are factually incorrect or ethically inappropriate. Human oversight is critical to:

- Interpret outputs in a clinical context
- Detect errors or omissions
- Protect patient privacy and dignity
- Ensure culturally competent communication

Together, these tools form your **AI toolkit**, but how you use them will determine their impact. As with a stethoscope or scalpel, these instruments of care require training, judgment, and professional responsibility.

Instructor's Guide: Chapter—The AI Toolkit

Chapter Overview

Purpose This chapter equips medical students with a practical understanding of generative AI technologies, focusing on their clinical applications, limitations, and responsible use. Students will learn to engage with these tools as critical, informed professionals rather than passive consumers.

Key Technologies Covered
- Natural language processing (NLP)
- Convolutional neural networks (CNNs)
- Retrieval-augmented generation (RAG)
- Prompt engineering techniques

Time Required: 90–120 min (can be split across two sessions)

Learning Objectives

By the end of this chapter, students should be able to:

1. **Explain** how NLP, CNNs, transformers, and RAG models function at a conceptual level relevant to clinical practice
2. **Identify** appropriate and inappropriate clinical use cases for each AI technology
3. **Craft** effective prompts for AI systems with attention to audience, context, and specificity
4. **Evaluate** AI-generated content for potential errors, limitations, or bias
5. **Reflect** on the ethical implications of using AI in clinical decision-making

Required Preparation

For Instructors

- Familiarize yourself with the chapter content.
- Test access to the AI tools you plan to demonstrate.
- Prepare clinical examples relevant to your students' specialty focus.
- Review the provided slides and supplementary materials.

For Students

- Read chapter before class.
- Bring a laptop or tablet for the interactive workshop.
- Complete the pre-class survey on current AI use (if assigned).

Teaching Structure

Opening Clinical Vignette (15 min)

Begin with the case vignette from Sect. 1:

Dr. Chu, an internal medicine resident, is preparing discharge instructions for a 76-year-old patient with newly diagnosed heart failure. Pressed for time, she asks an AI system to "write discharge instructions for heart failure."

Discussion Prompts

- What are the potential benefits and risks of Dr. Chu's approach?
- What critical information is missing from her prompt?
- How might the AI output mislead or help the patient?

Teaching Tip Use this discussion to establish the stakes—AI can either enhance or compromise care depending on how clinicians engage with it.

Core Technologies Walkthrough (25 min)

Natural Language Processing (NLP)

- Use the "language translation" analogy from the text.
- Emphasize: NLP enables machines to process and generate human language, but without true comprehension.

Convolutional Neural Networks (CNNs)

- Show visual examples of image recognition in dermatology or radiology.
- Emphasize: CNNs excel at pattern recognition but can't integrate broader clinical context.

Transformers

☐ **Use the "group discussion" analogy**

- Imagine a clinical team huddle where every member hears and responds to every other member's comment simultaneously, rather than waiting their turn. That's how self-attention works: each token in a sentence "listens" to all the others in parallel to build context.

☐ **Emphasize parallel context-building**

Transformers process entire patient notes at once, capturing long-range dependencies (e.g., linking a symptom mentioned at the top of the note with a medication adjustment at the bottom). They do this without true comprehension—statistical patterns, not understanding, drive their outputs.

Retrieval-Augmented Generation (RAG)

- Demo a RAG-powered tool if available (e.g., Elicit, Perplexity).
- Emphasize: RAG improves factual accuracy but isn't perfect; references should still be verified.

Active Learning Exercise Divide students into small groups. Assign each group one technology to research a published clinical application. Have them present a 3-min summary addressing:

- The clinical problem being solved
- How the AI technology was implemented
- Benefits and limitations observed

Prompt Engineering Workshop (30 min)

Introduction to Effective Prompting (10 min)

- Present the CRAFT framework from Sect. 5:
- Context: Provide relevant background information.
- Role: Specify the intended audience and purpose.
- Attributes: Define the desired characteristics of the response.
- Format: Indicate the preferred structure or organization.
- Task: Clearly state what you want the AI to do.

Interactive Exercise (20 min) Have students access a sandboxed AI tool to complete these tasks:

1. **Baseline Assessment:** Ask students to generate discharge instructions for heart failure (intentionally vague).
2. **Refinement:** Guide students to improve their prompts using the CRAFT framework.
3. **Role Adaptation:** Have students modify prompts for different audiences:
   - A patient with limited health literacy
   - A consulting specialist
   - A home health nurse

Debrief Compare outputs, highlighting how prompt structure dramatically affects quality and relevance.

Safety and Oversight (15 min)

AI Output Evaluation Activity

- Present students with a sample AI-generated clinical recommendation containing subtle errors or "hallucinations" (factually incorrect but plausible-sounding information).
- Have students work in pairs to identify problems.
- Use the ETHICAL framework from Sect. 7:
  - Evidence-based: Is the content consistent with current guidelines?
  - Transparent: Are limitations and uncertainties acknowledged?
  - Human-centered: Does it prioritize patient needs?
  - Inclusive: Does it account for diverse patient populations?
  - Context-aware: Is it appropriate for the specific clinical scenario?
  - Accurate: Are facts and recommendations correct?
  - Legal/regulatory compliance: Does it adhere to relevant standards?

Class Poll Ask students: "Would you implement this AI recommendation in patient care?" Discuss responses.

Reflection and Integration (15 min)

Small Group Discussion

- Divide students into groups of 3–4
- Have each group discuss one of the following questions:
  1. How might AI tools change the way you document patient encounters?
  2. What safeguards would you want in place before using AI for clinical decision support?

3. How might AI affect the doctor-patient relationship?
4. What skills will become more important for physicians as AI capabilities advance?

Whole Class Share-Out: Have each group summarize their key insights.

Assignment Introduction (5 min)

Review the reflection assignment (Sect. 8) and clarify expectations:

- 500–750-word written reflection OR 5-min presentation
- Personal experience using or observing AI in clinical settings
- Analysis of communication factors that affected the AI's performance
- Should demonstrate understanding of chapter concepts

Assessment Strategies

Formative Assessment

Workshop Feedback
- Provide real-time guidance on prompt structure during activities.
- Use peer review for prompt refinement exercises.

Comprehension Checks
- Brief multiple-choice questions on key concepts
- Example: "Which technology would be most appropriate for analyzing chest X-rays?"

Summative Assessment

Reflection Assignment Rubric

Criterion	Exemplary [5]	Satisfactory	Needs improvement
Clinical relevance	Connects AI concepts directly to specific clinical scenarios	Makes general connections to clinical practice	Limited connection to clinical applications
Technical understanding	Accurately applies chapter concepts	Shows basic understanding of concepts	Contains technical misconceptions
Critical analysis	Insightfully evaluates both benefits and limitations	Identifies some benefits and limitations	Uncritically accepts or rejects AI capabilities
Communication	Clear, concise, well-organized	Generally clear with minor issues	Difficult to follow

Knowledge Quiz (Ten Questions)

- Technical understanding (four questions)
- Safety evaluation (three questions)
- Prompt engineering (three questions)

Common Challenges and Solutions

Technical Issues

- **Problem:** Students unable to access AI tools during workshop.
- **Solution:** Prepare screenshots of sample interactions; have students work in pairs.

Varied Technical Background

- **Problem:** Students have widely different AI familiarity levels.
- **Solution:** Use peer teaching; pair technically confident students with those who have less experience.

Ethical Concerns

- **Problem:** Students express discomfort with AI in medicine.
- **Solution:** Acknowledge concerns as valid; emphasize AI as a tool that requires human oversight.

Additional Resources

For Instructors

- AI in Medical Education Resource Kit (available in faculty portal)
- Tutorial videos for setting up the workshop environment
- Sample prompts and outputs for demonstration

For Students

- Supplemental readings on clinical AI applications
- Access to practice sandboxes (provide institutional login details)
- Guide to evaluating AI-generated content

Adaptations for Different Teaching Contexts

For Large Classes

- Use polling software for interactive elements.
- Consider a flipped classroom approach with pre-recorded technology overviews.

For Clinical Settings

- Focus on real cases from your institution where AI could be applied.
- Invite clinical informatics specialists as guest speakers.

For Virtual Teaching

- Use breakout rooms for small group activities.
- Provide access to cloud-based AI tools that don't require local installation.

Note: This instructor's guide aligns with the current state of AI technology as of May 2025. As these technologies evolve rapidly, instructors are encouraged to update examples and applications with current research and use cases.

References

1. Starfield B. Is primary care essential? Lancet. 1994;344(8930):1129–33. https://doi.org/10.1016/s0140-6736(94)90634-3. PMID: 7934497
2. Wang Y, et al. Clinical information extraction applications: a literature review. J Biomed Inform. 2018;77:34–49. https://doi.org/10.1016/j.jbi.2017.11.011.
3. Epic Systems. NoteWriter AI documentation tool [Product site or whitepaper]. 2023
4. Chen, M., et al. DocsGPT: fine-tuning LLMs for patient messaging. arXiv preprint. 2023. https://arxiv.org/abs/2304.00040
5. Obermeyer Z, et al. Dissecting racial bias in an algorithm used to manage the health of populations. Science. 2019;366(6464):447–53. https://doi.org/10.1126/science.aax2342.
6. Rajpurkar P, Irvin J, Ball RL, Zhu K, Yang B, Mehta H, et al. Deep learning for chest radiograph diagnosis: a retrospective comparison of the CheXNeXt algorithm to practicing radiologists. PLoS Med. 2018;15(11):e1002686. https://doi.org/10.1371/journal.pmed.1002686.
7. Bai HX, et al. AI augmentation of radiologist performance in diagnosing COVID-19 pneumonia. Radiology. 2020;296(3):E156–65. https://doi.org/10.1148/radiol.2020201491.
8. Madani A, Arnaout R, Mofrad M, Arnaout R. Fast and accurate view classification of echocardiograms using deep learning. NPJ Digital Med. 2018;1:6. https://doi.org/10.1038/s41746-017-0013-1.
9. Hannun AY, Rajpurkar P, Haghpanahi M, Tison GH, Bourn C, Turakhia MP, Ng AY. Cardiologist-level arrhythmia detection and classification in ambulatory electrocardiograms using a deep neural network. Nature Med. 2019;25(1):65–9. https://doi.org/10.1038/s41591-018-0268-3.
10. Attia ZI, Noseworthy PA, Lopez-Jimenez F, Asirvatham SJ, Deshmukh AJ, Gersh BJ, et al. An artificial intelligence-enabled ECG algorithm for the identification of patients with atrial fibrillation during sinus rhythm: a retrospective analysis of outcome prediction. The Lancet. 2019;394(10201):861–7. https://doi.org/10.1016/S0140-6736(19)31721-0.
11. Vaswani A, et al. Attention is all you need. Adv Neural Inf Process Syst. 2017;30:5998–6008. https://papers.nips.cc/paper_files/paper/2017/file/3f5ee243547dee91fbd053c1c4a845aa-Paper.pdf
12. Alsentzer E, et al. Publicly available clinical BERT embeddings. In: Proceedings of the 2nd clinical natural language processing workshop; 2019. p. 72–8. https://aclanthology.org/W19-1909/.
13. Lewis P, et al. Retrieval-augmented generation for knowledge-intensive NLP tasks. Adv Neural Inf Process Syst. 2020;33:9459–74. https://arxiv.org/abs/2005.11401

Chapter 4
Image Recognition and Computer Vision Applications

Learning Objectives

By the end of this chapter, you will be able to:

1. Explain the basic principles of image recognition and computer vision in a clinical context.
2. Describe key applications of AI in radiology and histopathology.
3. Identify the benefits and limitations of integrating AI tools into imaging workflows.
4. Apply critical thinking to a clinical vignette involving the use of AI in image interpretation.
5. Answer targeted quiz questions to reinforce understanding.

Fundamentals of Image Recognition and Computer Vision

Before diving into clinical applications, it's essential to understand how AI systems "see" medical images. Computer vision is at the heart of many diagnostic tools. It is a field of AI that teaches machines to interpret visual information. Whether analyzing chest X-rays, retinal scans, or dermatologic photos, these systems rely on mathematical models to detect patterns, shapes, and abnormalities embedded in pixel data. In this section, we'll explore the foundational concepts that power medical image recognition, beginning with how algorithms extract meaning from raw images and building toward the sophisticated neural networks now used in clinical radiology.

Visualizations of research data or results in this manuscript were generated, refined, corrected, edited, or formatted with the assistance of artificial intelligence (AI) tools, specifically OpenAI's ChatGPT 4.0, 2024. All content has been thoroughly reviewed, revised, and approved by the author(s) to ensure scientific accuracy and preserve the integrity of the original material.

© The Author(s), under exclusive license to Springer Nature Switzerland AG 2025

C. Quinn, *Generative AI for the Medical Student*,
https://doi.org/10.1007/978-3-032-01613-3_4

Core Concepts

When you read a chest X-ray, your brain subconsciously assembles meaning from thousands of tiny squares, called pixels, that form the image. Computer vision works similarly, but instead of using clinical experience, algorithms analyze pixel patterns to detect features in the image [1].

One of the first steps in this process is identifying edges, or areas where the brightness of the pixels changes sharply. These often represent critical anatomical structures, such as the borders of the lungs or a suspicious nodule. Early computer vision tools, like the Marr-Hildreth edge detector, were designed to highlight these boundaries and make abnormalities more visible [2, 1] (see Table 4.1).

Modern systems take this a step further. Convolutional neural networks (CNNs) learn directly from raw image data (see section "Machine learning versus deep learning"). They apply small scanning filters, or kernels, across an image to detect patterns. These kernels are like digital "pattern detectors," each tuned to recognize features such as horizontal lines, sharp corners, or round shapes.

As a CNN processes an image through multiple layers, it builds feature maps. These are visual summaries that show how strongly each kernel responds to different parts of the image [1, 3]. Early layers detect basic features, like edges or textures. Deeper layers combine these to recognize complex structures, such as the shape of a lung, the outline of a heart, or even the irregular silhouette of a tumor [3].

This layered approach allows CNNs to move from basic anatomical shapes to complex diagnostic insights. Understanding how these networks learn from images helps clinicians appreciate both the strengths and limitations of AI-powered radiology tools.

Table 4.1 Traditional machine learning vs convolutional neural networks (CNNs)

Feature	Traditional machine learning (ML)	Convolutional neural networks (CNNs)
Input data type	Structured/tabular data (e.g., CSV files)	Unstructured image data (e.g., X-rays, MRIs)
Feature engineering	Requires manual feature extraction	Learns features automatically via filters
Spatial awareness	Limited (depends on engineered features)	High—detects patterns, edges, textures
Scalability to large datasets	Moderate—depends on preprocessing	Excellent—scales well with large image datasets
Performance on images	Poor to moderate unless paired with custom preprocessing	High—State-of-the-art in image classification
Model complexity	Lower (e.g., decision trees, logistic regression)	Higher (deep learning, GPU-intensive)
Typical use cases	Billing prediction, patient risk scoring, simple diagnostics	Tumor detection, lesion classification, radiology workflows

In the next section, we'll examine how CNNs are trained and how their performance depends on the quantity and quality of labeled clinical images used during model development.

However, beware: if your training images include noise (such as motion blur), artifacts (like grid lines), or sampling bias (due to an insufficient number of examples of small nodules), the model can "mislearn" and make unreliable predictions [4]. As a future physician using AI tools, you'll need to understand these limitations, so you know when to trust the AI's suggestion and when to rely on your own judgment [4].

Having covered how algorithms detect and map image features, we now compare traditional machine-learning methods with modern deep-learning approaches.

Sidebar: Core Image Recognition Concepts

Understanding these fundamental concepts is essential for grasping how artificial intelligence, particularly deep learning models like convolutional neural networks (CNNs), process and interpret images in fields like medical imaging.

- **Pixel**: Think of an image, such as a chest X-ray. It is made up of many tiny squares. Each one of these tiny squares is called a pixel. Every pixel contributes to the full image you see and interpret. Pixels are the most basic elements of a digital image.
- **Kernel**: In the context of computer vision, kernels are described as small filters. These filters are designed to scan across an image to detect specific patterns in groups of pixels. Early filters were developed to highlight features like edges. Modern CNNs use stacked layers of these small filters (kernels) to analyze images.
- **Feature Map**: A **feature map** is the output produced after a kernel scans an image. It essentially shows how strongly that specific kernel detected a particular pattern in each different location within the image. For instance, the kernels in the first layers of a CNN might detect simple patterns, and the resulting feature maps would indicate where these basic patterns (like lines or curves) are found in the image. Kernels in deeper layers combine these simple patterns to recognize more complex shapes, and their feature maps reflect the detection of these more intricate structures.

Machine Learning Versus Deep Learning

As a medical student learning to work alongside AI systems, it's vital to understand not just today's most powerful models but also the classical methods that paved the way. Before deep learning transformed computer vision, clinicians and engineers relied on models like support vector machines (SVMs) and random forests to interpret medical images. These systems are still used in certain clinical and research settings and offer key lessons in transparency, simplicity, and resource efficiency.

Classical machine learning methods depend on what's known as "feature engineering." This means converting an image into a set of simple measurements, such as brightness, texture, or shape size, chosen by humans. Each scan becomes a point in a multidimensional space, and the algorithm learns how to classify it based on these features.

Take SVMs, for example. Imagine plotting the features of healthy and diseased scans on a graph. An SVM draws the best line, or, in complex settings, a curved boundary, that separates the two groups with the widest possible margin. This "maximum margin" approach reduces the risk of overfitting and is particularly useful in early-stage studies with small datasets [5].

Random forests take a different route. They use an ensemble of decision trees, where each tree makes predictions based on simple rules (e.g., "Is brightness above a threshold?"). A single tree may overfit, but the system reaches a more balanced and robust conclusion when hundreds of trees each vote. Random forests also rank which features were most influential, offering a level of interpretability that builds trust [1].

These classical models were the foundation of early computer-aided detection (CAD) systems and remain in use today where interpretability, cost, or data limitations matter. They're still valuable in settings like global health, small clinical trials, or mobile applications that lack high-end computing.

But what if we remove the need for human-designed measurements entirely? That's the leap made by deep learning, especially with convolutional neural networks (CNNs). CNNs learn patterns directly from raw image pixels, stacking many layers to detect increasingly complex features—from simple edges to full anatomical structures. When trained on large labeled datasets, CNNs often outperform classical models, especially in accuracy and scalability [6].

However, CNNs often behave as "black boxes." Unlike random forests, they don't readily explain why they made a decision. This makes them powerful but sometimes opaque, an issue in safety-critical domains like medicine.

Understanding classical models prepares you to critically assess modern tools. It gives you language to collaborate with data scientists and helps you ask smarter questions about AI safety, fairness, and design. As AI continues to evolve, your ability to navigate both old and new methods will make you a stronger, more adaptable clinician.

To compare these approaches side by side, including their transparency, accuracy, and data requirements, refer to Fig. 4.1.

Generative adversarial networks (GANs) extend these capabilities, serving as a key technology for creating new, synthetic data 1. A GAN pairs a generator, which fabricates synthetic images, with a discriminator, which learns to distinguish real from fake; through this adversarial game, both improve in tandem [3]. But how does generating synthetic data help a radiologist? This synthetic data, generated by GANs, has several powerful applications in medical imaging:

- **Augmenting Training Data:** GANs can create realistic examples of rare findings, such as small liver lesions or subtle lung nodules. Using this synthetic data to augment training sets helps achieve rare-case balance, boosting model sensitivity by over 7% in one study [4].

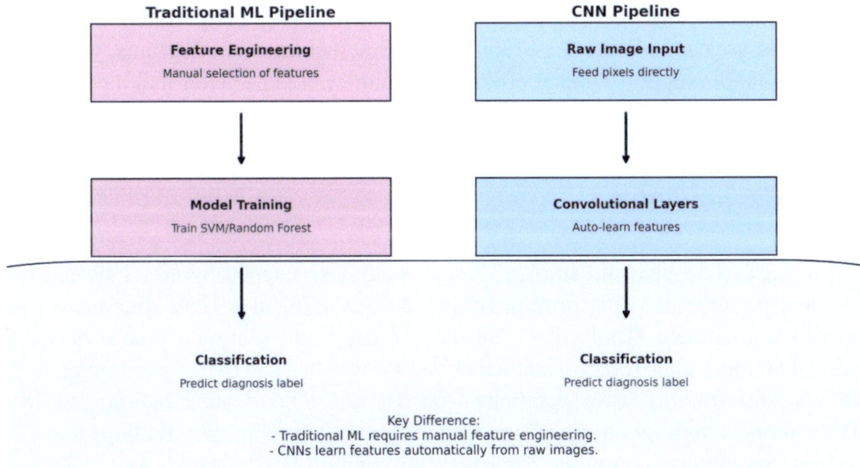

Fig. 4.1 Comparing ML vs CNN in image recognition

- **Super-resolution:** GAN-based super-resolution sharpens noisy or low-resolution scans, clarifying vessel contours and lesion margins, allowing for more confident tumor measurements [7].
- **Clinical Implication:** Synthetic image enhancement via GANs can improve the quality of low-dose scans, potentially reducing radiation exposure while preserving diagnostic detail.
- **Modality Translation:** GANs enable translating images from one modality to another, for instance, converting MRI into CT-style images. These translated images are another form of synthetic data that allows familiar CT reading protocols without additional patient radiation exposure [3]. See Sidebar 4.1: Synthetic Data in Clinical AI.

Radiologists don't directly review these synthetic scans in isolation. Instead, they interact with AI tools trained or enhanced using GAN data (which includes this synthetic data): highlighted regions, annotated measurements, and clearer reconstructions derived from or improved by GANs all inform more accurate diagnoses.

Having seen how GANs generate synthetic data, let's explore networks designed to segment real patient scans into meaningful regions.

Applications in Radiology

Radiology has been one of the earliest and most impactful frontiers for AI adoption in medicine. With the rise of deep learning and access to vast medical imaging datasets, AI systems now assist in detecting, classifying, and even prioritizing abnormalities across common imaging modalities. In this section, we explore how convolutional neural networks (CNNs) are transforming image interpretation in real-world use cases. From chest radiographs to screening mammograms, you'll see how these tools support clinical efficiency, accuracy, and decision-making.

Chest Radiography

In one case, a 58-year-old smoker's chest X-ray was flagged by an AI system for possible pneumonia. This prompt triggered early clinical review, diagnosis, and antibiotic treatment. Tools like CheXNet, a deep convolutional neural network trained on more than 100,000 labeled chest radiographs, can detect pneumonia with 76% sensitivity and 80% specificity—on par with experienced radiologists [8]. These models highlight areas of concern and generate preliminary findings that clinicians can confirm or revise. Their greatest strength lies in speed: AI accelerates review, especially during high-volume or after-hours periods.

Clinical Implication By matching radiologist-level performance in pneumonia detection, CNN tools like CheXNet can support faster triage and earlier intervention in emergency departments and urgent care settings.

Mammography

AI also enhances screening mammography, where the early detection of subtle abnormalities is critical. Deep learning models can detect microcalcifications and tiny calcium deposits that may signal early malignancy by analyzing subtle pixel variations across thousands of images. In a large multi-reader clinical study, AI-supported mammogram interpretation reduced false negatives by 20% and accelerated case review by highlighting suspicious regions for radiologist follow-up [9]. These AI tools do not replace human readers; instead, they triage images and direct your focus to high-priority cases, streamlining clinical workflow and potentially reducing diagnostic delays.

CT and MRI

One of the most time-consuming tasks in radiology is image segmentation, dividing a scan into meaningful regions like tumors, ventricles, or organs. Accurate segmentation is essential for measuring tumor size, planning radiation therapy, or assessing treatment response. Traditionally, this process required radiologists or radiation oncologists to manually outline structures frame by frame, a task that could take hours per patient.

U-Net, a neural network architecture designed for medical imaging, automates this task in seconds [10]. It works in two steps. First, the model "contracts" the image, compressing it to learn the general layout, like a bird's-eye view of where the lungs or liver is located. Then, it "expands" the image back to full resolution, adding finer details. To preserve accuracy, U-Net uses shortcut pathways, called skip-connections, which transfer essential spatial information from earlier layers to later ones. You can think of this like drafting a sketch: first, you block out the shape, and then add details, while referencing your original sketch to keep proportions accurate (see Fig. 4.2.).

The result is a precise contour map showing where structures begin and end. These segmentations can calculate tumor volume for radiation dosing, guide biopsies, or compare tumor size across follow-up scans.

Clinical Implication Automating image segmentation with U-Net reduces human error and saves valuable time, especially in oncology, where radiation planning often depends on precise tumor borders. For clinicians, it means faster turnaround, more reproducible measurements, and more time spent on patient care rather than pixel-by-pixel tracing.

Radiomics

Radiomics is a technique that transforms standard medical images, such as CT or MRI scans, into hundreds of measurable data points. Instead of relying solely on what the eye sees, radiomic algorithms extract features that describe the shape, texture, and brightness of tissues. These features act like noninvasive "biomarkers" that can help predict tumor biology, prognosis, or how likely a patient will respond to treatment [11].

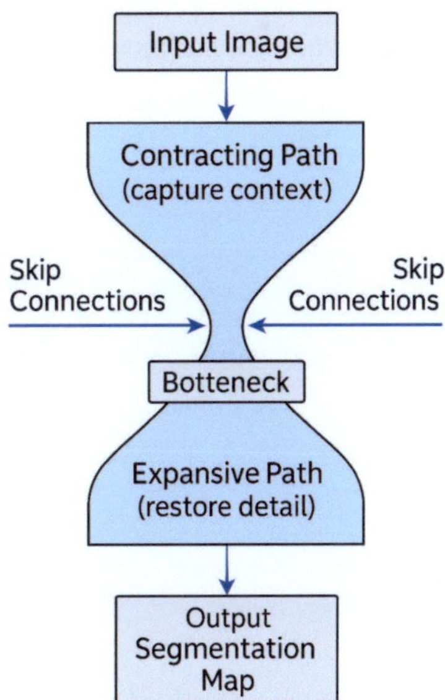

Fig. 4.2 AI image segmentation using U-Net's encoder-decoder structure and skip connections

For example, a lesion's shape can be quantified by descriptors like roundness or spiculation (the jaggedness of its edges). Its texture, or how uniform or varied it looks, can hint at tumor heterogeneity, while intensity features capture brightness levels using histogram analyses. See Fig. 4.3 for common radiomic features and what they reveal about disease.

In oncology, radiomics can identify subtle imaging patterns that correlate with outcomes such as recurrence risk or treatment response. These insights may not be visible to the naked eye. This can support clinical decision-making by adding an additional layer of quantitative evidence.

However, the method comes with important challenges. Images from different scanners or taken with slightly different protocols can vary in ways that affect radiomic measurements. This problem, known as batch effects, is similar to comparing lab tests done on different machines without proper calibration. A lesion might appear brighter or blurrier on one machine, even if it hasn't changed biologically.

To overcome this, researchers standardize the images, adjusting resolution, contrast, and other factors so all scans share consistent properties. They then select only the most stable and relevant features, removing any that are redundant or sensitive to technical noise. Finally, models are validated across multiple patient populations to ensure that the features actually reflect disease characteristics, not scanner quirks.

Clinical Implication
Radiomics adds depth to what imaging already offers. For future clinicians, understanding this approach means learning to integrate both visual impressions and quantitative image data to improve diagnostic precision and treatment planning.

With quantitative imaging biomarkers defined, we next apply these methods to digital pathology workflows. (Fig. 4.3)

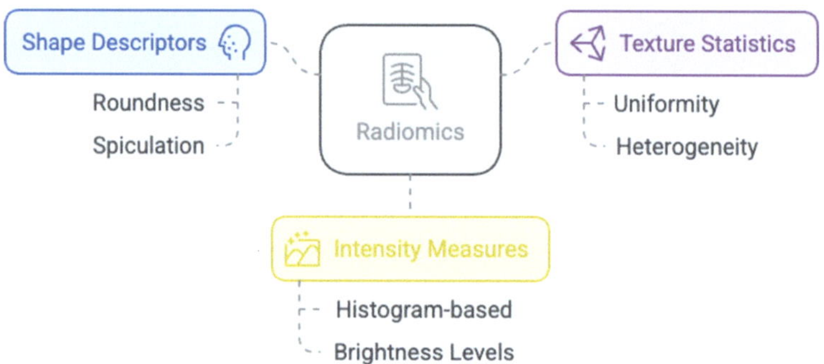

Fig. 4.3 Common radiomic features

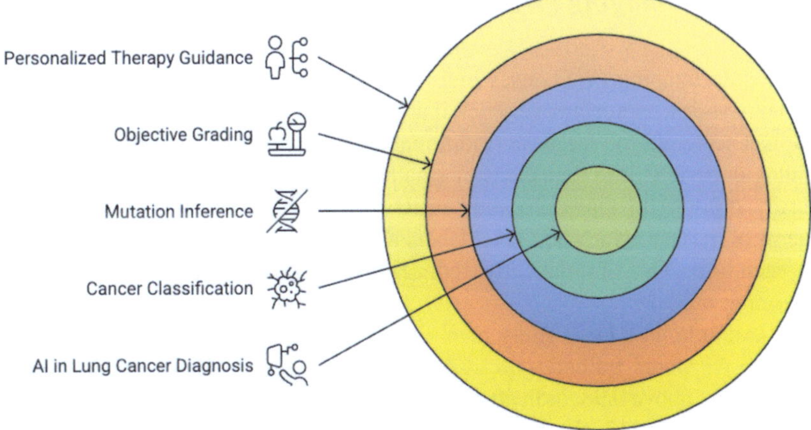

Fig. 4.4 AI in lung cancer diagnosis

Applications in Pathology

Digital pathology is undergoing a transformation thanks to AI, which enables faster, more accurate tissue analysis and diagnosis. Traditionally, pathologists examine glass slides under a microscope to identify cancer, infection, or inflammation. But now, whole slide imaging (WSI) allows those slides to be digitized, shared, and processed by AI models that can scan through gigapixel data to find patterns the human eye might miss. This section will explore how AI is used in pathology workflows, from image segmentation to diagnostic classification, and how it helps reduce review times while improving accuracy and consistency (see Fig. 4.4).

Sidebar: What Is Weak Supervision?

In traditional AI training, every image must be paired with detailed annotations. For example, a pathologist manually outlines the exact borders of each cancerous gland. This is called "strong supervision," which can be very time-consuming.

Weak supervision, on the other hand, allows models to learn from broader labels, such as "this slide contains cancer," without showing exactly where the cancer is. The AI breaks the slide into small tiles and determines which regions most likely explain the diagnosis. Over time, it learns to recognize patterns linked to cancerous changes, even without detailed instructions.

This approach saves pathologists time while still producing high-performing models, making it easier to train AI systems on large datasets lacking granular annotations.

Whole Slide Imaging (WSI)

Whole slide imaging (WSI) uses high-resolution scanners to digitize entire glass pathology slides, capturing every detail at the cellular level. These images can reach gigapixel scale, far too large for traditional image processing methods. AI helps by dividing each WSI into thousands of smaller image tiles and analyzing them individually. A powerful approach called *weakly supervised learning* allows AI to detect patterns of disease using slide-level labels instead of requiring pathologists to annotate each tile. This dramatically reduces the labor involved in training high-performing models.

For example, in a large study involving over 44,000 prostate and breast biopsy slides, an AI model trained with *weak supervision* achieved area under the curve (AUC) values above 0.98, indicating very high accuracy in distinguishing cancerous from benign tissue [12]. Rather than replacing the pathologist, these systems assist by producing heatmaps that highlight suspicious regions, guiding the human expert to areas most likely to require attention.

Clinical Implication AI-enhanced digital pathology improves efficiency by focusing the pathologist's attention on the most diagnostically relevant regions. This can reduce turnaround time, increase throughput, and help ensure consistent diagnostic quality across diverse patient populations.

Sidebar: Understanding AUC (Area Under the Curve)

The **area under the receiver operating characteristic curve (AUC)** is a single-number summary of a diagnostic test's overall accuracy. The ROC curve itself plots the true positive rate (sensitivity) against the false positive rate (1—specificity) across every possible decision threshold. The AUC quantifies how well the test discriminates between two states (e.g., disease vs. no disease):

- **AUC = 1.0** indicates perfect discrimination.
- **AUC = 0.5** implies no better than random chance.
- **Values between 0.5 and 1.0** reflect varying degrees of accuracy, with higher values indicating stronger diagnostic performance.

Clinical Relevance

An AUC above 0.8 is generally considered good for many medical tests, though acceptable thresholds depend on disease prevalence and the consequences of false positives versus false negatives. By comparing AUCs, clinicians and researchers can select the most effective predictive models or imaging algorithms for patient care.

Grading and Subtyping

AI technologies are increasingly capable of assisting with cancer grading and molecular subtyping, tasks traditionally performed by expert pathologists. In one study, a convolutional neural network (CNN), trained on routine H&E-stained lung cancer slides, achieved 97% accuracy in distinguishing adenocarcinoma from squamous cell carcinoma [13]. Even more remarkably, the model inferred the presence of clinically relevant mutations such as EGFR and KRAS with over 80% sensitivity, findings usually reserved for molecular testing [13]. This shows how AI can reveal subtle patterns in tissue architecture that may escape the human eye.

Rather than replacing pathologists, these tools offer standardized, reproducible grades by quantifying features such as nuclear pleomorphism and mitotic count. This objectivity helps reduce interobserver variability and may guide more precise, personalized therapy decisions [13].

The value of AI in pathology is further enhanced through the use of synthetic data. Synthetic data consists of computer-generated histology images, often referred to as "tiles" or "patches," that mimic real tissue samples. These are typically created using generative adversarial networks (GANs), as discussed earlier in section "Machine learning versus deep learning". GANs simulate realistic data by learning from real examples, producing new images resembling the originals [1, 3].

This is particularly useful in training AI systems to recognize rare tumor subtypes. Because these rare cases are underrepresented in most datasets, models can struggle to identify them reliably. By supplementing training datasets with GAN-generated synthetic patches, we can balance the data, improving model performance across diverse histologies [3, 4].

Clinical Implication AI-enhanced grading and synthetic data generation promise more equitable, reliable diagnostic support, especially in complex or rare cases, while keeping pathologists at the center of care decisions.

Sidebar 4.1: Synthetic Data in Clinical AI
Synthetic data are computer-generated patient records that mimic real clinical patterns without using any actual patient information. By producing realistic yet de-identified cases, synthetic datasets help developers prototype and validate AI tools more quickly and safely. Key benefits include:

- **Privacy Protection:** Eliminates identifiable details to comply with HIPAA.
- **Rare-Case Augmentation:** Generates additional examples of uncommon conditions, improving model sensitivity and reducing bias.
- **Rapid Testing:** Bypasses lengthy data-access approvals for prototyping and training.
- **Fairness Checks:** Allows controlled variation (age, demographics, labs) to evaluate model robustness.

Always confirm that synthetic cases accurately reflect true clinical scenarios before using them for model training or testing.

Integration into Clinical Workflow

Benefits

AI offers clear benefits when integrated thoughtfully into radiology and pathology workflows. First, efficiency gains arise as algorithms "pre-read" studies—triaging normal cases and flagging abnormalities so you can focus on the most critical images, reducing report turnaround times by up to 30% in pilot deployments [13]. Second, AI brings standardization: by applying consistent criteria, it diminishes interobserver variability that can arise among trainees or across institutions [14]. Finally, these tools serve an educational role—highlighting subtle findings for trainees and reinforcing pattern recognition, much like an expert mentor guiding your review.

Challenges

Nevertheless, challenges remain. Data bias can lead models to underperform on underrepresented populations, risking misdiagnosis if training datasets lack diversity [15]. Interpretability issues also arise: when AI functions as a "black box," it can erode clinician trust and hinder error detection. Efforts to develop explainable AI have yet to achieve clinical readiness [16]. Moreover, regulatory and ethical considerations—including patient privacy, liability, and adherence to evolving FDA guidelines for AI-based software—demand careful oversight and governance to ensure safe, equitable deployment [17].

Clinical Vignette: "AI-Assisted CT Interpretation"

A 65-year-old smoker undergoes a routine low-dose chest CT for lung cancer screening. His history includes a 40-pack-year smoking habit and controlled hypertension. No prior nodules were noted on previous scans.

The AI algorithm processes the volume and flags a 6 mm solitary pulmonary nodule in the right upper lobe. It annotates the axial slice and assigns a risk score based on size, shape, and attenuation. The recommendation cites the Fleischner Society guidelines—a set of expert consensus recommendations published by an international panel of thoracic radiologists and pulmonologists—to guide management of incidental solid nodules. For nodules between 6 and 8 mm in low-risk patients, these guidelines suggest a follow-up CT in 6–12 months to monitor growth [18, 21].

Discussion Prompts

1. What additional clinical details (symptoms, prior imaging, occupational exposures) would you gather before ordering follow-up?
2. How would you verify the AI's finding—what steps ensure the nodule isn't an artifact?
3. Under what circumstances might you override the AI and choose a different follow-up interval or diagnostic test?

Quiz 2

1. In one sentence, define the difference between classification and segmentation in medical imaging.
2. From section "Integration into clinical workflow", list three benefits of AI integration in radiology workflows.
3. Explain why data bias arises in deep-learning models and give one clinical example.
4. In two to three sentences, describe one scenario where AI might increase diagnostic error.
5. True or false: generative adversarial networks (GANs) can augment training datasets.

Conclusion

This chapter has shown how artificial intelligence is reshaping image-based specialties, from radiology to pathology, by detecting subtle patterns, speeding up workflows, and supporting more consistent, data-driven decisions. You learned how classical methods like support vector machines and random forests laid the groundwork for today's deep learning tools, and how models like CNNs and U-Nets now perform tasks ranging from pneumonia detection on chest X-rays to tumor segmentation and grading. We also introduced radiomics, a powerful technique that turns images into high-dimensional data, and explored how synthetic data can fill gaps in rare-case training. But imaging is only one part of patient care. In Chap. 5, we shift focus to chronic disease management, where AI's ability to track longitudinal data, predict deterioration, and support care coordination offers new ways to keep patients healthier, longer.

Instructor's Guide for This Chapter: Radiology and Pathology Applications of Generative AI

Overview

This chapter introduces medical students to the fundamentals of image recognition, compares traditional machine-learning and deep-learning approaches, surveys key applications in radiology and pathology, and explores integration into clinical workflows. This guide provides teaching strategies, discussion prompts, quiz answers, and supplementary resources.

Learning Objectives

By the end of this chapter, students should be able to:

1. Explain core image-processing concepts (pixels, features, patterns, edge detection, feature maps).
2. In medical imaging, distinguish between traditional algorithms (SVMs, random forests) and deep-learning (CNNs, GANs).
3. Describe AI applications in chest radiography, mammography, CT, and MRI.
4. Define U-Net segmentation and radiomics and discuss their clinical uses.
5. Summarize AI's benefits and challenges in workflow integration.
6. Apply critical reasoning in a clinical vignette and answer targeted quiz questions.

Teaching Strategies

- **Flipped Classroom**: Assign students to read sections "Fundamentals of image recognition and computer vision" and "Applications in radiology" in advance. Use class time to discuss real CT/X-ray examples.
- **Interactive Demonstration**: Show sample WSIs and have students annotate benign versus malignant regions before revealing an AI heatmap overlay.
- **Case Study Workshop**: In groups, analyze the AI-assisted CT vignette. Each group answers discussion prompts and presents reasoning.
- **Hands-On Exercise**: Provide students with a small open-source dataset (e.g., chest X-ray) and demo a simple CNN or GAN workflow using a web-based tool (e.g., Google Colab).

Discussion Prompts

1. After reviewing section "Core concepts", how does edge detection relate to early AI models?
2. In section "Machine learning versus deep learning", what are the trade-offs between interpretability and accuracy for SVMs versus CNNs?
3. For chest radiography and mammography (sections "Chest radiography" and "Mammography"), how might AI reduce health disparities or inadvertently worsen them?
4. In section "Applications in pathology", how does weak supervision in WSI accelerate model development, and what risks emerge?
5. Referencing section "Integration into clinical workflow", propose one policy change to address data bias in your future practice.

Quiz 2 Answer Key

1. **Classification Versus Segmentation**: Classification assigns a label to an entire image (e.g., pneumonia vs. no pneumonia). Segmentation delineates regions within the image (e.g., outlining a lesion).
2. **Three Benefits**: Efficiency gains (AI pre-reads and triages), standardization (reduces interobserver variability), and education (highlights findings for trainees).
3. **Data Bias**: Arises when training datasets lack diversity. Models learn features from overrepresented groups and underperform on underrepresented populations (e.g., racial bias in risk prediction) [15].
4. **Scenario of Increased Error**: AI may hallucinate features in noisy scans, resulting in false-positive detections in poor-quality images.
5. **True**: GANs can augment training data by synthesizing realistic images of rare pathologies.

Additional Resources

- **Online Tutorials**: Stanford's CS231n (Convolutional Neural Networks for Visual Recognition) lectures on segmentation and GANs.
- **Datasets**: NIH chest X-ray dataset, Camelyon16 WSI dataset.
- **Regulatory Guidelines**: FDA's AI/ML Software as a Medical Device (SaMD) action plan.

Timing Recommendations

- **Session 1 (90 min)**: Sections "Fundamentals of image recognition and computer vision" and "Applications in radiology", edge-detection demo, classification versus segmentation discussion.
- **Session 2 (90 min)**: Sections "Applications in pathology" and "Integration into clinical workflow", WSI heatmap exercise, clinical vignette workshop, quiz.

References

1. Breiman L. Random forests. Mach Learn. 2001;45(1):5–32.
2. Marr D, Hildreth EC. Theory of edge detection. Proc R Soc Lond Ser B Biol Sci. 1980;207(1167):187–217. https://royalsocietypublishing.org/doi/10.1098/rspb.1980.0020
3. Yi X, Walia E, Babyn P. Generative adversarial network in medical imaging: a review. Med Image Anal. 2019;58:101552. https://doi.org/10.1016/j.media.2019.101552.
4. Frid-Adar M, Klang E, Amitai M, Goldberger J, Greenspan H. GAN-based synthetic medical image augmentation for improved liver lesion classification. J Med Imaging. 2018;5(4):044502. https://doi.org/10.1117/1.JMI.5.4.044502.
5. Bishop CM. Pattern recognition and machine learning. New York: Springer; 2006.
6. LeCun Y, Bengio Y, Hinton G. Deep learning. Nature. 2015;521(7553):436–44. https://doi.org/10.1038/nature14539.
7. Wolterink JM, Dinkla AM, Savenije MHF, Seevinck PR, van den Berg CAT, Isgum I. Deep MR to CT synthesis using unpaired data. In: Descoteaux M, Maier-Hein L, Styner M, Tsaftaris S, editors. Medical image computing and computer-assisted intervention—MICCAI 2017. Cham: Springer; 2017. p. 14–23.
8. Rajpurkar P, Irvin J, Zhu K, Yang B, Mehta H, Duan T, et al. CheXNet: radiologist-level pneumonia detection on chest X-rays with deep learning. arXiv Preprint, *arXiv*:1711.05225. 2017.
9. Rodríguez-Ruiz A, Lång K, Gubern-Mérida A, et al. Detection of breast cancer in digital mammograms using deep learning: a multi-reader, multi-case study. Radiology. 2019;290(2):305–13. https://doi.org/10.1148/radiol.2018180785.
10. Ronneberger O, Fischer P, Brox T. U-net: convolutional networks for biomedical image segmentation. In: Descoteaux M, Maier-Hein L, Styner M, Tsaftaris S, editors. Medical image computing and computer-assisted intervention—MICCAI 2015, vol. 9351. Springer; 2015. p. 234–41. https://doi.org/10.1007/978-3-319-24574-4_28.
11. Lambin P, Rios-Velazquez E, Leijenaar R, et al. Radiomics: extracting more information from medical images using advanced feature analysis. Nat Rev Clin Oncol. 2017;14(12):749–62. https://doi.org/10.1038/nrclinonc.2017.141.
12. Campanella G, Hanna MG, Geneslaw L, et al. Clinical-grade computational pathology using weakly supervised deep learning on whole slide images. Nat Med. 2019;25(8):1301–9. https://doi.org/10.1038/s41591-019-0508-1.
13. Coudray N, Ocampo PS, Sakellaropoulos T, et al. Classification and mutation prediction from non–small cell lung cancer histopathology images using deep learning. Nat Med. 2018;24(10):1559–67. https://doi.org/10.1038/s41591-018-0177-5.
14. Topol EJ. High-performance medicine: the convergence of human and artificial intelligence. Nat Med. 2019;25(1):44–56. https://doi.org/10.1038/s41591-018-0300-7.
15. McBee MP, Awan O, Colucci AT, et al. Deep learning in radiology. Acad Radiol. 2018;25(11):1472–80. https://doi.org/10.1016/j.acra.2018.03.002.

16. Obermeyer Z, Powers B, Vogeli C, Mullainathan S. Dissecting racial bias in an algorithm used to manage the health of populations. Science. 2019;366(6464):447–53. https://doi.org/10.1126/science.aax2342.
17. Ghassemi M, Oakden-Rayner L, Beam AL. The false hope of current approaches to explainable artificial intelligence in health care. Lancet Digit Health. 2021;3(11):e745–50. https://doi.org/10.1016/S2589-7500(21)00208-9.
18. Morley J, Machado CCV, Burr C, Cowls J, Taddeo M, Floridi L. The ethics of AI in health care: a mapping review. Soc Sci Med. 2021;270:113554. https://doi.org/10.1016/j.socscimed.2020.113554.

Chapter 5
Primary Care and Chronic Disease Management

Learning Objectives
By the end of this chapter, you will be able to:

1. Describe the role of predictive analytics in identifying patients at risk for chronic disease exacerbations. Explain how remote patient monitoring (RPM) platforms integrate with clinical workflows to support ongoing care.
2. Develop an AI-enhanced care plan for a patient with a common chronic condition.
3. Critically evaluate the benefits and limitations of predictive models and RPM tools.
4. Apply chapter concepts in a collaborative group exercise.

Building on the previous chapter's focus on workflow integration, this chapter explores how AI enables proactive chronic disease management in frontline primary care.

Burden of Chronic Illness

Managing Chronic Disease in the Age of Generative AI

If you're training in primary care, you're stepping into the front line of chronic disease management. In the United States, over 60% of adults live with at least one long-term health condition, such as diabetes, hypertension, COPD, arthritis, or heart failure. These illnesses account for a staggering $3.8 trillion in healthcare spending

---

Visualizations of research data or results in this manuscript were generated, refined, corrected, edited, or formatted with the assistance of artificial intelligence (AI) tools, specifically OpenAI's ChatGPT 4.0, 2024. All content has been thoroughly reviewed, revised, and approved by the author(s) to ensure scientific accuracy and preserve the integrity of the original material.

© The Author(s), under exclusive license to Springer Nature Switzerland AG 2025

C. Quinn, *Generative AI for the Medical Student*,
https://doi.org/10.1007/978-3-032-01613-3_5

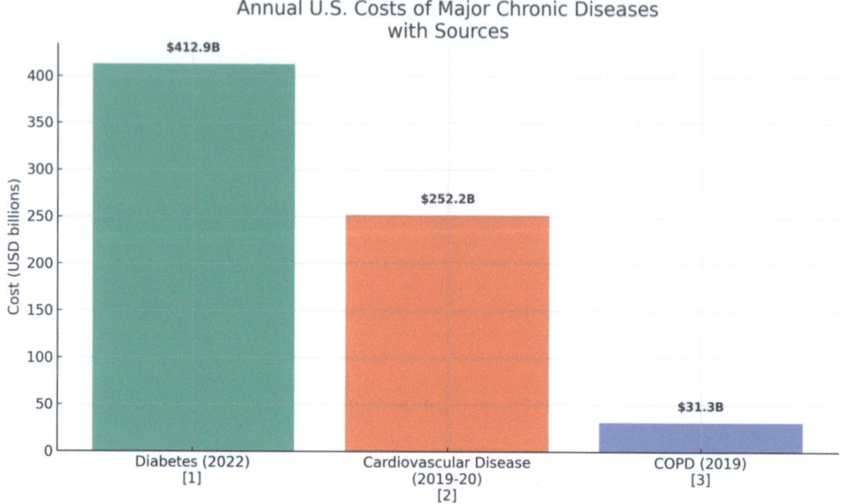

Fig. 5.1 Chronic diseases and their costs

annually [1] (see Fig. 5.1). Primary care teams handle over 90% of that burden. However, traditional models of care, brief, episodic visits focused on acute problems, aren't enough to manage complex, long-term conditions.

Healthcare systems are shifting toward the chronic care model (CCM), a framework developed by Dr. Edward Wagner and colleagues to close the gap. The CCM is designed to improve outcomes by transforming care from reactive to proactive. It emphasizes team-based planning, shared decision-making, patient education, and robust data systems. Instead of waiting for a patient with diabetes to develop complications, a CCM-based approach might include regular monitoring via digital glucometers, nurse-led coaching sessions, and early intervention when trends look concerning.

This sharply contrasts the episodic, or usual, care model, which often relies on short, physician-led visits that address immediate concerns but leave little time for preventive counseling or coordination. Under usual care, critical data, like symptom trends or medication adherence, can fall through the cracks (see Table 5.1).

That's where generative AI enters the picture. This chapter explores how these advanced tools can strengthen every component of chronic care, helping clinicians anticipate risk, personalize treatment plans, and extend the reach of the care team. From summarizing notes and predicting exacerbations to drafting tailored patient education, generative AI has the potential to make complex, coordinated care more efficient and more human.

Consider Maria, a 62-year-old with type 2 diabetes and heart failure: she takes seven different medications, a challenge known as polypharmacy (the use of multiple drugs, which increases risks of interactions), and relies on her primary physician to coordinate cardiology and endocrinology referrals. In a reactive care model, where intervention waits until symptoms worsen, patients like Maria often present

Table 5.1 Comparison of chronic care model and episodic (usual) care model

Domain	Chronic care model (CCM)	Episodic (usual) care model
Care approach	Proactive, continuous, team-based care	Reactive, intermittent, physician-centered
Primary focus	Long-term disease control, prevention, and quality of life	Immediate symptom relief or acute issue resolution
Care team	Multidisciplinary (physicians, nurses, care coordinators, pharmacists, social workers)	Primarily physician-led
Patient role	Active participant in self-management	Passive recipient of care
Use of data	Ongoing monitoring via registries, wearables, and clinical information systems	Limited to single-visit documentation
Visit structure	Structured follow-ups, group visits, virtual check-ins	Brief in-person visits when the patient seeks care
Technology integration	Emphasizes telehealth, remote monitoring, and decision-support tools	Often minimal or fragmented technology use
Goal orientation	Risk reduction, health maintenance, adherence, and early intervention	Problem resolution at time of presentation
Examples	Diabetes management program with nurse coaching and AI-generated trend analysis	Single appointment to adjust insulin dose without follow-up plan
Suitability for AI integration	High, AI tools support risk stratification, task automation, and personalized care pathways	Low, limited continuity reduces AI effectiveness and training data utility

in crisis. Nearly one in five Medicare beneficiaries is rehospitalized within 30 days of discharge, costing Medicare $17 billion annually; these readmissions worsen patient quality of life and expose them to hospital-acquired infections and functional decline [2]. Proactive outpatient management could prevent many of these costly, dangerous events.

Sidebar: Reactive Versus Proactive Healthcare

Reactive Healthcare: This aligns with traditional medical practice, which focuses on responding to illnesses or symptoms that have already occurred. Examples from the sources include using AI for analyzing clinical notes to identify present symptoms and findings, generating differential diagnoses based on a patient's narrative history or current presentation, recommending antibiotic treatment for infections, generating summaries of current patient encounters or discharge summaries, providing diagnostic support in fields like radiology, and managing schedules for current appointments. These tools are meant to improve efficiency and accuracy in managing existing conditions.

Proactive Healthcare: This aligns with approaches focused on predicting future risks, preventing illness, intervening early, and managing long-term

(continued)

health trajectories. Examples from the sources include using AI for identifying high-risk patients from written histories or datasets; predicting mortality or hospitalization risks; forecasting complications like sepsis or readmission; predicting no-shows to optimize scheduling; managing chronic conditions longitudinally over months or years, particularly in primary care; forecasting longer-term risks, such as fall risk 6–12 months ahead, particularly in primary care; generating personalized health messages and patient education materials tailored to health literacy or specific concerns; and real-time monitoring of digital signals (like social media) to detect emerging public health concerns earlier than traditional methods.

Why It's Important

Distinguishing between reactive and proactive applications is vital because AI can support healthcare in different ways depending on the goal:

Improving Efficiency in Reactive Care: AI tools can streamline tasks associated with reacting to illness, such as documentation, note-taking, and summarizing existing patient data, potentially reducing documentation time and administrative tasks, freeing up clinician time for patient care. Accurate clinical documentation has a direct impact on patient safety.

Enabling and Enhancing Proactive Care: AI's ability to analyze vast amounts of data, identify patterns, and make predictions is particularly powerful for proactive healthcare. It allows clinicians to move beyond simply treating existing conditions to identifying potential problems before they become severe, personalizing preventative strategies, and managing complex, chronic conditions more effectively over time. This potential shift from reactive to proactive models holds promise for improving patient outcomes, reducing complications, and addressing broader public health needs. AI can help synthesize complex material for students and support learning by helping them understand diagnosis and management, mirroring the process of systematically incorporating new information.

Understanding AI's role in both reactive and proactive contexts helps clinicians appreciate its capabilities and limitations, making informed decisions about when and how to integrate these tools responsibly. However, regardless of the application, human oversight is critical because AI tools can produce authoritative-sounding answers that are factually incorrect or ethically inappropriate, and they should augment, not replace, clinical judgment.

Sidebar: What Is Logistic Regression?

Logistic regression is a statistical technique used in medicine to predict whether something will happen, such as a patient being readmitted to the hospital or developing a complication. It does not give a simple yes or no answer. Instead, it calculates a probability between 0 and 1 (or 0–100%) based on the given information.

Here is how it works:

- The model looks at multiple risk factors, such as a patient's age, blood pressure, weight, medication history, or lab results.
- Each factor is assigned a numerical weight, based on how strongly it has been associated with the outcome in past data.
- The model adds these weighted factors and then runs them through a formula that converts the total into a probability. For instance, it might predict a patient has a 42 percent chance of being hospitalized in the next 30 days.

Clinicians or AI systems then set a decision threshold, such as 30 percent, to decide when to act. If a patient's predicted risk crosses that line, they may be flagged for additional follow-up or intervention.

You can think of logistic regression as a clinical scoring system, except that the weights are calculated from large datasets rather than assigned by expert opinion. Because logistic regression yields clear risk estimates and quantifies each predictor's impact, it remains a cornerstone tool for early warning systems, risk stratification, and timely clinical interventions.

Opportunities for AI

Chronic disease management is most effective when care is proactive, anticipating problems before they escalate, rather than reacting once a patient becomes acutely ill. Think of it like a smoke detector sensing danger before a fire breaks out. AI can play this anticipatory role by continuously scanning patient data for subtle warning signs.

Picture this: Gonzalo is a 72-year-old patient with heart failure and high blood pressure. An AI model reviews his electronic health record, home blood pressure readings, and social risk factors, such as living alone or recent missed appointments. It estimates that he has a 42% chance of serious health decline in the next 30 days. His care team is automatically alerted because this risk exceeds the system's preset threshold (e.g., 30%). They can intervene early with a telehealth check-in or a home visit from a community nurse, before Gonzalo ends up in the emergency department [3].

These kinds of predictions often rely on logistic regression, a statistical technique that estimates the probability of an event based on multiple patient characteristics. (See the "What is logistic regression?"sidebar for fuller explanation.)

But wait that's not all. AI doesn't stop at individual alerts. It can also give clinicians a panel-wide view through dashboards that visualize risk across an entire patient population. These interfaces often use color coding to highlight high-risk individuals, such as those with both diabetes and heart failure, and allow care teams to explore each case in detail. This dual view supports both public health goals (like reducing preventable hospitalizations) and personalized care planning, helping clinicians allocate time and resources where they're most needed.

Once high-risk patients are identified, remote patient monitoring (RPM) tools can support continuous tracking. These technologies include Bluetooth-enabled blood pressure cuffs, glucometers, and smart scales that transmit data directly to the care team. This allows clinicians to follow patients' progress in real time, even at home, and respond quickly to worrisome trends.

As a future clinician, you may encounter these tools embedded in population health platforms or integrated directly into the EHR. Understanding what these tools can and cannot do is critical for guiding safe, effective AI-assisted care.

Fundamentals of Predictive Modeling

Predictive modeling in healthcare works like a weather forecast for patient outcomes. You collect "meteorological data," such as EHR trends, pharmacy claims, and social factors such as housing stability, and feed them into an algorithm that learns which patterns precede flare-ups or hospitalizations [4] (see Fig. 5.2). A simple model like logistic regression assigns each risk factor (age, blood pressure, HbA_1c) a numerical weight and sums these to produce a single risk score. More sophisticated techniques, like gradient boosting machines and survival analysis models, layer many small, sequential predictions to improve accuracy and handle time-to-event data [5].

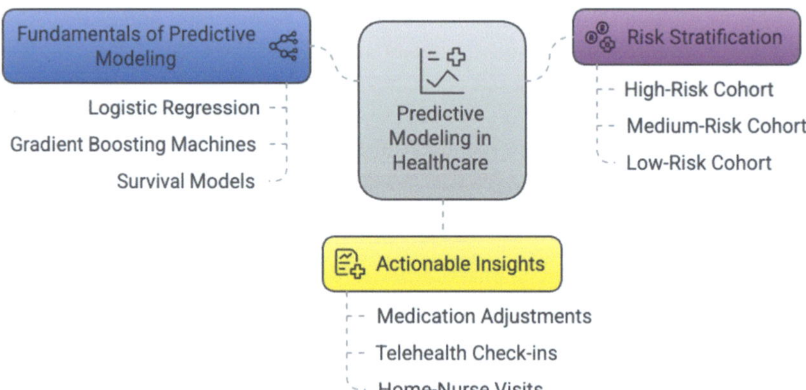

Fig. 5.2 Predictive modeling in healthcare

Clinical Vignette Imagine a patient whose rising HbA_1c, missed medication refills, and recent social service alerts combine to produce a high-risk score. That score serves as an early warning, prompting preemptive outreach before complications arise.

Risk Stratification

Risk stratification is akin to sorting your email by urgency: once each patient has a risk score, you group them into high-, medium-, or low-risk cohorts. For example, using the same gradient boosting techniques described earlier, a heart failure readmission model achieved an AUC of 0.78 in correctly ranking patients according to their 30-day rehospitalization risk [5]. Patients in the high-risk "bin" then receive prioritized outreach, such as nurse phone calls or expedited clinic visits, while lower-risk individuals follow standard monitoring schedules. This targeted approach ensures that limited resources focus on those most likely to benefit.

Actionable Insights

An actionable insight is a piece of information derived from data analysis that directly informs a specific, timely decision or intervention. In clinical practice, it goes beyond simply predicting risk; actionable insights turn risk scores into concrete clinical triggers. Imagine your car dashboard lighting up "Low Fuel" before you stall; in the EHR, an alert pops up when a patient's risk crosses a predefined threshold, prompting you to adjust treatments, schedule telehealth check-ins, or arrange home-nurse visits [6].

A panel-management dashboard acts as your clinical cockpit. It displays every patient, your panel, in a single view, color-coding them by risk level, flagging care gaps like overdue labs, and charting trends in key metrics (e.g., HbA_1c trajectories). This bird's-eye display ensures you spot and address high-need patients before crises emerge. Once high-risk patients are identified through risk models, the next step is continuous monitoring, a task increasingly supported by AI-enabled remote technologies.

Remote Patient Monitoring (RPM) Technologies

Remote patient monitoring extends care beyond clinic walls by continuously collecting health data and alerting care teams to emerging problems. Unlike telehealth, which involves live virtual visits between patients and providers, remote patient monitoring (RPM) refers to the continuous collection and analysis of health data from patients at home, often without real-time interaction. These tools allow care teams to detect changes in health status early, adjust treatment plans proactively, and reduce the risk of hospitalization.

Wearable sensors, such as Bluetooth-enabled blood pressure cuffs, glucometers, and pulse oximeters, automatically record vital signs and transmit them over cellular or Wi-Fi networks to secure cloud platforms. This seamless data flow mirrors how your fitness tracker syncs with a smartphone app, ensuring clinicians receive up-to-date readings without extra office visits [7].

Workflow Integration

Integrating RPM data into clinical workflows requires clear triage protocols and team roles. Automated systems generate two types of alerts: threshold alerts, for example, when a patient's systolic blood pressure exceeds 160 mm Hg, and trend alerts, which identify gradual changes such as a week-long rise in fasting glucose. Nurses typically perform the first review, assessing alert severity and contacting patients for clarification or coaching. They escalate critical issues, like sustained hypertension despite medication changes, to physicians via telehealth consultations, following predefined escalation pathways to ensure timely intervention [8].

Patient Engagement and Adherence

Patient engagement is the linchpin of RPM success. Devices alone won't improve outcomes unless patients consistently use them. RPM platforms address this by sending personalized behavioral nudges. These behavioral or adherence nudges are small, strategically timed prompts, such as text messages, app notifications, or phone calls, designed to encourage patients to take medications, record vitals, or follow care instructions consistently. These can be a morning text reminding patients to check their glucose and motivational messages celebrating adherence milestones. These prompts function like fitness apps that congratulate you for meeting step goals.

Yet barriers abound. Limited digital literacy can make device setup and data uploads confusing, while unreliable Internet access may interrupt data transmission. Privacy concerns may also deter participation. To mitigate these issues, choose devices with intuitive interfaces, provide brief training sessions or instructional videos, and offer connectivity support, such as cellular-enabled devices or subsidized broadband access. Transparent data policies reassure patients that their information remains secure, fostering trust and long-term adherence [9].

See Chap. 7 for prompt engineering and generative AI methods.

Clinical Use Case and Group Activity

Readers should review the following patient vignette before starting the group activity.

Patient: Maria Lopez, 72 years old
Chief Concern: Fatigue, mild dyspnea on exertion
Medical History: Hypertension, type 2 diabetes, stage 2 heart failure
Medications: Metformin, lisinopril, furosemide
Social History: Lives alone; daughter lives 45 min away; limited digital literacy
Recent Developments:

- Home blood pressure readings averaging 158/92 mmHg over the past 10 days.
- Remote weight monitoring shows a 4-pound gain over 5 days.
- Patient has missed two follow-up appointments due to transportation issues.

AI Output Predictive model flags Maria as having a 42% risk of hospital admission within 30 days.

Dashboard Indicators
- High-risk composite score for CHF + diabetes
- Yellow alert for reduced medication adherence
- Red alert for abnormal weight trend

Activity Prompt
Using the guiding question and rubric above, work with your group to create a care plan for Maria. Address how the AI outputs influenced your decisions and specify actions the care team should take in the next 72 hours. Be sure to include communication, follow-up strategies, and any interventions that address social or digital barriers.

Population Health Dashboard View for Maria Lopez: Composite risk score generated from an AI-enabled model integrating EHR, home monitoring, and social data. Red and yellow indicators flag weight gain and medication adherence concerns. This dashboard allows early intervention planning to prevent emergency escalation.

Objective
This team-based activity helps medical students apply AI-informed tools in the context of chronic disease management. Working through a real-world case, students will practice interpreting AI outputs, integrating social determinants, and formulating care plans that reflect patient needs and health system goals. The exercise emphasizes key clinical competencies, including collaborative planning, risk stratification, and ethical decision-making.

Relevant Entrustable Professional Activities (EPAs):

- **EPA 1**: Gather a history and perform a physical examination.
- **EPA 3**: Recommend and interpret common diagnostic and screening tests.

- **EPA 4**: Enter and discuss orders and prescriptions.
- **EPA 8**: Give or receive a patient handover to transition care responsibility.
- **EPA 9**: Collaborate as a member of an interprofessional team.

Framing Question
What makes a care plan "AI-informed," and how can clinicians balance algorithmic guidance with professional judgment?

AI-Informed Care Plan Rubric
Use the criteria below to guide your team's discussion and written care plan:

1. Data Use
   Does the plan incorporate AI-generated insights, such as a predictive risk score or adherence alert?
2. Clinical Interpretation
   How did the team use clinical reasoning to verify, modify, or challenge the AI recommendations?
3. Individualization
   Is the care plan tailored to the patient's health status, preferences, social circumstances, and comorbidities?
4. Actionability
   Are the proposed steps clear, feasible, and linked to specific AI outputs or dashboard indicators?
5. Ethical and Equity Considerations
   Does the plan account for digital access, algorithmic bias, and the patient's ability to participate in technology-enabled care?

Instructions for Student Groups
1. Review the patient case and dashboard visualization provided below.
2. As a group, develop a brief care plan that integrates:
   - The AI-generated risk and adherence alerts
   - The patient's clinical findings
   - Relevant social determinants of health
3. Prepare a 3–5 min presentation that includes:
   - Which AI outputs informed your decisions
   - The specific actions your team recommends
   - Any implementation or ethical concerns you encountered
4. Conclude by reflecting on how you integrated AI guidance with human clinical judgment and patient-centered reasoning.

Quiz 3
1. **In one sentence,** explain how risk stratification differs from diagnostic prediction in chronic disease management.
2. **Name three** data sources commonly used in predictive analytics for chronic care (e.g., lab trends, claims data, patient-reported outcomes).

3. **True or False:** RPM alerts should always trigger immediate clinical intervention.
4. **Multiple Choice:** Which algorithm type is best suited for time-to-event predictions (e.g., modeling time until hospitalization)?
   (a) Logistic regression
   (b) Random forest
   (c) proportional hazards model
   (d) k-Nearest neighbors
5. **In two to three sentences,** describe one potential pitfall of relying solely on RPM-generated alerts in your care plan.

Ethical and Operational Barriers

Even the most well-designed AI care plans face real-world challenges when translated into practice, especially when patients face social, digital, or systemic barriers.

AI-enabled chronic care tools promise earlier interventions, better resource targeting, and more personalized medicine. Yet realizing these benefits depends on addressing ethical risks and operational hurdles affecting how these tools are deployed, especially in underserved populations.

Data Equity and Algorithmic Bias
AI tools are only as equitable as the data on which they are trained. Suppose certain patient populations, such as those from rural areas, non-English speakers, or uninsured individuals, are underrepresented in training datasets. In that case, the model may systematically underestimate their risk or offer less appropriate care recommendations. This can worsen existing health disparities.

Digital Literacy and Access
Remote patient monitoring (RPM) and app-based adherence tools often assume patients have smartphones, Internet access, and the digital skills to use them. For older adults, patients with cognitive impairment, or those with limited health literacy, this assumption can create barriers rather than solutions. Clinics must pair digital interventions with human support, such as nurse educators or community health workers, to ensure equitable engagement.

Privacy and Trust
Continuous data streams from wearables, smart devices, and home sensors raise valid concerns about patient privacy. Patients may worry about who can access their data, how it will be used, or whether it could be shared with insurers or employers. Clinicians should explain how data are protected and used for clinical care, not surveillance, and should secure explicit consent where appropriate.

Reimbursement and Workflow Complexity
Operational barriers also shape whether AI tools can be scaled. While Medicare offers reimbursement codes for remote patient monitoring (RPM) and chronic care

management (CCM), billing rules are complex. RPM typically requires a minimum of 16 days of monitoring per month and documentation of at least 20 min of clinical interaction. These requirements can strain already burdened primary care workflows. Clinics need clear protocols, trained staff, and possibly third-party vendors to make these services sustainable.

Conclusion

Artificial intelligence is promising to improve chronic care by enabling earlier detection, smarter resource allocation, and more personalized interventions. But technology alone is not enough. Its success depends on clinical teams who can critically interpret AI outputs, engage patients with empathy, and navigate real-world care's ethical and logistical complexities. As you continue developing your skills, remember that algorithms will not lead the future of chronic disease management, but rather by clinicians who know how to use them wisely. In the next chapter, we'll explore how these same principles apply to acute care settings, where rapid decisions and evolving data streams test your ability to lead under pressure.

Instructor's Guide for This Chapter: Primary Care and Chronic Disease Management

Overview

This chapter explores how AI, including predictive analytics and remote patient monitoring (RPM), can transform chronic disease management in primary care. Students will apply concepts through a group exercise to build an AI-enhanced care plan.

Learning Objectives

By the end of this chapter, students should be able to:

1. Explain the burden of chronic illness in primary care and the limitations of reactive care models.
2. Describe how AI-driven predictive models identify patients at risk for exacerbations.
3. Outline RPM technologies and their integration into clinical workflows.
4. Address patient engagement and adherence challenges in RPM.
5. Collaboratively develop and defend an AI-enhanced care plan for a chronic care vignette.

Teaching Strategies

- **Case-Based Discussion**: Introduce Maria's case in section "Managing chronic disease in the age of generative AI" to illustrate polypharmacy and reactive care pitfalls.
- **Interactive Demo**: Show a live or recorded dashboard demo (predictive risk and panel management).
- **Simulation**: Use a mock EHR or spreadsheet to practice data review and risk score interpretation.
- **Role Play**: Assign students nursing versus physician roles for triaging RPM alerts in section "Workflow integration".
- **Group Workshop**: Guide teams through the activity in section "Clinical use case and group activity", with timed milestones and a rubric.

How to Use Discussion Prompts in This Chapter

The following discussion prompts are designed to deepen learners' understanding of how artificial intelligence enhances chronic disease management. Each question corresponds to a key section of the chapter and promotes application of theory to clinical scenarios.

Objectives

- Encourage critical thinking about AI's clinical utility and limitations.
- Foster dialogue around ethics, equity, and workflow integration.
- Develop students' ability to explain AI methods to clinical peers.
- Apply concepts like sensitivity/specificity, logistic regression, and risk prediction to real-world care decisions.

Instructional Strategies

1. **Small Group Breakouts (15–20 min)**
   Assign each group one question and ask them to analyze a relevant case example or create their own. For example:

   "Your group has been asked to evaluate an RPM protocol for rural heart failure patients. Based on Prompt 3, what challenges do you foresee and how would you address them?"

2. **Whole-Class Guided Discussion (10–15 min per Question)**
   Pose a prompt and ask for volunteers to respond. Encourage peers to build on, challenge, or refine the answer. Use probing follow-up questions:

"What if the patient doesn't trust AI tools—how should the care team respond?"
"Could a less interpretable model still be safe if it outperforms logistic regression?"

3. **Flip-Classroom or Asynchronous Assignments**
   Assign students to prepare written responses to one or more prompts before class. Use their answers to seed deeper in-person or online discussion.
4. **Clinical Simulation or Role Play**
   Use Prompt 4 during a simulated RPM case. Assign roles (nurse, resident, informaticist) and have each participant advocate for different RPM thresholds based on their perspective.

Assessment Suggestions

- Use a rubric for assessing the clarity, accuracy, and relevance of responses.
- Offer participation credit for thoughtful engagement.
- Incorporate discussion reflections into formative assessments or weekly journals.

Discussion Prompts with Answers

1. **In section "**Burden of chronic illness**", what are the downsides of waiting to intervene until after a patient decompensates?**
   Waiting to intervene until a patient decompensates often results in avoidable harm, higher costs, and diminished quality of life. Clinically, decompensation, such as acute heart failure exacerbation or diabetic ketoacidosis, usually signals missed warning signs that could have been addressed earlier. The patient may require hospitalization, invasive procedures, or prolonged recovery by that point. For health systems, reactive care leads to increased emergency department visits and readmissions, which strain resources and lower value-based care metrics. It can erode trust, limit autonomy, and worsen long-term outcomes for patients. Proactive intervention, supported by AI risk stratification, aims to shift care upstream, preventing deterioration before it starts.
2. **How would you explain the difference between logistic regression and gradient boosting to a colleague?**
   Logistic regression is one of the simplest and most established tools for clinical prediction. It looks at several input factors, say, a patient's age, blood pressure, and lab values, and assigns each a weight based on how strongly it's been associated with a particular outcome, like hospitalization. The model then combines those weighted factors into a single probability, giving you a clear sense of risk. Importantly, the relationships are assumed to be linear and additive, which makes the model transparent: you can easily see how much each factor contributes to the prediction.

Gradient boosting, by contrast, is a newer and more complex method. Instead of a single equation, it uses many small decision trees—simple rules based on yes/no questions (e.g., "Is the systolic BP over 160?"). These trees are built sequentially, with each one learning from the mistakes of the previous one. The result is a layered model that captures more complex, nonlinear patterns that logistic regression might miss. It often outperforms simpler models when the relationships between variables are messy or not obviously linear.

However, this added power comes at a cost: gradient boosting is harder to interpret. While it may be more accurate, it doesn't offer the same clarity about *why* a prediction was made. That makes it less ideal for situations where transparency matters, such as explaining risk to a patient or defending a clinical decision.

In clinical terms, think of logistic regression as a well-validated risk calculator, like $CHADS_2$ or ASCVD. It's straightforward and explainable. Gradient boosting is more like a black-box diagnostic assistant that integrates dozens of subtle patterns, very smart, often more accurate, but harder to unpack.

3. **In section** "Remote patient monitoring (RPM) technologies"**, what factors might limit RPM effectiveness in rural or underserved populations?**

   Several factors can undermine the effectiveness of remote patient monitoring (RPM) in rural or underserved settings:

   - **Limited broadband access**, which impairs the transmission of health data from devices to providers.
   - **Digital literacy gaps**, especially among older adults or non-English-speaking populations, can reduce proper device use and engagement.
   - **Device affordability**, where out-of-pocket costs or lack of insurance coverage may create access barriers.
   - **Cultural mistrust** or prior negative experiences with the health system may reduce patient willingness to participate in continuous monitoring programs.
   - **Provider shortages** in rural areas may limit the clinical workforce available to respond to RPM alerts in a timely, coordinated fashion.

   Addressing these challenges requires combining technology deployment with community-based outreach, patient education, and infrastructure investment.

4. **For the group activity (5.4), how do you balance sensitivity and alarm fatigue when setting RPM thresholds?**

   Balancing sensitivity and alarm fatigue requires calibrating thresholds to minimize false positives while still capturing clinically meaningful events. Setting the threshold too low may overwhelm care teams with alerts that require no action, contributing to desensitization and missed true positives. Conversely, setting it too high may delay necessary intervention. The optimal strategy involves:

   - **Using tiered alerts** (e.g., low-, medium-, and high-severity flags) to triage responses.
   - **Incorporating trend-based triggers**, such as rapid blood pressure escalation over days, rather than single-point outliers.

- **Engaging frontline clinicians** and patients in designing thresholds that reflect realistic care needs.
- **Periodically re-evaluating system performance**, using retrospective chart audits to assess how well thresholds are functioning in practice.

Ultimately, RPM alerts must be actionable, timely, and tailored to both the condition and the population being monitored.

This reflection promotes metacognition and helps identify areas for further teaching.

Quiz 3 Answer Key

1. **Risk stratification versus diagnostic prediction:** Risk stratification groups patients by future risk level; diagnostic prediction identifies current disease presence.
2. **Data sources:** Lab trends (e.g., HbA_1c), claims data (medication fills), patient-reported outcomes (home glucose logs).
3. **False:** Not all RPM alerts require immediate intervention; context and trends matter.
4. **C. Cox proportional hazards model** is suited for time-to-event predictions.
5. **Pitfall (example):** Overreliance on RPM alerts may cause false reassurance if devices malfunction or patients bypass readings.

Additional Resources

- **Tutorial:** Stanford CS229 lecture on predictive modeling.
- **Tool Demo:** Open-source RPM platforms (e.g., OpenAPS).
- **Guidelines:** American Diabetes Association standards on foot care and nephropathy risk.

Timing Recommendations

- **Session 1 (60 min):** Sections "Burden of chronic illness" and "Fundamentals of predictive modeling", case discussion, predictive-modeling exercise.
- **Session 2 (60 min):** Sections "Remote patient monitoring (RPM) technologies" and "Clinical use case and GROUP activity", RPM role play, group care plan workshop, quiz.

Optional Debrief

Close the session by asking:

"Which AI application from today's discussion do you feel most confident explaining to a patient or colleague? Which one still feels uncertain?"

References

1. Centers for Disease Control and Prevention. Chronic diseases in America. 2020. Retrieved from https://www.cdc.gov/chronicdisease/resources/infographic/chronic-diseases.htm
2. Jencks SF, Williams MV, Coleman EA. Rehospitalizations among patients in the Medicare fee-for-service program. N Engl J Med. 2009;360(14):1418–28. https://doi.org/10.1056/NEJMsa0803563.
3. Kueper JK, Terry AL, Zwarenstein M, Lizotte DJ. Artificial intelligence and primary care research: a scoping review. Ann Fam Med. 2020;18(3):250–8. https://doi.org/10.1370/afm.2560.
4. Goldstein BA, Navar AM, Pencina MJ, Ioannidis JPA. Opportunities and challenges in developing risk prediction models with electronic health records data: a systematic review. J Am Med Inform Assoc. 2017;24(1):198–208. https://doi.org/10.1093/jamia/ocw042.
5. Ahmad T, Desai N, Wilson FP, Wang G. Machine learning to predict hospital readmissions in heart failure patients. JACC Heart Fail. 2018;6(4):333–44. https://doi.org/10.1016/j.jchf.2018.01.014.
6. Bates DW, Saria S, Ohno-Machado L, Shah A, Escobar G. Big data in health care: using analytics to identify and manage high-risk and high-cost patients. Health Aff. 2018;37(7):1123–31. https://doi.org/10.1377/hlthaff.2017.1624.
7. Alhumud AZ, Alrowaily MH, Almudhefir AA. Mobile health in remote patient monitoring for chronic diseases: a review. J Med Internet Res. 2021;23(5):e26981. https://doi.org/10.2196/26981.
8. Noah B, Keller MS, Mosadeghi S, et al. Impact of remote patient monitoring on clinical outcomes: an updated meta-analysis of randomized controlled trials. NPJ Digit Med. 2018;1:Article 20172. https://doi.org/10.1038/s41746-017-0002-4.
9. Yaghubi A, Maeder A, O'Dwyer L. Remote patient monitoring strategies and wearable technology in chronic disease management: a review. Front Med. 2023;10:1236598. https://doi.org/10.3389/fmed.2023.1236598.
10. Tangri N, Stevens LA, Griffith J, Tighiouart H, Djurdjev O, Naimark D, et al. A predictive model for progression of chronic kidney disease to kidney failure. JAMA. 2011;305(15):1553–9. https://doi.org/10.1001/jama.2011.451.
11. Boulton AJM, Armstrong DG, Albert SF, Frykberg RG, Hellman R, Kirkman MS, et al. Comprehensive foot examination and risk assessment: a report of the Task Force of the Foot Care Interest Group of the American Diabetes Association. Diabetes Care. 2008;31(8):1679–85. https://doi.org/10.2337/dc08-9021.

Chapter 6
AI Utilization in Neurology

Learning Objectives

By the end of this chapter, students should be able to:

1. Explain the unique challenges of neuro data (3D volumes, electroencephalography (EEG)/EMG signals) and why specialized AI approaches are needed.
2. Describe key AI techniques (3D CNNs, recurrent neural network (RNN)/long short-term memory (LSTM), explainability methods) and their roles in neuroimaging and signal analysis.
3. Illustrate how AI accelerates stroke detection, perfusion mapping, and tumor segmentation in practice.
4. Discuss AI's impact on neurological emergencies (large-vessel occlusion (LVO) alerts, traumatic brain injury (TBI)/SCI triage, EEG prognostication).
5. Summarize AI-driven decision support for chronic neurologic and movement disorders, including autism screening.
6. Identify brain-machine interfaces and adaptive rehabilitation technologies, as well as their clinical benefits.
7. Evaluate neuro-specific workflow integration, ethical challenges, and regulatory pathways.
8. Analyze future innovations in multimodal fusion, generative reporting, and predictive care orchestration.
9. Critically assess case studies, recognizing both benefits and pitfalls of AI in neurology.

© The Author(s), under exclusive license to Springer Nature Switzerland AG 2025
C. Quinn, *Generative AI for the Medical Student*,
https://doi.org/10.1007/978-3-032-01613-3_6

Why Neurologic Data Challenges AI Systems

Neurological data present unique challenges for artificial intelligence systems. Unlike standard laboratory results or two-dimensional chest radiographs, neurologic imaging and electrophysiologic signals are multidimensional, noisy, and variable across individuals. These complexities demand advanced models and rigorous validation (see Fig. 6.1).

Volumetric imaging, such as MRI and CT, produces three-dimensional datasets composed of millions of tiny units called voxels. Detecting subtle abnormalities such as a 4 mm hemorrhage in the thalamus requires algorithms that can identify faint textural changes while preserving spatial relationships. These tasks initially overwhelmed early graphics processing units (GPUs) and continue to drive the development of modern three-dimensional convolutional neural networks [1].

Electrophysiologic data, such as electroencephalography (EEG), introduce an entirely different set of obstacles. A routine EEG records voltage fluctuations every few milliseconds across 19–32 scalp electrodes, generating hours of time-series data (see Fig. 6.1). Motion artifacts from eye blinks, ventilators, or even a vibrating ICU mattress can resemble epileptic spikes. Before seizure activity can be

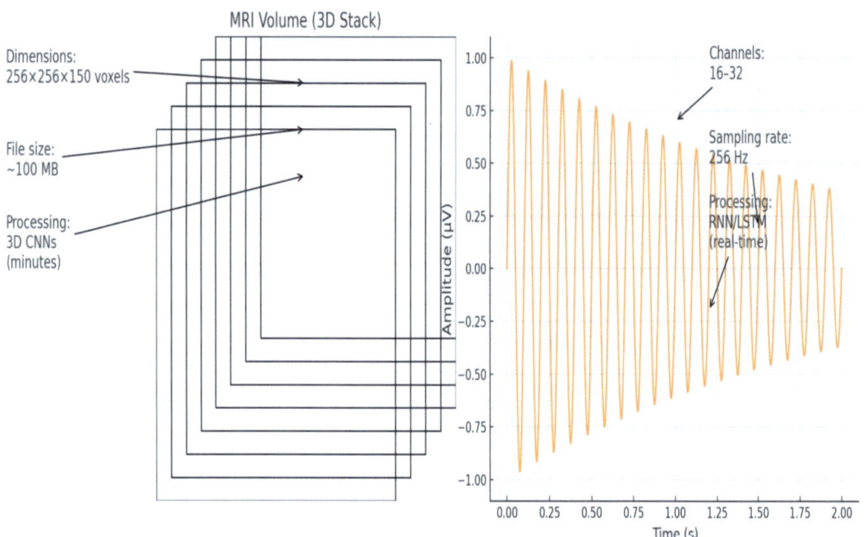
Comparison of MRI Volume and EEG Waveform Data
MRI Volume (3D Stack)
Dimensions:
256×256×150 voxels
File size:
~100 MB
Processing:
3D CNNs
(minutes)
Amplitude (µV)
1.00
0.75
0.50
0.25
0.00
−0.25
−0.50
−0.75
−1.00
0.00 0.25 0.50 0.75 1.00 1.25 1.50 1.75 2.00
Time (s)
Channels:
16-32
Sampling rate:
256 Hz
Processing:
RNN/LSTM
(real-time)
This graphic compares two types of neurological data: a three-dimensional MRI volume, which represents structural brain information as stacked voxel slices processed by 3D convolutional neural networks (CNNs) over minutes, and an EEG waveform, which captures real-time electrical activity processed by RNN/LSTM models. Understanding these formats helps clinicians appreciate how AI handles diverse data in neurology.

Fig. 6.1 Neurological data comparison

identified, deep-learning models must first clean this signal and then detect events that may last only a few seconds [2].

Anatomical variation among patients further complicates the training of generalizable models. For example, a middle cerebral artery stroke may affect Broca's area and result in aphasia in one patient, yet spare language entirely in another due to collateral blood flow or individual differences in neuroanatomy. As a result, an algorithm trained on lesion patterns from one hospital may fail when applied to unfamiliar patient populations [3].

Rare neurologic conditions pose yet another challenge. Disorders like pediatric epileptic encephalopathies or autoimmune limbic encephalitis occur infrequently, limiting the size of usable datasets. Moreover, privacy laws constrain the ability to share raw imaging across institutions. In response, researchers have begun using privacy-preserving methods such as federated learning, which allows model training across hospitals without transferring patient images. Only encrypted model updates are shared across institutions.

These factors help explain why neurologic AI has developed more slowly than applications in fields like dermatology or ophthalmology. Progress will depend on more innovative models and collaborative dataset curation and regulatory frameworks that support responsible data sharing.

Now that we've explored why neurologic data presents such technical hurdles, we turn to the AI tools built specifically for analyzing three-dimensional imaging and time-series signals and the ways these tools are transforming neurovascular care.

Sidebar 6.1: Understanding Electrophysiologic Time-Series Waveforms

Electrophysiologic waveforms are continuous recordings of the body's electrical signals plotted over time. In neurology, we most often see electroencephalogram (EEG) traces, where each line represents voltage fluctuations caused by neuronal firing. In cardiology, electrocardiogram (ECG) waveforms display the heart's depolarization and repolarization cycles. These time-series plots allow clinicians (and AI models) to detect characteristic patterns, such as the P-QRS-T complex in ECGs or the alpha, beta, and delta rhythms in EEGs, that correspond to normal function or specific pathologies.

Key features to recognize include the following:

- **Amplitude and Frequency:** The height and spacing of peaks reveal signal strength and rate (e.g., a fast, low-amplitude beta rhythm vs. a slow, high-amplitude delta wave).
- **Morphology:** The shape of each waveform component (e.g., the sharp QRS spike in ECG or the rhythmic alpha peak in EEG) helps distinguish normal activity from arrhythmias or epileptiform discharges.

Milestones in Neuro-AI Approval

When a large-vessel occlusion (LVO) blocks a major brain artery, every minute of delay costs neurons. Computed tomography angiography (CTA) is an emergency scan that shows these vessels. Still, a radiologist may need several minutes to open the study, scroll through hundreds of images, and phone the stroke team. Two FDA-cleared algorithms now shoulder that triage burden:

1. **ContaCT (Viz.ai)**—the first stroke-AI system to receive **De Novo clearance** (DEN170073, February 2018). The software automatically reviews each CTA, highlights voxels consistent with an LVO, and sends a secure push notification, with the key slice, to the on-call neurologist's phone in **<6 min**. In the pivotal trial, it detected proximal LVOs with **87% sensitivity and 87% specificity** compared with expert consensus [4].
2. **Rapid LVO (iSchemaView)**—cleared via the **510(k) pathway** in April 2020 (K200941) as substantially equivalent to ContaCT. Tested on 1245 CTAs from 12 US hospitals, Rapid LVO flagged occlusions in **2.7 min mean processing time** with **97% sensitivity and 96% specificity** for the internal carotid and first segment of the middle cerebral artery [5].

For medical students, the take-home is simple: by screening every CTA in real time and alerting the team before the radiologist can scroll to the culprit artery, these algorithms shave tens of minutes off decision-making, often converting a "too late" thrombectomy candidate into a salvageable one. Their clear regulatory pathway—De Novo for a first-in-class device, then 510(k) for a similar successor—paved the way for dozens of neuro-AI tools now entering practice.

Neuro-specific AI Methods

Handling Volumetric Data: Convolutional Approaches for MRI/CT

Before modern neural networks, lesion volume was measured by manual region-of-interest tracing: a radiologist or technologist outlined the abnormal area on every slice of the scan and then multiplied the total number of highlighted voxels by the voxel dimensions to obtain volume. Even with semiautomated threshold tools, the clinician still adjusted each contour, a process that could take 20–30 min for a single brain MRI and varied significantly between readers [6]. Convolutional neural networks (CNNs) replace that labor-intensive "pixel counting" with small, learnable filters that slide through the three-dimensional volume and mark voxels showing tumor borders, edema, or acute ischemia in seconds [7]. Studies comparing manual to CNN-based segmentation report time savings of 9% or more and inter-reader agreement improving from moderate ($\kappa \approx 0.6$) to near-perfect ($\kappa > 0.9$) [8].

For medical students, the key point is that CNNs deliver rapid, reproducible lesion volumes, critical when decisions such as thrombolysis hinge on knowing whether an infarct is below a treatment threshold. Radiologists can therefore focus on clinical interpretation rather than slice-by-slice tracing, enabling faster, more accurate care in acute neuro-imaging scenarios.

Rapid Signal Processing: AI for EEG/EMG Interpretation

Electrophysiology traditionally involves hours of strip-chart review to spot spikes, slowing neurologic assessment. Recurrent neural networks (RNNs) and their variant long short-term memory (LSTM) models excel at learning patterns over time, flagging seizure activity or muscle burst potentials within seconds [9, 10]. For example, an AI-assisted EEG reading can alert a clinician to subclinical seizures without obvious clinical signs, prompting early treatment and preventing secondary injury. By automating routine analysis, these models accelerate decision-making in the EEG lab and reduce cognitive load on trainees still mastering the intricacies of waveform morphology.

Explainability in Neuro-models: Why "Black Boxes" Matter in Patient Care

Suppose a deep-learning system marks a faint abnormality in the motor cortex as malignant. Before referring the patient to oncology or neurosurgery, the neurologist needs to understand why the model reached that conclusion. Explainability techniques, such as saliency or heat maps, overlay color on the MRI or CT scan to reveal exactly which voxels drove the prediction. When the colored region aligns with the lesion suspected by the neurologist, the neurologist gains confidence in acting on the result; if the map instead highlights an unrelated artifact, the alert can be questioned and the model reviewed [11]. Explainability techniques allow the clinician to verify that the AI focused on the lesion, not an imaging artifact or electrode noise, before guiding treatment decisions. For students, understanding these safeguards underscores how trustworthy AI can become an integrated member of the care team rather than an opaque oracle.

With these AI methods in mind, let's examine their practical applications in neuroimaging tasks, including stroke detection, perfusion analysis, and tumor segmentation.

Clinical Pearl: Verify AI Focus with Saliency Maps
Saliency maps help you see exactly where an AI model "looks" when it analyzes an image. Think of a saliency map as a color overlay that highlights the pixels most responsible for the model's decision. For example, a tumor-detection algorithm should light up the lesion itself, not unrelated objects such as surgical clips or motion artifacts. Always review these overlays in your practice: if the heatmap points to the wrong area, it signals that the AI may be learning the wrong features, so further validation or model adjustment is needed.

Neuroimaging Applications

Neuroimaging is a cornerstone of neurologic diagnosis, particularly in time-sensitive conditions like stroke and hemorrhage. Artificial intelligence tools are increasingly used to support faster interpretation, reduce diagnostic variability, and guide urgent clinical decisions.

Automated Stroke Detection (ASPECTS Scoring; Hyperdense Vessel Alerts)

In acute ischemic stroke, time is critical. The Alberta Stroke Program Early CT Score (ASPECTS) is a 10-point scale used to assess early ischemic changes within the middle cerebral artery (MCA) territory on non-contrast CT scans. Each region showing signs of infarction—such as loss of gray-white differentiation or sulcal effacement—reduces the score, indicating more extensive damage.

Manual ASPECTS scoring is time-consuming and often varies between readers, especially under the pressure of an evolving stroke code. AI tools using convolutional neural networks now automate this process, rapidly identifying subtle areas of hypoattenuation (reduced tissue density) and calculating ASPECTS in seconds [12]. These models also detect the hyperdense vessel sign, which may suggest an occluded artery and signal the need for emergent thrombectomy evaluation.

For medical students and early learners, this means the care team can receive immediate, standardized alerts that support the activation of a "code stroke." Early notification helps accelerate imaging review, expedite transfer to thrombectomy-capable centers, and reduce door-to-needle times. By minimizing both delay and variability, AI-driven stroke detection tools have the potential to improve neurologic outcomes for patients presenting with large vessel occlusion [12].

Clinical Pearl: Rapid ASPECTS Interpretation
AI-generated ASPECTS scores highlight ten specific brain regions on CT that may show early signs of stroke. When you see an AI flag, for example, a shaded area in the right lentiform nucleus, make sure to cross-check that finding with the patient's NIHSS exam (e.g., facial droop or arm weakness) before calling a "code stroke." This correlation ensures you act on true positives and understand how imaging findings map to clinical deficits.

Perfusion Mapping for Penumbra Identification (RAPID; CBF/ADC Thresholds)

In the setting of acute ischemic stroke, identifying which brain tissue is already infarcted and which is still salvageable, the ischemic penumbra, is essential for guiding treatment decisions. This process relies on perfusion imaging, using either CT or MRI, to estimate blood flow and cellular integrity.

The core infarct represents brain tissue that is already irreversibly damaged. The penumbra surrounds this core and is at risk, but potentially recoverable if blood flow is restored. Two imaging metrics help differentiate these zones: cerebral blood flow (CBF) and the apparent diffusion coefficient (ADC). Severely reduced CBF suggests infarction, while moderate reductions may indicate penumbra. Low ADC values reflect cytotoxic edema and cellular injury.

AI-powered software platforms such as RAPID automate the analysis of these maps. They segment regions of interest, apply validated thresholds, and generate color-coded overlays that highlight infarcted and at-risk areas [13]. The software outputs quantitative volume estimates in just a few minutes and eliminates the need for manual region-of-interest placement.

For clinicians, this allows faster decision-making about intravenous thrombolysis or endovascular thrombectomy, particularly in patients who arrive beyond the conventional 4.5- or 6-h treatment windows. RAPID has been FDA-cleared and is routinely used in comprehensive stroke centers to support evidence-based intervention planning [13].

Clinical Pearl: Perfusion Threshold Nuances
Automated perfusion maps color-code brain tissue based on blood flow (CBF) and water diffusion (ADC). Most platforms mark the core infarct as the area where CBF is less than 30% of normal, and the penumbra as the area where ADC is below 620×10^{-6} mm^2/s. If you see a thin blue rim barely meeting the threshold, review the raw numeric values. Some vendors calibrate differently, and small variances can change treatment eligibility, especially in late-presenting strokes.

Tumor and Lesion Segmentation in Neuro-oncology

Accurately defining the borders of brain tumors on MRI is essential for safe surgical resection, precise radiation targeting, and longitudinal treatment planning. Traditionally, this task requires time-consuming manual contouring by neuroradiologists or neurosurgeons, and the results may vary between readers.

Deep learning models trained on expert-annotated datasets now offer automated solutions. These systems can segment both enhancing tumor regions, which typically show up as contrast-avid on T1-weighted images, and non-enhancing components, which may reflect edema or infiltrative disease [14]. The AI generates three-dimensional volumetric masks that closely match expert-defined contours and are overlaid on standard imaging sequences (see Fig. 6.2).

This technology illustrates how AI can streamline imaging workflows for medical students while improving consistency. Automated segmentation tools also provide reproducible metrics such as tumor volume, shape, and growth rate. These outputs assist with prognosis, inform treatment response, and support shared decision-making across multidisciplinary teams.

As we've seen, AI improves static imaging interpretation in oncology. Next, we turn to its role in high-acuity situations, examining how these tools support urgent workflows in stroke, trauma, and seizure management.

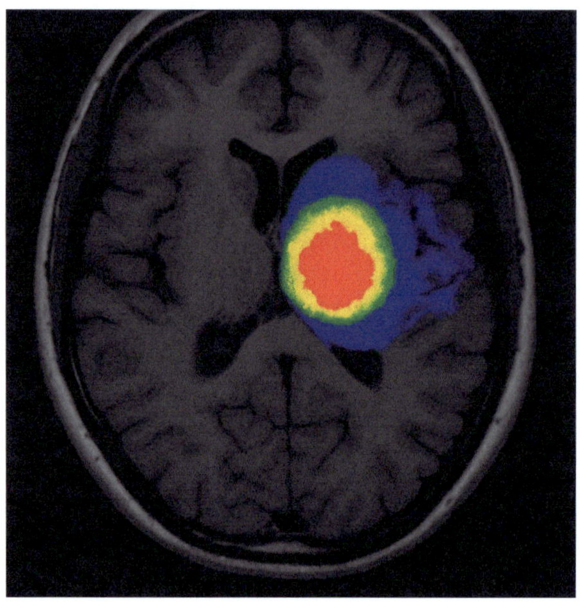

Fig. 6.2 Axial T1-weighted post-contrast MRI image showing automated segmentation of a glioblastoma using a deep learning model. Color overlays indicate the tumor subregions: red for enhancing core, yellow for non-enhancing infiltrative tissue, and blue for surrounding edema. The model-generated volumetric mask provides reproducible measurements of tumor burden, which assist with surgical planning, radiation therapy targeting, and longitudinal disease monitoring

AI in Neurological Emergencies

In emergencies where every second counts, AI accelerates recognition and response, starting with the detection of large-vessel occlusions (LVOs).

LVO Alert Systems and "Code Stroke" Integration

Large vessel occlusion (LVO) strokes are among the most time-sensitive neurologic emergencies. Prompt recognition and transfer to a thrombectomy-capable center can significantly improve outcomes. AI tools such as **Viz.ai** support this process by automatically analyzing CT angiograms to detect suspected occlusions in large arteries, including the internal carotid and proximal middle cerebral arteries.

The system processes images in under 3 min and has demonstrated a sensitivity of 90.6% and specificity of 87.5% for LVO detection [15]. The software sends secure alerts to the stroke team via a mobile application when an occlusion is identified, including radiologists, neurologists, and interventionalists. This automated notification reduces the median time to clinical activation by approximately 10 min, a meaningful gain in acute stroke care.

For medical students, the key takeaway is that AI can serve as an early warning system, expediting "code stroke" activation. This protocol mobilizes stroke resources rapidly, shortens door-to-needle and door-to-groin puncture intervals, and increases the chances of timely thrombectomy, directly impacting neurologic recovery and functional independence.

Sidebar 6.2: Door-to-Needle Interval in Acute Stroke Care

The **door-to-needle interval** measures the time from a patient's arrival at the hospital ("door") to the administration of intravenous thrombolytic therapy ("needle"). Every minute counts when treating ischemic stroke [16]. In one study that used data from 58,353 patients in the US Get-With-The-Guidelines-Stroke registry, the authors showed that every 15-min reduction in door-to-needle time increased the odds of the patient walking independently at discharge and decreased the odds of in-hospital mortality and symptomatic intracranial hemorrhage [17]. The American Heart Association/American Stroke Association recommends a target of ≤60 min for at least 50% of eligible patients, with an aspirational goal of ≤45 min when possible [18].

Clinically, shortening this interval involves streamlined triage, rapid imaging (CT or MRI), immediate lab processing, and pre-notification of the stroke team. When these steps are tightly coordinated, patients gain critical minutes of brain perfusion, translating directly into saved neurons and improved recovery.

Triage Support in Traumatic Brain Injury and Spinal Cord Injury

In trauma settings, intracranial hemorrhages are sometimes missed or delayed in busy emergency departments, particularly when imaging backlogs compete with time-sensitive triage. Traumatic brain injury (TBI) and spinal cord trauma require rapid radiologic interpretation to guide critical neurosurgical decisions.

AI triage tools, such as **Aidoc's** hemorrhage detection algorithm, automatically screen non-contrast head CTs for signs of acute bleeding. These systems can identify epidural, subdural, subarachnoid, and intraparenchymal hemorrhages, flagging suspicious cases for prioritized review. In one study, this approach reduced the average turnaround time for positive CT cases from 53 to 46 min, a statistically significant improvement ($p < 0.001$) [19, 20].

For medical students, it is essential to recognize that early hemorrhage detection can determine the urgency of neurosurgical consultation and affect patient outcomes. Whether managing a patient with TBI or evaluating possible spinal cord compression, AI-supported triage systems help ensure that the most critical scans are reviewed first, potentially saving lives when minutes matter.

Seizure Detection and Prognostication with AI-Enhanced EEG

Continuous electroencephalogram (EEG) monitoring generates vast amounts of data, and hundreds of voltage waveforms are captured every second across multiple channels. Analyzing these patterns manually can be time-consuming and delay critical decisions. Deep learning has opened new possibilities in two major areas of EEG interpretation: seizure detection and neurologic outcome prediction.

1. **Real-Time Seizure Detection**

In critically ill patients, seizures often occur without visible convulsions, a phenomenon known as nonconvulsive status epilepticus. These events can go unnoticed for hours and lead to irreversible neuronal damage if untreated. Continuous EEG monitoring is the gold standard for detecting these seizures, but human technologists usually review data intermittently, such as every 30 min. This delay can postpone treatment.

AI models, including convolutional and recurrent neural networks, offer a solution. These systems are trained to recognize characteristic EEG patterns, such as spike-and-wave discharges seen in both focal and generalized seizures. In a multicenter validation study using data from the Temple University Hospital (TUH) corpus and private ICU sources, a hybrid model that combined long short-term memory (LSTM) layers with transformer blocks achieved 92% sensitivity, with only 1.2 false alarms per 24 h [21]. This level of accuracy allows for near-instantaneous seizure alerts, enabling clinicians to intervene quickly with antiseizure medications, potentially improving neurologic outcomes and reducing ICU length of stay.

2. **Prognostication After Cardiac Arrest**

Comatose patients who survive cardiac arrest present a unique challenge. Families and clinicians must make critical decisions about continuing life-sustaining care, often within the first 48 h. Traditional tools for neurologic prognosis, such as the absence of brain stem reflexes or bilateral N20 wave absence on somatosensory evoked potentials (SSEPs), can be insensitive or only become reliable several days post-arrest.

Recent advances in AI offer earlier and potentially more accurate predictions. By analyzing EEG recordings from the first 24 h after cardiac arrest, deep learning models can estimate the likelihood that a patient will regain meaningful neurologic function. In a multicenter study involving 1038 EEG recordings, such models achieved an area under the receiver operating characteristic curve (AUC) of 0.92 [22]. This means the AI could distinguish favorable from poor outcomes with high accuracy, outperforming many established prognostic markers. Used appropriately, this information can help guide family discussions, clarify goals of care, and support ethically grounded decision-making.

Why this matters for future clinicians:

- **Faster intervention**: AI-powered seizure alerts allow for quicker administration of intravenous benzodiazepines or adjustment of antiseizure medications, potentially limiting neuronal damage.
- **Improved family communication**: Early, objective predictions about neurologic recovery can help frame sensitive conversations about prognosis and end-of-life care.
- **Resource efficiency**: Overnight, AI can screen hours of EEG recordings and triage for review, freeing neurophysiologists to focus on complex or ambiguous cases.
- **Standardized interpretation**: Algorithms apply consistent criteria across institutions, which can reduce the variability in EEG readings that often challenges learners.

As with all clinical AI tools, outputs must be interpreted within the full clinical picture. Motion artifacts, muscle activity, ventilator rhythms, and other noise can still lead to false positives. Prognostic predictions should complement, not replace, ongoing neurologic exams and clinician judgment.

Sidebar: Traditional Coma Markers Versus Post-arrest EEG

Classic bedside tests for prognosis after cardiac arrest look for signs that the brain stem and cortex have shut down irreversibly:

- **Brain stem reflexes**—pupillary light response, corneal blink, and gag/cough. If these are absent 72 h after re-warming, the chance of meaningful recovery is very low.

(continued)

- **Somatosensory Evoked Potentials (SSEPs)**—electrodes record a cortical wave, the **N20**, after the median nerve is electrically stimulated at the wrist. **Bilateral absence of the N20** suggests the primary sensory cortex is nonfunctional.

Limitations: sedatives, hypothermia, or metabolic disturbances can temporarily suppress these signals, risking a falsely pessimistic outlook.

Why add continuous EEG?

- Captures real-time cortical activity over hours, not a single snapshot.
- Detects "reactivity" (EEG changes to sound or pain) that predicts better outcomes even when reflexes seem absent.
- Allows automated algorithms to calculate recovery probabilities (AUC $\approx$ 0.9 in recent studies), providing a more nuanced forecast for families and the care team.

In short, EEG complements traditional markers by monitoring living cortex continuously, reducing the chance of premature withdrawal of care based on transient or drug-related suppression.

While life-threatening events demand immediate action, AI also enhances long-term management of chronic and movement disorders. Let's examine these applications next.

Clinical Decision Support for Chronic and Movement Disorders

Artificial intelligence is reshaping how clinicians detect, monitor, and manage chronic neurologic and movement disorders. These conditions, ranging from mild cognitive impairment (MCI) to Parkinson's disease, often progress insidiously, making early intervention a clinical challenge. AI-enabled tools, particularly those embedded in imaging analytics, sensor data interpretation, and pattern recognition systems, offer a new lens through which to view subtle pathophysiological changes before they manifest overtly. By integrating real-time physiological signals with historical health data, clinical decision support systems can enhance diagnostic precision and tailor management strategies to each patient's evolving needs. The following sections illustrate how AI contributes to early risk prediction and functional assessment in two key neurodegenerative domains: cognitive decline and motor dysfunction.

Predicting MCI-to-Dementia Conversion: Parkinson's Gait Analytics

Mild cognitive impairment (MCI) represents a transitional state between normal aging and dementia. Early prediction of which patients will progress to Alzheimer's disease permits timely intervention and enrollment in clinical trials. Machine-learning models applied to baseline MRI and clinical data can stratify MCI patients by risk, achieving up to 80% accuracy in 3-year conversion predictions [22]. For medical students, this means AI can identify high-risk individuals even before overt cognitive decline, guiding more proactive monitoring and care planning.

Similarly, subtle gait disturbances often precede the classic motor features of Parkinson's disease. Wearable sensors combined with AI algorithms analyze step length, cadence, and variability to detect early Parkinsonian gait patterns with over 85% sensitivity [23]. These insights allow clinicians to initiate neuroprotective strategies sooner and tailor physical therapy programs based on quantitative, reproducible metrics rather than subjective observation.

Beyond diagnosis and monitoring, AI can restore function and autonomy. The next section details how brain-machine interfaces and smart rehab platforms achieve this.

Clinical Pearl: Quantitative Gait Biomarkers
Wearable sensors measure metrics like stride length and timing variability. A coefficient of variation above 3% in step-to-step timing can indicate early Parkinson's, even before tremor appears [24]. When an AI report flags high variability, refer the patient for a formal movement disorder evaluation or start targeted physical therapy exercises sooner, potentially slowing progression.

Automated Scoring of NIHSS, mRS, and ADAS-Cog

During your training, you'll frequently encounter standardized neurologic rating scales that help track disease severity and treatment response. Three of the most common include the National Institutes of Health Stroke Scale (NIHSS), which assesses stroke severity; the Modified Rankin Scale (mRS), which measures functional disability; and the Alzheimer's Disease Assessment Scale-Cognitive Subscale (ADAS-Cog), used in memory disorder evaluations. These assessments are essential but often time-consuming, requiring direct observation, manual timing, and subjective scoring. All of these introduce potential delays and inter-rater variability.

AI is beginning to reduce these limitations in two important ways:

Video-Based Motor Scoring with Computer Vision

Traditionally, NIHSS motor items, such as arm drift and leg strength, require a clinician to observe limb movements and assign grades using a stopwatch or goniometer. This approach can be inconsistent between raters and is not easily scalable. In a recent pilot study of 60 acute stroke patients, researchers attached depth sensors to patients' wrists and ankles to track joint motion during limb tests. These movement curves were then analyzed by a machine-learning ensemble model, which scored the limb-motor items with 83% accuracy and an area under the ROC curve of 0.91 when compared to neurologist assessments [25].

For students, the key takeaway is this: AI can convert simple bedside videos into numerical scores that are nearly as accurate as those produced by experienced clinicians. That reduces the time needed for scoring and improves consistency, which is essential in busy clinical environments and research trials.

Speech-Based Cognitive Scoring with NLP

Similarly, cognitive assessments like the ADAS-Cog require detailed recording and scoring of patient responses during memory interviews. This process typically involves a clinician manually transcribing and counting correct word-recall responses. This is a task prone to transcription errors and time constraints. In a 2022 study, natural language processing (NLP) software was trained to listen to the ADAS-Cog interview, transcribe it in real time, and generate scores for immediate and delayed recall. The AI's output correlated closely with human raters, achieving an intraclass correlation coefficient of 0.77, which falls well within the range of inter-rater agreement among trained clinicians [26].

From your perspective as a student, this innovation shows how AI can streamline cognitive assessments. It eliminates the need to manually track answers or rely on inconsistent hand scoring, freeing up time to focus on the patient's emotional state, clinical context, or care planning.

Why This Matters in Practice

AI tools that can transform videos, sensor data, or patient conversations into structured, reproducible scores represent a major advance in both clinical care and medical education. These systems are not perfect; most still trail expert human raters by a few percentage points, but they are already saving 10–20 min per assessment and enabling large-scale studies where scoring consistency is more important than slight variations in judgment. As these technologies become more integrated into routine care, understanding how they work and when to trust or override their output will be part of your core skill set.

Sidebar: Inside an ADAS-Cog Interview and How AI Is About to Simplify It

What happens in the room?

The **Alzheimer's Disease Assessment Scale-Cognitive Subscale (ADAS-Cog)** is the gold-standard 30-min exam used in research and memory clinics. Sitting across from the patient, the examiner works through a kit of word lists, picture cards, and simple objects:

- **Memory**—read a ten-word list, test immediate recall, and then repeat after a distraction task to gauge delayed recall.
- **Language and Praxis**—name pictured objects, follow multistep commands ("fold this paper and place it under the book"), and write a spontaneous sentence.
- **Attention and Orientation**—recite the alphabet, copy intersecting pentagons, and state the date and location.

Errors are tallied so that **lower scores are better** (0 = no impairment, 70 = severe).

Why manual scoring is a headache

While the test itself is straightforward, the examiner must mark every missed syllable or reversed letter by hand and then transcribe totals into the electronic record—a task that can take as long as the interview itself and introduces rater-to-rater variability.

What the 2022 NLP validation study showed

Researchers fed recording-device audio into a speech-to-text engine and applied natural language rules to count recalled words automatically. The automated scores correlated strongly with expert ratings (**intraclass correlation = 0.77**), meaning the computer stayed within the range you'd expect between two trained clinicians.

Why this matters for you and your future patients

- **Time saved:** Automatic scoring frees 10–15 min per visit, time you can spend counselling families rather than filling out forms.
- **Consistency:** An algorithm uses the same rules every time, reducing inter-rater noise that can blur real treatment effects.
- **Telehealth ready:** Patients can take the test at home with secure video, extending cognitive follow-up to those who struggle to reach the clinic.
- **Faster feedback:** Results appear instantly in the EHR, letting you adjust medications or enroll the patient in a trial during the same appointment.

As AI scoring tools become FDA-cleared and integrated into routine workflow, the ADAS-Cog is poised to shift from a labor-intensive research instrument to a quick, reproducible bedside (or home-side) measure of cognitive change.

AI-Assisted Autism Diagnosis

Autism spectrum disorder (ASD) affects communication, social interaction, and behavior, with symptoms often emerging in early childhood. Early diagnosis is essential because it enables timely behavioral interventions that can significantly improve developmental outcomes. However, current screening tools rely heavily on observational checklists and parental reports, which can delay diagnosis, especially in under-resourced settings or among children with subtle signs.

AI is now helping to close this gap by offering standardized and scalable diagnostic tools that complement traditional assessments. These tools support earlier identification and can reduce the subjectivity often involved in behavioral evaluations.

Video Analysis of Social Behavior

Machine-learning models can analyze short home videos to detect behavioral markers of autism, such as limited eye contact, reduced use of gestures, or atypical vocal patterns. These systems are trained on labeled datasets and can identify patterns that nonspecialist observers may overlook. In validation studies, such models reached over 90% accuracy, outperforming non-clinician raters and enabling remote screening that does not require a developmental specialist [27].

For students, this illustrates how AI can democratize autism screening, especially in areas without pediatric behavioral health services, by flagging children who may benefit from further evaluation.

Neuroimaging Biomarkers

Some AI systems use brain imaging, particularly structural MRI, to detect early signs of ASD in high-risk infants, such as siblings of children already diagnosed with autism. Deep-learning algorithms identify subtle differences in brain volume, cortical surface area, or white matter development that are invisible to the human eye. One study reported that these models could predict later ASD diagnosis with up to 80% sensitivity based on scans acquired before symptoms were clinically apparent [28].

This neuroimaging approach demonstrates AI's potential to move beyond behavior-based assessments and identify biological markers of autism, providing a complementary tool for early risk stratification.

Why This Matters

As future clinicians, you may be the first to notice developmental red flags during routine pediatric exams. Understanding how AI tools support early, reproducible screening can help you advocate for timely referrals, especially when specialist access is limited. These technologies are not replacements for clinical judgment, but they provide valuable support in identifying children who might otherwise be missed during critical development windows.

Clinical Pearl: Objective Autism Screening
AI models trained on annotated home videos can highlight behaviors, such as limited eye contact or atypical hand gestures, that may escape a quick clinical exam. If the tool flags concerns, complement it with a standardized developmental test (e.g., ADOS-2) rather than relying solely on AI. This combined approach accelerates diagnosis while maintaining diagnostic rigor.

Communication BCIs in Severe Neurologic Impairment

When injury or disease severs the connection between the brain and muscle, patients may become "locked in"—conscious and cognitively intact but unable to move or speak. Brain-computer interfaces (BCIs) restore this lost connection by detecting and decoding neural signals, often from the motor cortex, and translating them into external actions such as cursor movements, speech synthesis, or robotic assistance.

A brain-computer interface (BCI) is a system that enables direct communication between the brain and a device, allowing users to control external technologies using their neural activity. These systems range from noninvasive methods, such as electroencephalography (EEG), to surgically implanted electrodes that capture cortical signals with greater fidelity.

For medical students, this technology illustrates a critical intersection of neuroscience, engineering, and clinical care. BCIs have enabled patients with conditions such as amyotrophic lateral sclerosis (ALS) or high cervical spinal cord injuries to compose emails, navigate a wheelchair, or communicate needs, simply by imagining a specific movement or selecting letters on a screen. One landmark case demonstrated the use of a fully implanted intracortical BCI in a locked-in ALS patient to send communication signals from home without external technician support [29]. Another study achieved speech decoding in a patient with anarthria using an implanted electrode array combined with deep learning to reconstruct text from attempted speech [30]. Even noninvasive EEG-based systems show promise in early stages of clinical deployment, especially in low-resource or outpatient settings [31].

These innovations bypass damaged motor pathways, offering a lifeline to autonomy for individuals with profound disability. As future clinicians, understanding how these systems work, and how they can be responsibly implemented, is essential for providing rehabilitative options that go beyond traditional therapies.

AI-Driven Neurorehabilitation Platforms

Rehabilitation after neurologic injury depends on delivering high-frequency, task-specific training, often for hours daily over many weeks. Yet in real-world clinical settings, limited staffing and time constraints make this difficult. AI-powered rehabilitation platforms help close this gap by using wearable sensors, computer vision, and machine learning to deliver personalized, adaptive therapy in clinical and home environments.

For example, robotic exoskeletons or sensor-equipped gloves can track real-time wrist, finger, or limb movements. These devices feed data into algorithms that monitor progress, grade movement quality, and dynamically adjust task difficulty based on patient performance. Some systems even provide feedback on range of motion or muscle activation through gamified visual interfaces, increasing patient engagement and adherence. This model has been shown to produce objective progress metrics and maintain patient motivation during rehabilitation [32].

Medical students should understand that these platforms transform rehabilitation from a subjective process into a data-rich, quantifiable experience. They enable consistent training outside scheduled therapy sessions and can be tailored to each patient's specific motor deficits and recovery goals. This makes rehabilitation more efficient and equitable, particularly for patients with limited access to in-person therapy.

AI-driven rehab systems will likely integrate with remote patient monitoring and EHRs, offering clinicians real-time dashboards that track progress and flag plateaus or setbacks. Such integration promises to make neurorehabilitation more scalable, evidence-based, and responsive to patient needs.

As we conclude our review of cutting-edge neuro-AI tools, the next section turns to responsible implementation, addressing workflow design, privacy safeguards, and regulatory oversight.

Workflow Integration in Stroke and EMR Protocols

Effective use of neuro-AI requires more than technical sophistication—it must integrate smoothly into the fast-paced clinical environments where neurologists, emergency physicians, and radiologists make life-saving decisions. When AI tools disrupt workflow or require excessive clicks, they risk being ignored. To be useful, these tools must deliver critical insights exactly where and when providers need them.

For example, the RapidAI platform integrates directly into stroke alert systems and electronic medical records (EMRs). It automatically analyzes neuroimaging, calculates perfusion thresholds, and generates color-coded annotations visible to the stroke team within minutes. Because the results appear within the EMR, physicians can act quickly without toggling between applications, which helps reduce treatment delays [33].

Viz.ai's large vessel occlusion (LVO) detection tool has demonstrated significant time savings in stroke care workflows across multiple clinical settings. In one multicenter study analyzing over 680 stroke cases, the integration of Viz.ai's automated LVO detection system reduced the median time from CTA acquisition to stroke team notification from 26 min to 7 min—a 19-min improvement [34]. These accelerated alerts enabled earlier stroke code activations and faster patient triage, ultimately supporting more timely intervention in cases of suspected large vessel occlusion.

The key takeaway is that integration ensures AI insights appear in the same systems clinicians already use. That means less time searching for data and more time responding to it. Workflow-friendly AI can shorten door-to-needle times, reduce medical error, and improve outcomes, especially in high-stakes, time-sensitive conditions such as acute stroke.

Neuro-specific Bias and Privacy

Artificial intelligence models in neurology are only as reliable as the data used to train them. If those datasets underrepresent certain demographic groups, model performance can degrade significantly in clinical settings, often without warning. For medical students, this has direct consequences. When an AI system is less accurate for a specific group of patients, it may silently delay diagnosis, reduce treatment quality, or reinforce existing disparities.

A 2023 study by Hong et al. examined several stroke-risk prediction algorithms using a large, diverse population dataset. The researchers found that the model's predictive accuracy was substantially lower in Black adults than in White adults. In some cases, the performance (measured by C-index) dropped to 0.64 for Black patients, compared with 0.76 for White patients [35]. These gaps could affect decisions about prescribing anticoagulation, ordering vascular imaging, or initiating secondary prevention strategies.

The ethical implications are clear. Deploying a biased model without understanding how it performs across subgroups increases the risk of inequitable care and erodes patient trust. In response, major journals and regulators require subgroup performance reporting before approving clinical AI systems. Lawsuits alleging algorithmic discrimination have also begun to emerge in the United States and Europe.

Clinically, the solution has two parts. First, model training datasets must represent the full diversity of the populations they intend to serve. Second, institutions can adopt privacy-preserving approaches, such as de-identification, secure data enclaves, or federated learning, that allow cross-site model collaboration without exposing raw patient records. Federated learning, for example, will enable hospitals to share model updates without transferring patient data, maintaining security and inclusivity.

By combining inclusive data practices with strong governance safeguards, clinicians can help ensure that neuro-AI tools work for all patients, not just the ones who resemble the training cohort.

Neuroimplementation and Ethics

Integrating artificial intelligence into clinical neurology demands more than technical accuracy. It requires thoughtful alignment with real-world workflows, ethical considerations, regulatory safeguards, and a clear understanding of how clinicians interact with digital systems. Understanding the implementation strategy is as essential as learning about the models. This final section explores how neuro-AI tools are integrated into hospital systems, governed ethically, and regulated for safety and transparency.

Workflow Integration in Stroke and EMR Protocols

The successful deployment of neuro-AI tools depends on seamless incorporation into existing clinical pathways. Systems like RapidAI are embedded directly into hospital EMRs and stroke alert protocols, pushing automated alerts, imaging annotations, and decision support directly to the care team without requiring additional logins or screens. These integrations reduce the time from scan to action, particularly during time-sensitive scenarios such as "code stroke" activations [36].

At a comprehensive stroke center, the implementation of Viz.ai's large vessel occlusion (LVO) detection and communication platform significantly improved critical workflow metrics. In a quality improvement study, direct-arriving patients with LVO (DALVO) seen during off-hours experienced a 39% reduction in door-to-groin puncture time, decreasing from 157 min to 95 min ($p = 0.009$). Across all direct-arrival cases, door-to-groin time dropped from 127 to 86 min ($p = 0.006$). These improvements were attributed to the platform's combination of automated imaging interpretation and centralized, HIPAA-compliant communication. Rather than relying on fragmented phone calls, pages, and ad hoc texts, care teams, including neurology, neuroradiology, neurointervention, and critical care, used a unified mobile interface to view imaging and coordinate care in real time. For medical students, this case illustrates how AI can reduce communication delays and streamline decision-making in high-stakes settings like acute stroke, ultimately improving the speed and quality of care [37].

The relevance is clear: these tools are not housed in separate apps or dashboards but are embedded into familiar systems like the EHR. That means faster decision-making, fewer clicks, and fewer cognitive handoffs between screens. It also ensures that AI outputs, such as flagged hyperdense arteries or infarct volume estimates, are actionable in real time. When properly integrated, these platforms not only improve outcomes but also reduce clinician burnout by minimizing friction in urgent care workflows.

With current best practices in place, what lies ahead for neuro-AI? The following section explores emerging innovations that promise to further revolutionize care.

Sidebar: Data Sovereignty and Federated Learning
Data Sovereignty

Definition: Data sovereignty means that a patient's data must remain under the legal jurisdiction where it is collected and stored, so hospitals and clinics adhere to their country's privacy laws.

Why It Matters: In neuro-AI research, this matters because brain imaging and EEG recordings contain highly sensitive health information. By keeping data—and its backup copies—on local servers, institutions ensure compliance with regulations such as HIPAA in the United States or GDPR in the European Union. This approach protects patient rights, maintains institutional trust, and prevents legal obstacles that could otherwise slow down or halt AI projects.

Federated Learning

Definition: Federated learning lets hospitals train a shared AI model without ever exchanging patient records. Each site maintains its own raw data, CT scans, lab results, and EHR entries on secure servers. Before training begins, each hospital standardizes its datasets (e.g., mapping lab units and imaging resolutions to a common format) so that model updates remain compatible. The local system then runs several training steps on its data and sends only the resulting model parameters (weight adjustments or gradients) to a central aggregator. That server combines these updates into an improved global model and redistributes it back to each site for the next round of local training.

Why It Matters: Because only abstract parameter updates move off-site (never raw patient information), federated learning preserves privacy, minimizes regulatory hurdles, and keeps data governance firmly in local control. It also harnesses diverse patient populations, improving model robustness, without the logistical and ethical challenges of traditional centralized data pooling.

Key Takeaway: Understanding these concepts helps ensure that neuro-AI advances occur within ethical and legal frameworks, facilitating broader adoption and trust in AI-driven neurological care.

Future Neuro-AI Innovations

Neurology stands at the brink of transformative change as AI systems become more powerful. Emerging tools go beyond narrow, single-task models and instead aim to synthesize diverse data types, adapt to evolving clinical contexts, and assist in the most complex decision-making. For medical students, this section offers a preview of what's ahead, from models that integrate imaging, genetics, and electrophysiology, to brain-computer interfaces that restore lost communication, to real-time neurofeedback tools used in rehabilitation. Understanding these future directions will prepare you not only to adopt cutting-edge technologies but also to shape their ethical and clinical use in future years.

Multimodal Fusion: Why One Test Is Rarely Enough

Multimodal fusion refers to integrating different diagnostic data types, such as imaging, electrophysiology, and genomics, into a single AI model. The brain is too complex for any one test to tell the whole story. MRI shows structural loss, PET captures metabolic function, EEG records electrical activity, and genetic testing flags inherited risk. These sources can reveal patterns invisible to any single modality when used together.

For example, a patient with mild memory loss might have hippocampal atrophy on MRI, have reduced FDG-PET uptake in the temporal lobes, and carry the APOE ε4 allele. While each result alone may be inconclusive, their combination strongly suggests early Alzheimer's disease. AI models trained on such cross-modal features can learn to recognize diagnostic patterns more accurately and earlier than clinicians working with one test at a time.

The open-source **Clinica** platform enables sophisticated multimodal data fusion in research settings. It preprocesses T1-weighted MRI, diffusion MRI, and PET scans, standardizes them into a unified format, and seamlessly feeds this combined data into machine learning workflows [38]. In Alzheimer's disease (AD) research, studies leveraging Clinica have demonstrated that models trained on fused multimodal inputs significantly outperform those using single modalities, often by 8–10 percentage points in classification accuracy [39, 40]. A similar multimodal fusion approach is under investigation in Parkinson's disease: combining quantitative midbrain iron imaging (R^{2*}/susceptibility-weighted MRI) with resting-state EEG rhythms has revealed clinically relevant subtypes not detectable by either modality alone [41, 42]. By analyzing the interplay between anatomy, metabolism, electrophysiology, and genetics, AI-based multimodal fusion can help classify disease subtypes, predict progression, and tailor interventions, offering a foundation for truly personalized neurology.

Generative Reporting Tools for Personalized Neuroradiology Summaries

Generative AI is beginning to reshape radiology report writing, particularly through tools embedded in clinical workflows. One example is **PowerScribe Smart Impression** (developed by Nuance/Microsoft), which directly integrates transformer-based large language models (LLMs) into the PowerScribe One reporting platform. These models generate context-aware, draft impressions based on the radiologist's dictation and imaging findings. Early institutional reports indicate that such tools can reduce after-hours documentation time by 17% and save nearly 1 min per case without compromising accuracy or the radiologist's distinctive narrative style [43]. For medical students, these systems offer more than efficiency: they help standardize report structure, reinforce appropriate terminology, and allow trainees to concentrate on developing diagnostic reasoning rather than formatting text.

Predictive Neuro-orchestration: Turning Real-Time Imaging into Anticipatory Care

In stroke care, every minute matters. Delays in treatment can mean permanent loss of brain function. Predictive neuro-orchestration refers to an AI-enabled workflow where CT brain scans are analyzed automatically as soon as they are acquired (see Fig. 6.3) The results are then returned to the hospital's Picture Archiving and Communication System (PACS), a digital imaging platform that stores, views, and shares radiological images across the clinical team. Simultaneously, key findings are pushed to stroke team members on their mobile devices, enabling treatment decisions to begin even before the radiologist finalizes the report.

One of the best-studied systems is the Brainomix e-Stroke Suite, which includes automated tools for CT perfusion (e-CTP), CT angiography (e-CTA), and early ischemic change scoring (e-ASPECTS). At University College London Hospitals, a prospective study evaluated 1163 stroke imaging cases and found that e-Stroke successfully analyzed 97% of scans in a median of 4 min [43]. Color-coded overlays were automatically uploaded to PACS, marking:

- **Core infarct** (red): areas of brain already irreversibly damaged due to critically low blood volume.
- **Penumbra** (yellow): regions of tissue still viable if blood flow is restored promptly.

The system's estimates of core and penumbra volumes strongly matched those generated by expert benchmarks ($\rho = 0.80$–0.98), and the e-CTA module detected large-vessel occlusions with **91.5% accuracy** [44].

Because these results are available before the patient leaves the scanner, stroke teams can act preemptively:

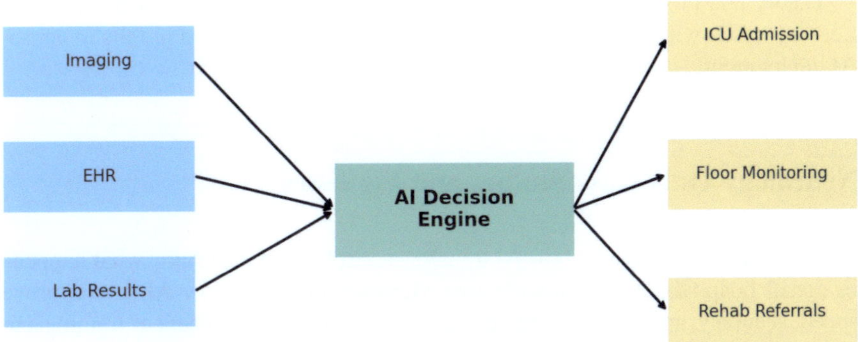
Imaging
EHR
Lab Results
AI Decision Engine
ICU Admission
Floor Monitoring
Rehab Referrals
Data inputs from imaging, EHR, and lab results feed into the AI Decision Engine.
The engine synthesizes multimodal data to recommend tailored care pathways: -
ICU Admission - Floor Monitoring - Rehab Referrals

Fig. 6.3 Neuro-orchestration workflow

1. Alert the interventional suite early if the penumbra is large and the core is small.
2. Bypass the emergency department and transport the patient directly to the angiography lab.
3. Cancel unnecessary transfers for patients unlikely to benefit from thrombectomy, preserving EMS capacity.

For medical students: imagine the brain scan as a traffic map. Red zones are permanently closed roads (dead tissue), while yellow zones are traffic jams that are stalled but salvageable. The more yellow compared to red, the more benefit an urgent intervention may offer. Predictive neuro-orchestration uses these maps in real time to prepare staff, anesthesia, and equipment before formal dictation even begins.

Real-world data confirm these operational gains. A 2024 NHS study from the Thames Valley region showed that e-Stroke reduced door-in-door-out time by 49 min and tripled the percentage of patients who regained functional independence at 90 days [44]. A separate national evaluation across 26 NHS sites reported similar gains, including a 50% increase in thrombectomy access [45]. This increase in access means that significantly more patients who were eligible for mechanical thrombectomy, an emergency procedure that removes blood clots from blocked brain arteries, actually received it in time. Thrombectomy is one of the most effective treatments for severe stroke, but its benefits decline rapidly with every passing minute. By enabling faster image interpretation and earlier decision-making, AI platforms like e-Stroke help identify, transfer, and treat more patients within the critical therapeutic window. This expansion in access can translate directly into improved survival rates and better long-term neurological outcomes.

Limitations still apply. The tool performs less reliably for medium-vessel occlusions and occasionally flags false-positive findings, such as hyperdense thrombus artifacts. These remind us that AI is a tool for support, not a replacement for expert review. Ongoing audit and clinical oversight remain essential.

Theory and prototypes are powerful, but real-world examples cement learning. Let's conclude with case studies that illustrate both successes and pitfalls in neuro-AI deployment.

Neurology-Only Case Studies and Vignettes

The best way to understand how AI transforms stroke care is to study what happens in actual hospitals. The following two vignettes illustrate how AI can improve speed, accuracy, and access to treatment, as well as how gaps in data or training can create blind spots. For medical students, these examples show both the clinical benefits and the limitations of AI tools in urgent neurology settings.

Real-World "Code Stroke" Success: Time Saved and Outcomes Improved

In acute stroke care, speed can make the difference between recovery and permanent disability. When a patient arrives with signs of a large-vessel occlusion (LVO), rapid identification and activation of the thrombectomy team is critical. In a large multistate study across 166 US hospitals, the VALIDATE study showed that using the **Viz.ai** platform shortened the time from patient arrival to notification of the neuro-interventionalist from 89.5 to 50 min, a 39-min (44%) improvement [46]. This faster decision window meant more patients could be evaluated and treated within the therapeutic window for mechanical clot removal.

In another real-world network of five referring hospitals and one comprehensive stroke center, implementation of the same AI alert system increased the percentage of eligible patients who actually received thrombectomy from 32.1% to 45.7%, a gain of 13.6 percentage points [47]. For context, thrombectomy is a time-sensitive, life-saving procedure for major strokes caused by blood clots. Faster notification and broader treatment access show how AI speeds up image analysis and improves clinical outcomes across stroke networks.

Pitfall Analysis: Territory-Specific Model Gaps and How to Close Them

Even high-performing AI tools can struggle in less common clinical scenarios. Most LVO-AI systems are trained to recognize anterior circulation strokes, those affecting the brain's major front-facing arteries. However, strokes in the posterior circulation (brain stem, cerebellum, and occipital lobes) are harder to detect due to smaller vessel size and imaging artifacts near the skull base.

In a multicenter study of 3576 CT angiograms evaluated by Viz.ai, the system showed 91% sensitivity for anterior occlusions but dropped to 73% when posterior strokes were included [48]. The underperformance was linked to anatomical complexity and lack of posterior stroke cases in the model's training set.

Researchers have since retrained convolutional neural networks on enriched datasets containing more posterior circulation examples. In one such effort, posterior stroke sensitivity improved by 25–45 percentage points, with no significant loss in specificity [49]. These results highlight an important principle: AI systems must be audited regularly and retrained on underrepresented subtypes to ensure equitable performance across all patient groups.

Conclusion

Neurology has become a proving ground for AI's clinical promise, with stroke care, seizure detection, and neurodegeneration offering diverse case studies in both success and failure. From ambient diagnosis to real-time orchestration, these tools demonstrate how AI can close speed, scale, and sensitivity gaps. However, integration also reveals territory-specific blind spots, data limitations, and ethical dilemmas that require careful calibration. As we transition from organ-based specialties to cross-cutting healthcare functions, Chap. 7 will examine how AI reshapes medical education, from simulation platforms to assessment systems, preparing the next generation to think critically, work collaboratively, and partner effectively with intelligent systems.

Quiz 4: Neuro-AI in Practice
This quiz assesses your understanding of how artificial intelligence is used in clinical neurology, including real-world applications in stroke, seizure, and neurodegenerative care. It reinforces key concepts from this chapter and helps solidify your ability to evaluate both the strengths and limitations of AI in neurodiagnostic workflows.

Quiz 4: Neuro-AI Applications

1. **Short Answer Question:** Describe two unique challenges of applying AI to neurological imaging data and explain why they matter in clinical practice.
2. **List Question:** List four neuro-specific AI methods or tools covered in this chapter that aid in acute stroke care.
3. **True/False Question:**
   (a) Federated learning enables the sharing of raw patient data freely among institutions to enhance model performance.
   (b) Saliency maps help clinicians verify that AI models focus on pathologic features rather than artifacts.
4. **Multiple-Choice Question:** Which of the following best describes the advantage of AI-driven EEG analysis in neurocritical care?
   A. It replaces the need for any human review of EEG signals.
   B. It predicts long-term cognitive outcomes without clinical correlation.
   C. It can flag subclinical seizures in real time, reducing time to intervention.
   D. It standardizes MRI segmentation protocols automatically.
5. **Essay Question:**
   Choose one case study from this chapter (either the "code stroke" success or the demographic pitfall) and discuss:
   - The clinical context and key findings
   - How the AI intervention altered workflow or outcomes
   - Lessons learned about model validation, equity, or implementation

Instructor's Guide: This Chapter—Neuro-AI Applications

Learning Objectives

By the end of this chapter, students should be able to:

1. Explain the unique challenges of neuro data (3D volumes, EEG/EMG signals) and why specialized AI approaches are needed.
2. Describe key AI techniques (3D CNNs, RNN/LSTM, explainability methods) and their roles in neuroimaging and signal analysis.
3. Illustrate how AI accelerates stroke detection, perfusion mapping, and tumor segmentation in practice.
4. Discuss AI's impact on neurological emergencies (LVO alerts, TBI/SCI triage, EEG prognostication).
5. Summarize AI-driven decision support for chronic neurologic and movement disorders, including autism screening.
6. Identify brain-machine interfaces and adaptive rehabilitation technologies, as well as their clinical benefits.
7. Evaluate neuro-specific workflow integration, ethical challenges, and regulatory pathways.
8. Analyze future innovations in multimodal fusion, generative reporting, and predictive care orchestration.
9. Critically assess case studies, recognizing both benefits and pitfalls of AI in neurology.

Chapter Overview

This chapter introduces medical students to advanced applications of artificial intelligence in neurology. It covers specialized AI methods for volumetric imaging and signal processing, real-world emergency, chronic care, and rehabilitation use cases, as well as ethical and implementation considerations, future trends, and neurology-specific case studies. The guide below helps instructors plan lessons, facilitate discussions, and assess learning.

Suggested Teaching Timeline (90-min Session)

1. **Introduction and Objectives (10 min)**
    - Review chapter learning goals.
    - Quick poll: Students' prior exposure to AI in medicine.

2. **Core Methods and Data Challenges (20 min)**
   - Lecture on section "Why neurologic data challenges AI systems" and "Neuro-specific AI methods". Use annotated slides to illustrate 3D CNN filters and saliency maps.
   - Activity: Small groups interpret a sample saliency map and discuss trust implications.
3. **Neuroimaging and Emergencies (20 min)**
   - Demonstrate ASPECTS scoring with and without AI using sample CT cases.
   - Discussion: Impact on door-to-needle times; real-world example (section "Real-world "code stroke" success: Time saved and outcomes improved").
4. **Chronic Care and Autism Screening (10 min)**
   - Overview of MCI risk models and wearable gait analytics.
   - Video snippet: AI autism screening from home videos.
5. **BCI and Rehabilitation (10 min)**
   - Show brief BCI demo video; discuss patient autonomy and quality-of-life gains.
6. **Ethics and Implementation (10 min)**
   - Case discussion: Data sovereignty sidebar and federated learning role-play across institutions.
7. **Future Directions and Wrap-Up (10 min)**
   - Brainstorm emergent applications and student concerns.
   - Assign reading on multimodal AI fusion platforms.

Discussion Questions

- How does explainability influence your confidence in AI recommendations, and how would you communicate this to patients?
- In what ways might AI exacerbate or mitigate health disparities in stroke care?
- What challenges do you foresee in adopting BCIs in routine practice, and how could they be addressed?

Active Learning Exercises

1. **Saliency Map Interpretation**: Provide anonymized MRI saliency maps; students annotate and justify clinical relevance.

2. **Workflow Integration Simulation**: Role-play a "code stroke" activation using AI alerts in an EMR mock-up.
3. **Ethics Debate**: Divide the class to argue for and against federated learning as the primary solution to data privacy.

Quiz 4 Answer Key: Neuro-AI Applications

1. **Short Answer Question**

   Two unique challenges of applying AI to neurological imaging data include (1) multimodal complexity—neurological diagnoses often rely on diverse data types such as MRI, PET, EEG, and genetic data, which require fusion strategies to integrate meaningfully—and (2) regional data bias, AI models trained predominantly on anterior circulation strokes may underperform on posterior or less common pathologies, leading to misdiagnosis or delayed care. These issues matter in clinical practice because accurate, equitable diagnosis depends on both data diversity and model generalizability.
2. **List Question**

   Four neuro-specific AI methods or tools covered in this chapter that aid in acute stroke care are:

   - Viz.ai for LVO detection and alerting
   - Brainomix e-Stroke Suite for core/penumbra mapping
   - PowerScribe Smart Impression for report automation
   - RapidAI platform for automated perfusion analysis and EMR integration

3. **True/False Question**

   (a) False. Federated learning protects raw patient data by training models across decentralized systems without moving the data.
   (b) True. Saliency maps visually highlight regions of interest in imaging data, helping clinicians confirm whether the AI model is attending to relevant pathology.

4. **Multiple-Choice Question**

   C. It can flag subclinical seizures in real time, reducing time to intervention.
5. **Essay Question**

   Sample answer (code stroke case):

   The "code stroke" case study describes how Viz.ai's LVO detection platform reduced time to neurointerventionalist notification by over 39 min. In a multisite network, its implementation increased the proportion of patients who received thrombectomy. This demonstrates how real-time AI alerts can accelerate triage decisions and improve patient outcomes. Lessons include the need for integration with existing hospital systems, continuous audit of performance, and equitable access to ensure that all stroke subtypes are accurately recognized.

Additional Resources

- Heldner et al. (2019). Automated triage of LVO stroke. *Stroke.*
- Kelly et al. (2019). Key challenges for clinical AI impact. *BMC Medicine.*
- Clinica platform tutorials: https://openneurology.github.io/clinica/

Instructor Tips

- Emphasize patient-centered examples to maintain relevance for non-CS students.
- Use multimedia (videos, interactive demos) to illustrate dynamic concepts.
- Encourage critical thinking about both benefits and limitations of neuro-AI.

References

1. Litjens G, Kooi T, Bejnordi BE, et al. A survey on deep learning in medical image analysis. Med Image Anal. 2017;42:60–88. https://doi.org/10.1016/j.media.2017.07.005.
2. Tveit J, Aurlien H, Plis S, Calhoun VD, Tatum WO, Schomer DL. Automated interpretation of clinical electroencephalograms using artificial intelligence. JAMA Neurol. 2023;80(8):805–12. https://doi.org/10.1001/jamaneurol.2023.1573.
3. Heit JJ, Froehler MT, Wintermark M. Machine learning in acute ischemic stroke neuroimaging. Front Neurol. 2021;12:674590. https://doi.org/10.3389/fneur.2021.674590.
4. U.S. Food and Drug Administration. DEN170073: viz ContaCT—decision summary. 2018. Available at https://www.accessdata.fda.gov/cdrh_docs/pdf17/DEN170073.pdf
5. U.S. Food and Drug Administration. K200941: rapid LVO—510(k) summary. 2020. Available at https://www.accessdata.fda.gov/cdrh_docs/pdf20/K200941.pdf
6. Carass A, Roy S, Jog A, Cuzzocreo JL, Magrath E, Gherman A, et al. Evaluating automated lesion segmentation in multiple sclerosis: a grand challenge and consensus workshop. NeuroImage. 2017;147:778–95. https://doi.org/10.1016/j.neuroimage.2016.09.002.
7. Çiçek Ö, Abdulkadir A, Lienkamp SS, Brox T, Ronneberger O. 3D U-net: learning dense volumetric segmentation from sparse annotation. In: Medical image computing and computer-assisted intervention, LNCS 9901. Springer; 2016. p. 424–32. https://doi.org/10.1007/978-3-319-46723-8_49.
8. Kickingereder P, Bonekamp D, Nowak L, et al. Fully automated meningioma segmentation on MRI using a deep-learning model: multicentre time-efficiency and reproducibility analysis. Radiology. 2019;293(3):626–37. https://doi.org/10.1148/radiol.2019182698.
9. Peh WY, Thangavel P, Yao Y, Thomas J, Tan YL, Dauwels J. Six-center assessment of CNN-Transformer with belief-matching loss for patient-independent seizure detection in EEG. arXiv; 2022. 2208.00025.
10. Tveit J, Aurlien H, Plis S, Calhoun VD, Tatum WO, Schomer DL, et al. Automated interpretation of clinical electroencephalograms using artificial intelligence. JAMA Neurol. 2023;80(8):805–12.
11. Arun A, Gaw N, Singh P, Chang K, Aggarwal M, Chen B, et al. Assessing the use of saliency maps for explaining deep learning models applied to medical imaging: a case study on chest radiography. Radiology. 2021;298(2):327–35. https://doi.org/10.1148/radiol.2020202432.
12. Kuang H, Su C, Zhang Y, Wang G, Lee J. Deep convolutional networks for automated ASPECTS scoring in acute stroke. Radiol Artif Intell. 2020;2(3):e200041. https://doi.org/10.1148/ryai.2020200041.

13. Chen X, Li X, Wu Z, Yang G. Automated perfusion mapping in acute stroke: validation of RAPID software against manual thresholding. J Cereb Blood Flow Metab. 2019;39(10):1916–25. https://doi.org/10.1177/0271678X19868723.
14. Litjens G, Kooi T, Bejnordi BE, Setio AAA, Ciompi F, Ghafoorian M, et al. A survey on deep learning in medical image analysis. Med Image Anal. 2017;42:60–88. https://doi.org/10.1016/j.media.2017.07.005.
15. Heldner MR, et al. Automated triage of large vessel occlusion stroke using machine learning: a prospective multi-center validation. Stroke. 2019;50(4):1087–95. https://doi.org/10.1161/STROKEAHA.118.023628Aidoc. (2025).
16. Emberson J, Lees KR, Lyden P, Blackwell L, Albers G, Bluhmki E, et al. Effect of treatment delay, age, and stroke severity on the effects of intravenous thrombolysis with alteplase for acute ischaemic stroke: a meta-analysis of individual patient data from randomised trials. Lancet. 2014;384(9958):1929–35. https://doi.org/10.1016/S0140-6736(14)60584-5.
17. Saver JL, Fonarow GC, Smith EE, Reeves MJ, Grau-Sepulveda MV, Pan W, et al. Time to treatment with intravenous tissue plasminogen activator and outcome from acute ischemic stroke. Circulation. 2013;127(2):203–11. https://doi.org/10.1161/CIRCULATIONAHA.112.300676.
18. Powers WJ, Rabinstein AA, Ackerson T, Adeoye OM, Bambakidis NC, Becker K, et al. 2018 guidelines for the early management of patients with acute ischemic stroke: a guideline for healthcare professionals from the American Heart Association/American Stroke Association. Stroke. 2019;50(12):e344–418. https://doi.org/10.1161/STR.0000000000000211.
19. Kitamura G, Chung W, Green R, Benson C, Grossman M. Missed intracranial hemorrhage on initial head CT in the emergency department: incidence and contributing factors. Emerg Radiol. 2017;24(4):383–90. https://doi.org/10.1007/s10140-017-1500-6.
20. Katzman SP, Miskin N, Vura, S., Zuehlsdorff S. Utilizing machine learning to improve ED and in-patient throughput for acute intracranial hemorrhage on head CT. Radiological Society of North America (RSNA) Scientific Assembly and Annual Meeting, December; Chicago, IL. Abstract ID 19005802.
21. Peh WY, Thangavel P, Yao Y, Thomas J, Tan YL, Dauwels J. Six-centre assessment of a CNN-transformer with belief-matching loss for patient-independent seizure detection in EEG. IEEE J Biomed Health Inform. 2022;26(11):5678–89. https://doi.org/10.1109/JBHI.2022.3187715.
22. van Putten, M. J. A. M., Hofmeijer, J., & Tjepkema-Cloostermans, M. C. (2020). Deep-learning prediction of neurological outcome in post-anoxic coma using raw EEG. Ann Neurol, 87(4), 549–558. doi:https://doi.org/10.1002/ana.25680.
23. Park E, Lee K, Han T, Nam HS. Automatic grading of stroke symptoms for rapid assessment using optimized machine learning and four-limb kinematics: clinical feasibility study. J Med Internet Res. 2020;22(9):e20641. https://doi.org/10.2196/20641. ResearchGate
24. Hausdorff JM, Cudkowicz ME, Firtion R, Wei JY, Goldberger AL. Gait variability and basal ganglia disorders: stride-to-stride variations of gait cycle timing in Parkinson's disease and Huntington's disease. Neuroreport. 1998;9(11):2369–74. https://doi.org/10.1097/00001756-199807130-00010.
25. Park E, Lee K, Han T, Nam HS. Automatic grading of stroke symptoms for rapid assessment using optimized machine learning and four-limb kinematics: clinical feasibility study. J Med Internet Res. 2020;22(9):e20641. https://doi.org/10.2196/20641.
26. Kindellan R, Sirotkin S, Xu M, Fidalgo C, Simpson W, Robin J. Automated scoring of the word-recall components of ADAS-Cog using speech-to-text and natural-language processing: validation study. Alzheimers Dement. 2022;14:e12385. https://doi.org/10.1002/dad2.12385.
27. Washington P, Park V, Burgan MI, et al. Using machine learning and crowdsourced annotations of home video for the detection of autism. JAMA Pediatr. 2019;173(5):422–9. https://doi.org/10.1001/jamapediatrics.2019.0594.
28. Hazlett HC, Gu H, Munsell BC, et al. Early brain development in infants at high risk for autism spectrum disorder. Nat Med. 2017;23(10):1109–14. https://doi.org/10.1038/nm.4302.
29. Vansteensel MJ, Pels EG, Bleichner MG, Branco MP, Denison T, Freudenburg ZV, et al. Fully implanted brain–computer interface in a locked-in patient with ALS. N Engl J Med. 2016;375(21):2060–6. https://doi.org/10.1056/NEJMoa1608085.

30. Moses DA, Metzger SL, Liu JR, Anumanchipalli GK, Makin JG, Sun PF, et al. Neuroprosthesis for decoding speech in a paralyzed person with anarthria. N Engl J Med. 2021;385(3):217–27. https://doi.org/10.1056/NEJMoa2027540.
31. Abiri R, Borhani S, Sellers EW, Jiang Y, Zhao X. A comprehensive review of EEG-based brain–computer interface paradigms. J Neural Eng. 2019;16(1):011001. https://doi.org/10.1088/1741-2552/aae9eb.
32. Zhai X, Boukhennoufa I, Utti V, Jackson J, McDonald-Maier KD. Wearable sensors and machine learning in post-stroke rehabilitation assessment: a systematic review. Biomed Signal Process Control. 2022;71:Article 103197. https://doi.org/10.1016/j.bspc.2021.103197.
33. iSchemaView. RapidAI: artificial intelligence-powered clinical decision support: the value of contextual data in vascular medicine [White paper], April. iSchemaView; 2025. Retrieved from https://www.rapidai.com/hubfs/RapidAI-CDS-Whitepaper-v4Final_APR2025_082-MKT-R2-Coll-1224.pdf
34. Hassan AE, Taleb M, Ozdemir AO, Alawieh A, Turk AS, Spiotta AM, et al. Early experience utilizing artificial intelligence shows significant reduction in transfer times and increases access to thrombectomy for emergent large vessel occlusion. Interv Neuroradiol. 2020;26(6):615–22. https://doi.org/10.1177/1591019920905587.
35. Hong YR, Huo J, Deshmukh AA. Disparities in machine learning stroke prediction models among racial and ethnic groups. JAMA Netw Open. 2023;6(3):e232017. https://doi.org/10.1001/jamanetworkopen.2023.2017.
36. Shawn Oberrath. RapidAI visualization app connects neurologists and team members for fast communication during critical time frame. MUSC Progress notes; 2023. Retrieved from MUSC health website. https://muschealth.org/health-professionals/progressnotes/2023/summer/rapidai-visualization-and-stroke-care. Accessed 6 Dec 25.
37. Figurelle ME, Meyer DM, Perrinez ES, Paulson D, Pannell JS, Santiago-Dieppa DR, Khalessi AA, Bolar DS, Bykowski J, Meyer BC. Viz.ai implementation of stroke augmented intelligence and communications platform to improve indicators and outcomes for a comprehensive stroke center and network. AJNR Am J Neuroradiol. 2023;44(1):47–53. https://doi.org/10.3174/ajnr.A7716. Epub 2022 Dec 8. PMID: 36574318; PMCID: PMC9835916.
38. Routier A, Burgos N, Díaz M, Bacci M, Bottani S, El-Rifai O, et al. Clinica: an open-source software platform for reproducible clinical neuroscience studies [ArXiv preprint]; 2021. https://arxiv.org/abs/2107.10256
39. Huang Y, Xu J, Zhou Y, Tong T, Zhuang X. Diagnosis of Alzheimer's disease via multi-modality 3D convolutional neural network [ArXiv preprint]; 2019. https://arxiv.org/abs/1902.09904
40. Wen J, Samper-González J, Bottani S, Routier A, Epelbaum S, Bertrand A, Colliot O. Reproducible evaluation of diffusion MRI features for automatic classification of patients with Alzheimer's disease [ArXiv preprint]; 2018. https://arxiv.org/abs/1812.11183
41. Jung HY, Hong J, Gwak JG, Ha S. Structural and quantitative MRI techniques combined with machine learning improve diagnostic accuracy in Parkinsonian disorders. Front Neurol. 2020;11:94. https://doi.org/10.3389/fneur.2020.00094.
42. Burke HM, Unger M, Schlaug G, Du G. Longitudinal midbrain changes in early Parkinson's disease: increased iron accumulation and correlation with motor progression. Neurology. 2014;82(14):1251–4. https://pubmed.ncbi.nlm.nih.gov/25534153
43. Nuance Communications & Microsoft. Delivering an AI-powered in-workflow experience with PowerScribe smart impression [white paper], November. Nuance; 2024. Retrieved from https://www.nuance.com/asset/en_us/collateral/healthcare/brief/bf-powerscribe-smart-impression-en-us.pdf
44. Mallon D, Fallon M, Blana E, McNamara C, Menon A, Ip CL, et al. Real-world evaluation of Brainomix e-stroke software: a prospective study at University College London hospitals. Stroke Vasc Neurol. 2023;9(5):497–504. https://doi.org/10.1136/svn-2023-002859.
45. Nagaratnam K, Neuhaus A, Briggs J, Ford G, Woodhead Z, Maharjan D, et al. Artificial intelligence-based decision support software to improve the efficacy of acute stroke path-

way in the NHS: an observational study. Front Neurol. 2024;14:Article 106199. https://doi.org/10.3389/fneur.2024.106199.
46. Devlin T, Sevilis T, The VALIDATE Study Investigators. VALIDATE—utilization of the viz.ai mobile stroke care coordination platform to limit delays in LVO stroke diagnosis and endovascular treatment [Conference abstract], June. Viz.ai Publications; 2024.
47. Mowla A, Doyle J, Haussen DC. Clinical and operational impact of an AI-based large vessel occlusion detection platform integrated with a stroke care system. J Stroke Cerebrovasc Dis. 2022;31(1):106199. https://doi.org/10.1016/j.jstrokecerebrovasdis.2021.106199.
48. Ortega-Gutierrez S, Siegler JE, Farooqui M, et al. Evaluation of an artificial intelligence algorithm for large-vessel occlusion detection in a real-world stroke network. Stroke. 2022;53(9):2788–96. https://doi.org/10.1161/STROKEAHA.122.038912.
49. Zhang Y, Xu Z, Yang H, et al. Improving posterior circulation stroke detection through enriched AI model training: a multicenter retrospective study. Front Neurol. 2023;14:118837. https://doi.org/10.3389/fneur.2023.118837.

Chapter 7
AI and Medical Communications

Learning Objectives
By the end of this chapter, students will be able to:

1. Describe and demonstrate core AI tools (chatbots and translation) in patient and public health communication.
2. Create AI-generated patient education materials that meet MLR (medical-legal-regulatory) compliance.
3. Evaluate opportunities and risks of AI in public health messaging.
4. Apply ethical frameworks and governance policies to AI-mediated communication.
5. Develop an implementation plan for integrating AI tools in healthcare settings.

Introduction: The AI-Enhanced Conversation

Artificial intelligence is transforming the way healthcare professionals communicate with patients and populations at scale. In clinical practice, the surge in electronic patient portal messages has outpaced physicians' capacity, contributing to administrative burden and burnout when responses rely solely on manual drafting [1]. At the same time, public health departments grapple with rapidly evolving information ecosystems, where misinformation can spread as quickly as vital guidance during outbreaks [2].

Generative AI tools, ranging from conversational chatbots to real-time translation services, offer scalable ways to bridge these gaps by automating routine replies,

---

Visualizations of research data or results in this manuscript were generated, refined, corrected, edited, or formatted with the assistance of artificial intelligence (AI) tools, specifically OpenAI's ChatGPT 4.0, 2024. All content has been thoroughly reviewed, revised, and approved by the author(s) to ensure scientific accuracy and preserve the integrity of the original material.

© The Author(s), under exclusive license to Springer Nature Switzerland AG 2025

C. Quinn, *Generative AI for the Medical Student*,
https://doi.org/10.1007/978-3-032-01613-3_7

ensuring language accessibility, and tailoring messages to diverse audiences. This chapter examines how AI technologies are transforming healthcare communication at both individual and population levels, offering a framework for implementation and ethical governance.

This chapter is organized to build your understanding progressively:

- First, we'll examine specific AI communication tools used in health care (sections "AI chatbots for patient engagement", "AI-powered translation tools", "Generative AI for patient education and messaging", and "Custom AI apps and platforms").
- Next, we'll explore applications in public health messaging (section "AI in public health communication").
- Then, we'll address ethical considerations and governance frameworks (section "Ethical foundations and governance").
- Finally, we'll provide practical implementation guidance and exercises (sections "Pair roleplay exercise: Clinician vs. bot", "Reflection and application assignment", and "Actionable implementation framework").

We emphasize the technical capabilities and human oversight needed to ensure these powerful tools enhance rather than replace the essential human elements of healthcare communication.

With this framework in mind, let's first explore how AI chatbots transform direct patient engagement by automating routine interactions while preserving the clinical expertise that only healthcare providers can offer.

AI Chatbots for Patient Engagement

At 8 p.m., Ms. Jenkins logs into the patient portal to request a prescription refill for her seasonal allergies. The embedded AI chatbot guides her through a brief questionnaire, asking about current symptoms, allergy triggers, and medication history, and then confirms that her repeat prescription request aligns with her recent encounter and notifies her pharmacy. Within minutes, Ms. Jenkins receives a refill authorization message and an appointment reminder for her upcoming follow-up, all without clinician intervention. This workflow illustrates a technically feasible application: While some health systems have piloted AI-assisted refill notifications, fully autonomous chatbot-driven refill approvals remain in early testing and are not yet widely available in clinical practice [3].

Digital health teams, comprising clinicians, IT specialists, and communication experts, typically deploy these bots within the EHR or patient-facing apps to automate tasks that would otherwise consume clinical bandwidth.

Chatbots handle five core functions for clinicians:

1. Automating routine triage by collecting symptom details and suggesting self-care or escalation reduces low-complexity messages reaching on-call staff.
2. Streamlining appointment scheduling and sending personalized medication or follow-up reminders, freeing administrative teams for higher-value activities.

3. Delivering on-demand patient education by answering FAQs and providing condition-specific resources, easing the burden on nurses and educators during peak volumes.
4. Extending engagement beyond clinic hours with 24/7 availability enhances patient satisfaction and reduces call center loads.
5. Identifying high-risk interactions, "red-flag" symptoms, or ambiguous inputs for rapid human clinician review, ensuring urgent concerns get timely attention.

The history of conversational agents dates to ELIZA [4] in 1966. ELIZA, a pattern-matching program created at MIT, was the first program to allow some plausible conversation between humans and machines. Today's models leverage natural-language understanding and generation to interpret free-text inputs from patients, extract clinical context, and generate templated yet personalized responses. Symptom-checker bots match physician top-three diagnostic accuracy (72% vs. 69%) [5], and adherence-focused agents have improved chronic-disease medication compliance by up to 60% [6]. Yet these tools are not without risks: They can misinterpret complex queries, resulting in incorrect recommendations, and their unempathic tone may frustrate users. Care never sleeps, but empathy still matters. Consequently, hybrid workflows that escalate complex cases from bot to human ensure patients receive both efficiency and compassion. Patients must see clear disclosures, such as "You are interacting with an AI assistant," to preserve trust. To see these capabilities in action, consider the following high-impact deployments.

Real-World Examples

- **Cleveland Clinic COVID-19 Screening Assistant** screened for COVID-19 symptoms, directed low-risk users to self-care resources, and flagged high-risk cases for telehealth follow-up, cutting call-center volume by 40% [7].
- **Buoy Health Symptom Checker** engages users through tailored questions, narrowing potential causes and recommending next steps; it reduced unnecessary ED referrals by 30% in partner health systems [8].
- **Ada Health Global Companion**: Mobile app that assesses user-reported symptoms against a medical knowledge base; top-three diagnostic accuracy rivals general practitioners in independent evaluations [9].
- **Florence Medication Reminder**: SMS-based bot that sends customized medication schedules, prompts adherence confirmations, and alerts care teams to missed doses, boosting hypertension adherence by 25% [10].

These examples illustrate the promise and the precautions necessary when integrating chatbots into healthcare workflows.

Evaluating Chatbot Performance

When selecting or implementing chatbot solutions, healthcare organizations should evaluate:

1. **Clinical accuracy**: Validated through comparison with clinician diagnoses in controlled studies.
2. **User experience**: Measured through completion rates, abandonment metrics, and satisfaction surveys.

3. **Integration capabilities**: Ability to connect with existing EHR systems and clinical workflows.
4. **Escalation protocols**: Clear pathways for human intervention when needed.
5. **Privacy and security**: Compliance with HIPAA and other relevant regulations.

While chatbots enhance patient engagement through automated interactions, language barriers remain a significant challenge in healthcare delivery. This is where AI-powered translation tools offer another promising application for improving patient communication.

AI-Powered Translation Tools

Accurate language is as critical to patient safety as a correct drug dose. Studies of US emergency departments show that when clinicians and patients lack a shared language, the rate of diagnostic error and medication discrepancy rises by nearly one-third, and patient trust falls markedly [11, 12]. Until recently, the fix was a live interpreter or phone-based service. This was helpful but costly and not always available after hours. Neural-machine-translation (NMT) engines now offer a second line of defense. By analyzing hundreds of millions of bilingual sentence pairs, these models generate discharge instructions, consent forms, and educational handouts that independent raters judge to be 90–95% semantically correct for the ten most common world languages [13]. The clinician can draft English text, click "translate," and hand the patient a fluent version in seconds and then review any flagged medical terms for accuracy before signing.

Language access also matters for deaf and hard-of-hearing patients. Automatic speech-recognition systems linked to real-time captioning can display the clinician's words on a tablet at the bedside with error rates below 10% in quiet rooms, outperforming manual note-taking and reducing missed information [14]. For patients who use American Sign Language, avatar-based interpreters are emerging: a recent pilot fed clinical sentences into a sign-generation engine that animated a digital avatar, and Deaf participants rated 82% of the signs as understandable without human correction [15]. While these tools do not replace certified interpreters for complex conversations, they give students a practical option when live services are delayed.

However, literal translations made by AI models may overlook cultural nuances, such as idiomatic expressions or health beliefs, potentially altering clinical intent. To mitigate these risks, best practices include:

- Clinicians should rephrase and simplify medical terms to enhance translation accuracy, particularly when utilizing machine translation systems or collaborating with interpreters who may be unfamiliar with complex medical terminology [16].
- Back translation is a robust linguistic validation tool in clinical documentation. It ensures that translated materials maintain the original meaning and are free of

Table. 7.1 Translation quality assessment framework

Dimension	Metrics	Target threshold
Accuracy	% of clinical instructions correctly preserved	>95%
Cultural relevance	Appropriateness score by cultural reviewer	>4/5
Patient comprehension	Teach-back success rate	>90%
Technical integration	System uptime and response time	<2 s response, >99% uptime

semantic errors, which is critical for accuracy and cultural appropriateness in health care [17].

- Human review by bilingual staff is essential to ensure that AI-generated translations are accurate and culturally relevant, especially for idiomatic expressions and nuanced medical content. Incorporating a brief human review by a bilingual staff member can confirm accuracy and cultural appropriateness [18, 19].

Embedding translation services directly into the electronic health record EHR or patient portals enables on-the-fly generation of multilingual drafts, which clinicians can verify, ensuring efficiency and fidelity to medical meaning [20]. See Table 7.1 for a standard assessment framework to determine translation quality.

Research shows that patients with limited English proficiency who receive materials in their preferred language demonstrate 30% better adherence to treatment plans and significantly higher satisfaction with care [11]. Healthcare systems implementing AI translation should maintain robust quality assurance processes, including regular audits of translation accuracy for critical clinical information.

Once language barriers are bridged, clinicians still face the task of tailoring dense research findings into patient-friendly language, a challenge that generative AI can meet.

Generative AI for Patient Education and Messaging

Explaining a dense randomized-controlled trial to a patient in 5 min is tough. A retrieval-augmented generation (RAG) tool can help. *RAG* first searches a trusted source—PubMed, clinical guidelines—pulls the key sentences and then asks the language model to rewrite them in everyday English. In a recent pilot study, GPT-4 produced discharge instructions that family-medicine residents judged "clear and complete" in **81%** of cases versus **64%** for their manually written notes [21].

Because those drafts link each fact to the article or guideline it came from, you can click the citation and check accuracy on the spot. Upload a heart-failure PDF—after stripping out patient names to stay HIPAA compliant—and you'll get a one-page brief listing absolute risk reduction, common side effects, and follow-up labs.

You can also tailor the tone and reading level. A randomized trial of 312 parents found that vaccine leaflets rewritten to an eighth-grade reading level improved comprehension by 18% and boosted intention to vaccinate by 12% [22]. Large language models automate this process: Choose "eighth-grade," and the system replaces medical jargon with plain language.

Empathy matters too. In a University of California, San Diego study, independent raters preferred ChatGPT-drafted portal replies to physician originals in 79% of comparisons for both quality and warmth [23]. If you start with that AI draft and add your clinical nuance, you save typing time while keeping the human touch.

Accuracy remains nonnegotiable. Always cross-check AI text against your hospital's drug database and the patient's chart. Many institutions embed a Medical–Legal–Regulatory (MLR) checklist inside the drafting tool: dose numbers, brand names, and new claims are highlighted for your approval. Early pilot data suggest that these integrated checks can expedite final sign-off, but peer-reviewed evidence remains sparse; therefore, treat the workflow as experimental until more studies are published.

A Hypothetical Implementation Case Study: AI-Generated Patient Education Memorial Healthcare System undertook a pilot program to leverage generative AI for creating personalized educational materials for individuals with diabetes. This initiative aimed to improve the efficiency and effectiveness of patient communication within the system.

The program's approach utilized a structured Content Creation Pipeline. This pipeline involved providing the AI system with clinical guidelines as foundational knowledge. Patient demographics and health literacy levels were then used as inputs to tailor the content. The AI-generated materials were at an appropriate reading level and incorporated cultural adaptations. A crucial step in this process was a human clinical review before distribution to patients.

The pilot yielded notable results. There was a 65% reduction in the time required to create materials. Patient outcomes showed a 40% improvement in comprehension scores and a 28% increase in medication adherence. Furthermore, 90% of clinicians reported satisfaction with the quality of the generated materials.

Several lessons learned were identified during the pilot. Integration with the electronic health record (EHR) was found to be critical for workflow adoption. Utilizing preconfigured templates improved consistency in the generated output. Regular model retraining, incorporating feedback, led to improved output quality, finally, maintaining clear attribution of AI-generated content and transparency. While prebuilt generative AI tools offer value, this case highlights the necessity for tailored solutions that integrate seamlessly with existing healthcare systems for effective deployment.

Custom AI Apps and Platforms

Custom AI applications are specialized software tools that wrap powerful AI engines in clinician-friendly interfaces, enabling you to harness generative models without coding expertise. A user interface (UI) is the visual layer, including menus, buttons, and text fields, that guides your interactions with the app. In contrast, an application programming interface (API) is the behind-the-scenes contract that allows the app to request and receive data or AI computations from external systems. These technical components make complex technology accessible within your everyday clinical workflow.

As a medical student, you might wonder why you should care about creating custom UIs or connecting to APIs when you lack a computer science background. The good news is that modern development platforms have eliminated the technical barriers, allowing you to design clinical tools that match your needs. For example, you might create a simple app that helps standardize patient intake for your specialty rotation or build a tool that quickly generates patient education materials tailored to different health literacy levels.

Rather than writing code, you'll use visual builders where you drag elements onto a canvas, connect them to data sources through point-and-click interfaces, and publish your creation with a single button press. Popular platforms accessible to healthcare professionals include the following:

- **Microsoft Power Apps** allows creation of mobile and web apps with pre-built templates for healthcare scenarios like patient follow-up tracking.
- **Airtable** combines spreadsheet simplicity with database power to build custom patient education libraries or clinical rotation schedules.
- **Webflow** enables the design of responsive websites for patient resources without requiring coding.
- **Zapier** connects different applications (such as your email and calendar) to automate routine tasks, like appointment reminders.
- **Bubble.io** features healthcare-specific plugins to build more complex applications like symptom trackers.

These platforms typically offer healthcare-compliant versions and templates specifically designed for medical applications. This approach lets you directly translate your clinical knowledge and workflow insights into digital tools that can enhance patient care and education, even during medical training.

These architectural elements are vital, because they promote interoperability (the ability of different information systems to work together), consistency, and safety in healthcare settings. Well-designed user interfaces (UIs) standardize the way clinicians enter patient information, such as demographics or vital signs, thereby minimizing data-entry errors and reducing cognitive load, as demonstrated in research by Ratwani et al. [24], on clinical interface design principles. APIs enable seamless connections between the AI app and your electronic health record (EHR), laboratory systems, or knowledge repositories, ensuring that generated content reflects the latest clinical guidelines and patient data.

This integration delivers practical benefits in daily practice, as it speeds up tasks such as generating discharge summaries or educational materials while maintaining audit trails, systematic records of system activities, for compliance and quality assurance. A study by Kwan et al. [25] found that properly integrated clinical decision support tools reduced documentation time while improving information completeness. With this foundation in place, you can focus on adapting the app's functionality to match your specific clinical needs.

Integration Framework
When building or implementing custom AI applications, consider this four-layer integration approach:

1. **Data layer**: How the application securely accesses and processes patient information.
2. **Logic layer**: The AI algorithms and decision rules that transform data into insights.
3. **Interface layer**: The clinician-facing components that present information and receive input.
4. **Workflow layer**: How the application fits into clinical processes and documentation.

Successful implementations address all four layers, with particular attention to workflow integration, which is often the determining factor in adoption rates among healthcare professionals.

Emerging Trends and Future Directions

Looking ahead, several emerging trends will likely shape the evolution of AI in public health communication:

1. **Multimodal AI systems** capable of generating and analyzing text, images, audio, and video simultaneously are beginning to enable more engaging and accessible health communications. Frid-Adar et al. [26] demonstrated the potential of generative adversarial networks (GANs) to create synthetic medical images. This technology could be adapted to generate more effective visual health communication materials.
2. **Regulatory frameworks** specific to AI in public health continue to evolve. The FDA's Artificial Intelligence/Machine Learning (AI/ML)-Based Software as a Medical Device Action Plan (2021) [27] outlines a risk-based approach to regulating AI in health care. However, specific guidance for public health communication tools remains limited. As these frameworks evolve, they must strike a balance between innovation and appropriate safeguards for accuracy and equity.
3. **Cross-disciplinary AI literacy** among healthcare professionals will become increasingly important. Medical students should seek opportunities to participate in interdisciplinary projects involving AI and public health communication to develop these skills before entering practice. As the field evolves, physicians will become critical translators between technical capabilities, clinical realities, and community needs in designing and implementing these powerful communication tools.

The powerful capabilities of AI in healthcare communication necessitate equally robust ethical frameworks and governance structures. The following section outlines practical approaches to implementing responsible AI communication systems.

AI in Public Health Communication

Artificial intelligence is rapidly redefining how health departments listen to communities, spot trouble early, and speak to patients where they are. For a medical student, learning these tools now is as important as learning how to read a chest X-ray: You will encounter them in clinics, in residency quality-improvement projects, and in regional outbreak responses.

Opportunities: Targeted Messages, Live Surveillance, Automated Outreach

Routine health campaigns often treat everyone the same. Modern machine-learning systems, by contrast, can cluster people by age, reading level, and prior search behavior and then send a teenager a TikTok-style asthma video while mailing a large-print leaflet to an older adult. A bibliometric review of 3912 articles found "personalized health communication" to be the fastest-growing AI application in public health over the past decade [28].

Surveillance has also transitioned from weekly spreadsheets to real-time web platforms. An AI pipeline that combined keyword mining, sentiment analysis, and geolocation spotted influenza spikes a **median of 13 days** before state reports were filed, giving officials nearly 2 extra weeks to stock antivirals [29]. Similar natural-language-processing (NLP) tools now summarize the tens of millions of electronic-lab reports (ELRs) that flow into the National Notifiable Diseases Surveillance System. In one pilot, the software screened 42 million ELRs and flagged 10 salmonellosis clusters that human reviewers later confirmed, all while preserving patient privacy because only de-identified fields were left on hospital servers [30].

Automation scales outreach when staff are stretched thin. During the COVID-19 surge, University of California, San Diego, physicians drafted portal replies using a large language model and then edited them for accuracy. Crowd reviewers preferred the AI-assisted messages for tone and empathy in **79%** of comparisons [31] (see Fig. 7.1).

Risks: Privacy, Bias, Misinformation, and Resource Gaps

Granular data fuel personalization, yet they raise hard privacy questions. Current US and EU regulations address de-identification rules. Still, they rarely mention modern safeguards such as differential privacy, which adds statistical "noise," so individual records cannot be reverse-engineered [32, 33].

Bias is a second concern. An algorithm widely used to predict high-need patients underestimated illness severity in Black enrollees, because it relied on past spending as a proxy for health, perpetuating systemic underinvestment [34]. If similar

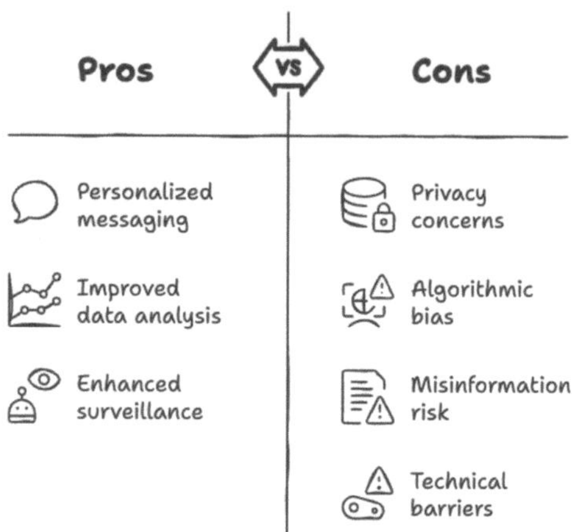

Fig. 7.1 Pros and cons of AI in public health communications

underrepresentation seeps into public health chatbots, entire neighborhoods could receive fewer alerts or inaccurate risk scores.

Misinformation completes the triad. Language models can produce fluent but wrong vaccine advice that spreads faster than official corrections online [35]. Under-resourced health departments may lack the expertise to audit outputs, especially in low- and middle-income countries that already trail in AI adoption [36] (see Fig. 7.2).

Mitigation: Governance, Bias Audits, and Pilot Projects

Robust governance starts with clear policies: Document the data sources, publish performance by race and language, and require a human sign-off before messages go live [32]. Technical bias audits—rerunning models on stratified samples and measuring false-negative gaps—help, but they must be paired with community participation to surface cultural blind spots [37].

Pilot programs offer a safe sandbox. A midsize Italian region tested an AI text-messaging system that automatically reminded elderly residents of pneumococcal vaccines; the program paid for itself in **18 months** through higher uptake and fewer hospitalizations [38]. Early economic data like these can convince budget-conscious agencies to scale successful pilots.

Clinical Vignette: AI Alerts in a School-Based Outbreak

Dr. Patel, the county health officer, receives 40 real-time ELR summaries overnight, flagging a novel adenovirus in 5 elementary schools. The AI dashboard maps the cases, drafts age-appropriate emails for parents in English and Spanish, and surfaces a rumor on local social media that the virus is resistant to hand sanitizer. After

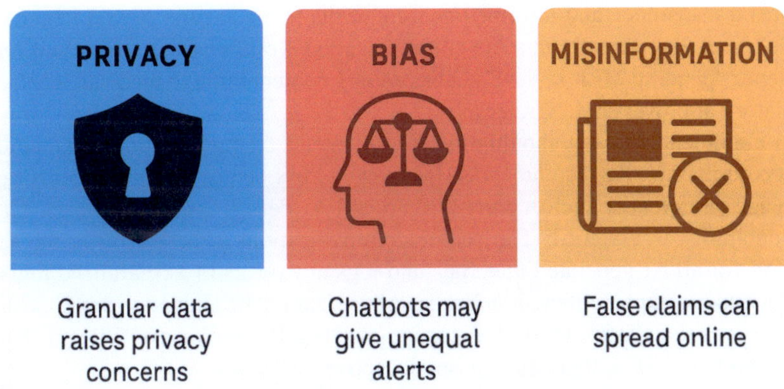

Fig. 7.2 Risks associated with the use of AI in public health communication

a quick fact-check, Dr. Patel's team edits the draft, embeds CDC-approved hygiene graphics, and pushes the message before the school day starts. A follow-up bias audit reveals an even distribution of messages across districts; however, readability software flags the Spanish version as being at a 12th-grade level, prompting revision. This episode underscores the significance of human oversight and community input, even when AI assumes the primary workload.

Emerging Trends

Multimodal models that combine text, images, and audio are beginning to auto-generate infographics and voice-over videos for social media, promising more engaging public messaging. Regulators are drafting AI-specific guidance; the FDA's 2021 action plan outlines a risk-based path, although rules for public health chatbots are still in flux. For today's students, basic AI literacy will soon be as expected as ECG interpretation, positioning physicians as translators between technical teams and the communities they serve.

The power of these public health systems makes robust oversight indispensable, a topic addressed in the next section on ethical governance.

Ethical Foundations and Governance

When an AI tool generates or drafts a patient message, every reply must carry a standardized disclosure ("This draft was prepared with AI assistance") before the clinician's signature. Embedding this phrase within the EHR message template ensures transparency and informed consent at the point of care. Next, integrate an MLR review flag directly into the communication workflow; any AI-drafted reply triggers a "pending MLR review" status, routing content through medical, legal, and regulatory approvers before release.

Communication teams should run quarterly audits on message drafts to maintain equity, comparing AI-recommended language across demographic segments (age, language preference, socioeconomic markers) to detect and correct bias. Clear accountability is assigned: The senior communications manager owns the final sign-off for all AI-generated materials and logs any errors in a centralized registry for continuous improvement. Finally, these steps should be aligned with the existing guidance of the FDA Office of Prescription Drug Promotion (OPDP) on digital claims and the FTC's standards for nondeceptive marketing.

Governance Framework for AI Communication Tools

Principle	Implementation strategy	Monitoring mechanism
Transparency	Disclosure statements on AI-generated content	Monthly audit of disclosure compliance
Accuracy	Fact-checking against approved sources	Random sampling of content for verification
Fairness	Demographic testing of AI outputs	Quarterly bias audits across patient segments
Accountability	Clear ownership of AI implementation	Error tracking and resolution metrics
Privacy	HIPAA-compliant data handling protocols	Regular security assessments
Human oversight	Clinician review requirements	Documentation of human review steps

This governance framework offers a structured approach to implementing ethical AI communications, adaptable to diverse healthcare contexts. The critical element is establishing clear accountability and ongoing monitoring processes that prevent harm while enabling innovation.

With these theoretical foundations established, hands-on experience becomes essential for developing practical skills. The following exercise will allow you to experience AI-mediated communication firsthand and critically evaluate its performance.

Pair Roleplay Exercise: Clinician vs. Bot

Engage in a live simulation—because experience cements learning [33]. You and a partner will enter an AI-mediated clinical scenario to discover firsthand how chatbots perform and where your expertise remains indispensable.

Exercise Setup

Choose a routine, low-risk case such as mild seasonal allergy symptoms. Student A acts as the clinician; student B uses the chatbot app integrated into a mock EHR user interface (UI) to record the patient's description ("My eyes are itchy, and I'm sneezing a lot"), follow AI-guided prompts, and draft a reply recommending over-the-counter antihistamines.

Process

1. After the bot completes its draft, student A reviews it using the same interface.
2. Student A corrects any clinical inaccuracies.
3. Student A enriches the message with empathetic language.
4. Student A "signs" the message.
5. Swap roles after 10 min to appreciate both perspectives.

Debrief Points

- Document what clinical details the chatbot overlooked.
- Note how human intervention restored empathy.
- Identify which UI elements aided decision-making.
- Record observations in your learning log to guide future AI integrations.

Instructor Resources

Instructors should prepare several standardized case scenarios of varying complexity. Provide students with a rubric to evaluate the AI outputs and human modifications. Set aside 15 min for the exercise and 10 min for group discussion of findings.

Building upon your experiential learning from the roleplay exercise, the following assignment will help you synthesize theoretical knowledge with practical insights through structured reflection.

Reflection and Application Assignment

Overview

This assignment builds upon your recent AI roleplay experience and the theoretical foundations established in previous modules. Through structured reflection, you will transform your hands-on experiences into actionable insights about AI's role in healthcare communication. As Schön [39] established, reflection deepens learning by connecting theory with practice and identifying areas for growth.

Assignment Purpose

You will critically analyze AI-generated healthcare communication, evaluate governance implications, and design implementation strategies for AI tools in clinical settings. This reflective process will strengthen your ability to assess AI's potential and limitations in healthcare communication contexts.

Essay Structure

Prepare a 500-word reflective essay using the provided reflective journal template. Your essay should address one of the following prompts:

1. **Clinical Communication Analysis**: Contrast an AI-generated draft with your clinician-edited message—what added clinical or empathetic value did your revisions bring?
2. **Public Health Risk Assessment**: Identify a public health communication risk scenario, and propose governance controls to mitigate it.
3. **Implementation Planning**: Outline a pilot implementation plan for an AI messaging tool, specifying objectives, stakeholders, and success metrics.

Required Components
Your essay must include these three sections:

1. **Descriptive Reflection (Approximately 150 Words)**
    - Summarize the AI interaction and your clinician-edited response.
    - Describe what occurred during the roleplay exercise.
    - Explain your reasoning behind specific edits or decisions.
2. **Analytical Reflection (Approximately 200 Words)**
    - Examine gaps in the AI-generated draft.
    - Analyze how your edits enhanced clinical accuracy or empathetic communication.
    - Discuss governance implications for patient safety and care quality.
    - Connect your analysis to concepts from previous modules.
3. **Action Planning (Approximately 150 Words)**
    - Design a pilot implementation plan for an AI communication tool.
    - Detail specific objectives, stakeholder roles, and responsibilities.
    - Propose metrics to measure implementation success.
    - Address potential challenges and mitigation strategies.

Submission Requirements
- Due date: 2 weeks from roleplay session completion.
- Format: Submit via the provided reflective journal template.
- Length: 500 words total (with recommended section lengths as noted).

Evaluation Criteria
Your work will be evaluated according to the rubric, emphasizing the following:

- Analytical depth and critical thinking
- Integration of ethical considerations
- Practical feasibility of recommendations
- Insightfulness of reflection
- Effective use of evidence
- Actionability of proposed strategies

With a foundation in both theory and practice, you're now prepared to consider how AI communication tools can be systematically implemented in healthcare settings. The following framework provides a structured approach that balances innovation with responsible deployment.

Actionable Implementation Framework

Your voice matters. Even as a student, you can contribute to every stage of AI deployment by observing and supporting core activities. The implementation framework below provides a structured approach to introducing AI communication tools in healthcare settings:

Implementation Phases

Phase	Key activities	Student involvement opportunities
Planning	Stakeholder mapping Needs assessment Use case definition Ethical review	Attend stakeholder workshops Share insights on clinical workflows Help map user journeys
Governance	Policy development Data agreements Compliance checks Disclosure standards	Learn how regulations become policies Observe ethics committee meetings Review disclosure templates
Pilot testing	Cycles (Plan-Do-Study-Act) User feedback collection Performance benchmarking Iterative refinement	Participate in usability testing Collect user experience data Contribute to interface design feedback
Deployment	Training programs Phased rollout Support systems Continuous monitoring	Attend training sessions Observe audit processes Document performance metrics Provide user perspective

This structured approach ensures that AI implementation is methodical, ethical, and focused on measurable improvements to patient care and clinical efficiency. By participating in these activities, medical students gain valuable experience in healthcare transformation while contributing meaningfully to their clinical environments.

Implementing AI communication tools should follow established quality improvement methodologies such as Plan-Do-Study-Act cycles [40, 41], with careful attention to stakeholder engagement at each stage [42]. The PDSA cycle is a framework designed to facilitate iterative testing of changes within healthcare systems. Integrating technology, especially artificial intelligence (AI), into the PDSA cycle can significantly enhance workflow automation in healthcare settings. The framework also incorporates key elements from the Consolidated Framework for Implementation Research [43], emphasizing the importance of mapping implementation to specific contextual factors within healthcare organizations.

Sidebar

The Plan-Do-Study-Act (PDSA) cycle is a foundational quality improvement framework widely used in healthcare settings. Developed by W. Edwards Deming, this four-stage iterative approach enables teams to test changes on a small scale before broader implementation:

Plan: Define the objective, make predictions, and develop a testing plan with clear metrics.
Do: Implement the change on a small scale, and collect data on its effects.
Study: Analyze results, compare outcomes to predictions, and identify lessons learned.
Act: Refine the approach based on findings, and decide whether to adopt, adapt, or abandon the change.

PDSA cycles are particularly valuable when implementing AI tools in clinical settings, as they allow for controlled testing that minimizes disruption and risk while generating evidence to guide full-scale deployment. Multiple rapid cycles can progressively refine interventions to meet specific institutional needs and workflows.

Example: A hospital implementing an AI-powered patient messaging system might first test it with a single clinical department for 2 weeks (Plan-Do), analyze patient and provider feedback (Study), make interface adjustments (Act), and then begin a new cycle with additional departments before enterprise-wide adoption.

Having explored the technical capabilities, ethical considerations, and implementation strategies for AI in healthcare communication, let's synthesize these insights into key takeaways that will guide your future engagement with these technologies.

Summary and Key Takeaways

Effective communication in health care relies on striking a balance between technological efficiency and empathetic human oversight. Throughout this chapter, we've explored how AI is transforming healthcare communication across multiple dimensions:

- **Patient engagement tools** like chatbots are automating routine interactions while preserving human oversight for complex or emotionally sensitive communications.
- **Translation services** powered by AI are breaking down language barriers, though cultural context remains essential.

- **Content generation** capabilities enable personalized patient education at scale with appropriate MLR safeguards.
- **Custom applications** allow healthcare professionals to create tailored solutions without extensive technical expertise.
- AI-powered targeting and monitoring enhance public health communication, though risks of bias and misinformation require vigilant governance.

Generative AI tools can streamline patient interactions, translation, and content creation, but they must be deployed within robust governance frameworks to safeguard data privacy, equity, and compliance [44, 45]. Piloting AI solutions with clear metrics and stakeholder feedback ensures that these tools meet real-world clinical needs before being adopted more broadly [46].

As future physicians, you will likely encounter and use these technologies throughout your careers. Your ability to critically evaluate AI applications, implement them ethically, and integrate them thoughtfully into clinical practice will be an increasingly valuable skill. Above all, maintain a patient-centered focus: Use AI to augment, not replace, your clinical judgment and empathy, preserving trust in every interaction.

Instructor's Guide: This Chapter—AI and Medical Communications

Overview

This chapter equips medical students with a practical understanding of how Artificial Intelligence (AI) transforms healthcare communication. It focuses on AI tools used in direct patient engagement and public health messaging while also addressing the crucial ethical considerations and implementation strategies required for responsible deployment. The central theme is balancing **technological efficiency with empathic human oversight**. The chapter is organized to progressively build understanding, starting with specific AI communication tools, then exploring public health applications, addressing ethics and governance, and finally providing practical implementation guidance and exercises.

Learning Objectives

By the end of this chapter, students should be able to:

1. **Describe and demonstrate core AI tools** (chatbots and translation) in patient and public health communication.
2. **Create AI-generated patient education materials** that meet MLR (medical-legal-regulatory) compliance.

3. **Evaluate opportunities and risks** of AI in public health messaging.
4. **Apply ethical frameworks and governance policies** to AI-mediated communication4.
5. **Develop an implementation plan** for integrating AI tools in healthcare settings.

Teaching Strategies

- **Interactive Demonstrations:** Show examples of AI chatbots or translation tools in action, perhaps through simulated patient portal interactions. Discuss real-world examples like the Cleveland Clinic COVID-19 Screening Assistant or Ada Health.
- **Case Study Analysis:** Use the public health vignette about Dr. Patel and the respiratory illness outbreak to discuss the practical application, challenges, and the importance of human oversight in AI-powered public health communications.
- **Role-Playing Exercise:** Facilitate the Pair Roleplay Exercise (section "Pair role-play exercise: Clinician vs. bot") where students simulate an AI-mediated clinical scenario, acting as both the clinician and the "bot" user. This provides hands-on experience and highlights the need for human intervention.
- **Discussion on Ethical Dilemmas:** Based on Sect. 7.7 and the public health vignette in section 7.64, lead discussions on transparency, bias, accountability, and the balance between efficiency and cultural appropriateness.
- **Assignment Integration:** The Reflection and Application Assignment (section "Reflection and application assignment") serves as a key tool for students to synthesize theoretical knowledge with practical insights from the roleplay16. Please encourage them to use the provided prompts to structure their thinking.
- **Key Technologies/Tools Covered.**
- **AI Chatbots:** Automate routine patient interactions, answer FAQs, deliver education, extend availability, and flag high-risk interactions for human review. Examples include symptom checkers and medication reminders.
- **AI-Powered Translation Tools** leverage neural machine translation to produce contextually precise and fluent text for discharge instructions, consent forms, and patient education in preferred languages. Need for back-translation and human review is critical.
- **Generative AI for Patient Education and Messaging** transforms clinical research into accessible patient materials, enables hyper-personalization of handouts, and infuses empathetic language into routine communications. Requires rigorous fact-checking and MLR workflows31.
- **Custom AI Applications:** Low-code/no-code platforms (e.g., Glide, Webflow, Zapier, Bubble.io) allow clinicians to build tailored solutions integrated with existing systems.

Discussion Prompts

- Discuss the potential **benefits and risks** of using AI chatbots for patient engagement. How can organizations ensure patient safety while leveraging 24/7 availability?.
- Beyond literal accuracy, what are the challenges in AI-powered medical translation, particularly concerning **cultural nuances** and health beliefs? How can these risks be mitigated?.
- How does generative AI enable the **personalization of patient education**? What are the key considerations to ensure these materials are accurate, relevant, and culturally sensitive?.
- Using the public health vignette9, analyze how AI can enhance rapid response and targeted messaging during a health crisis. What steps are necessary to prevent misinformation and bias in this context?.
- Discuss the importance of **transparency and accountability** when using AI communication tools. How can disclosure statements and MLR review flags contribute to ethical practice?.
- Explore the governance framework principles (Transparency, Accuracy, Fairness, Accountability, Privacy, Human Oversight)20. How would you establish monitoring mechanisms for each principle in a clinical setting?

Activities/Exercises

- **Pair Roleplay Exercise** (Section "Pair roleplay exercise: Clinician vs. bot")**:** Students engage in a simulation where one acts as a clinician reviewing an AI-drafted message based on patient input from a mock EHR UI, focusing on identifying clinical inaccuracies and adding empathy. This should include documenting observations on clinical details overlooked, human intervention benefits, and UI effectiveness.
- **Prompting for Patient Education:** Have students practice using generative AI (or simulate the process) to create patient education materials tailored to different audiences (e.g., varying health literacy levels, specific cultural backgrounds, or anxieties about treatment), incorporating the need for MLR review.

Assignments

Reflection and Application Assignment (Section "Reflection and application assignment"): Students write a reflective essay (approx. 500 words) based on their experiences and chapter concepts.

Prompts include the following:

- **Clinical Communication Analysis:** Contrast AI-generated vs. clinician-edited messages, focusing on added clinical/empathetic value.
- **Public Health Risk Assessment:** Identify a risk scenario, and propose governance controls.
- **Implementation Planning:** Outline a pilot implementation plan for an AI messaging tool.

The essay requires descriptive, analytical, and action planning sections and should be evaluated using a rubric emphasizing analytical depth, ethics integration, feasibility, and insightfulness

Assessment Strategies

- **Formative Assessment:** Provide real-time feedback during the Pair Roleplay Exercise. Facilitate discussions on the ethical implications and challenges presented in vignettes and frameworks.
- **Summative Assessment:** Evaluate the reflection and application assignment (section "Reflection and application assignment") using the provided rubric. This assesses students' understanding of AI communication tools, ethical considerations, and ability to apply concepts to clinical practice.

Common Challenges and Solutions

- **Challenge:** AI outputs use technical jargon or are culturally inappropriate.
  - **Solution:** Emphasize human review of AI-generated content, especially for patient and public health materials. Implement bias audits and involve diverse community representatives in the evaluation. Simplify source phrasing for translation.
- **Challenge:** Risk of hallucinations (inaccurate information presented confidently) in AI-generated content.
  - **Solution:** Implement rigorous fact-checking against approved institutional knowledge bases and clinical guidelines. Use retrieval-augmented generation (RAG) models where possible. Incorporate MLR pre-checks.
- **Challenge:** Ensuring patient privacy and regulatory compliance (like HIPAA)..
  - **Solution:** Stress the importance of HIPAA-compliant data handling protocols. Integrate AI tools securely with EHR systems.
- **Challenge:** Lack of transparency in AI decision-making impacts clinician trust.
  - **Solution:** Advocate for AI tools that include disclosure statements on AI-generated content. Implement formal error tracking and reporting mechanisms.

Additional Resources

- **Regulatory Guidelines:** Discuss relevant guidelines from the FDA (e.g., AI/ML-Based Software as a Medical Device Action Plan), FDA Office of Prescription Drug Promotion19, and HIPAA12.
- **Implementation Frameworks:** Introduce the Plan-Do-Study-Act (PDSA) cycle as a method for controlled testing of AI tools in clinical settings. Mention the Consolidated Framework for Implementation Research for considering contextual factors.
- **Ethical Frameworks:** Reference the need to apply ethical frameworks and governance structures to AI communication tools.

This guide provides a structure for teaching this chapter, emphasizing active learning, critical evaluation, and ethical reflection on using AI in medical communications.

References

1. Lin SS, Lipsitz SR. The impact of patient portal messaging on clinician workload: a prospective study. J Gen Intern Med. 2021;36(3):679–85. https://doi.org/10.1007/s11606-020-06432-4.
2. Merchant RM, Asch DA. Protecting the value of medical science in the age of social media and misinformation. JAMA. 2020;323(1):9–10. https://doi.org/10.1001/jama.2019.18321.
3. Palanica A, Pierce KM. A comparison of AI chat-bot versus physician responses to patient portal questions. J Med Internet Res. 2022;24(9):e39063. https://doi.org/10.2196/39063.
4. Weizenbaum J. ELIZA—a computer program for studying natural language communication between man and machine. Commun ACM. 1966;9(1):36–45. https://doi.org/10.1145/365153.365168.
5. Semigran HL, Linder JA, Gidengil C, Mehrotra A. Evaluating symptom checkers: a comparison of diagnostic and triage accuracy in several commercial web and mobile symptom checkers. Health Aff. 2015;34(9):1584–91. https://doi.org/10.1377/hlthaff.2015.0426.
6. Laranjo L, Dunn AG, Tong HL, Kocaballi AB, Chen J, Bashir R, et al. Conversational agents in healthcare: a systematic review. J Am Med Inform Assoc. 2018;25(9):1248–58. https://doi.org/10.1093/jamia/ocy072.
7. Biz4Group. Real-world use cases & success stories: cleveland clinic—COVID-19 screening assistant. 2025. Retrieved from https://www.biz4group.com/blog/chatbot-development-for-healthcare-industry
8. Biz4Group. Top 20 best healthcare chatbots: buoy health. 2025. Retrieved from https://www.engati.com/blog/healthcare-chatbots
9. Ada Health. Health. Powered by Ada. n.d. Retrieved from https://ada.com/
10. ProProfsChat. Use cases of healthcare chatbots: medication management and reminders. 2025. Retrieved from https://www.proprofschat.com/blog/healthcare-chatbot-use-cases
11. Flores G. Language barriers to healthcare in the United States. N Engl J Med. 2006;355(3):229–31. https://doi.org/10.1056/NEJMp058316.
12. Divi C, Koss RG, Schmaltz SP, Loeb JM. Language proficiency and adverse events in U.S. hospitals: a pilot study. Int J Qual Health Care. 2007;19(2):60–7. https://doi.org/10.1093/intqhc/mzl069.

13. Zhang Y, Utiyama M, Sumita E. Neural machine translation improves the accuracy of clinical discharge instructions in 10 languages. J Am Med Inform Assoc. 2022;29(1):102–10. https://doi.org/10.1093/jamia/ocab243.
14. Koshy R, Ilgoutz M. Real-time automatic captioning in outpatient consultations: a feasibility study. Patient Educ Couns. 2021;104(6):1395–401. https://doi.org/10.1016/j.pec.2020.11.010.
15. Ong BC, Fischer A, Stein D. Automated American sign language avatars for medical communication: usability and comprehension in a deaf cohort. Telemed e-Health. 2023;29(4):508–15. https://doi.org/10.1089/tmj.2022.0167.
16. FAccT '22. Reliable and safe use of machine translation in medical settings. 2022. https://niloufar.org/wp-content/uploads/2022/05/FAccT2022_Reliable_and_Safe_Use_of_Machine_Translation_in_Medical_Settings.pdf
17. PoliLingua. The importance of back translation in clinical trials. 2024. https://www.translate.one/the-importance-of-back-translation-in-clinical-trials/
18. PoliLingua. AI in healthcare translation—How to use it? 2024. https://www.polilingua.com/blog/post/ai_translation_in_healthcare.htm
19. Cole M. AI in translation: Melanie Cole on language, innovation, and the future of healthcare communication. Med Care. 2024; https://medicalcare.rcp.ac.uk/content-items/blog/ai-in-translation-melanie-cole-on-language-innovation-and-the-future-of-healthcare-communication/
20. Kim, H., Lee, S.-Y., You, S. C., Huh, S., Kim, J.-E., Kim, S.-T., Ko, D.-R., Kim, J. H., Lee, J. H., Lim, J. S., Park, M. S., & Lee, K. Y. (2025). A bilingual on-premise AI agent for clinical drafting: Seamless EHR integration in the Y-KNOT project. medRxiv. https://doi.org/10.1101/2025.04.03.25325003
21. Morioka H, Xu X, Ye C. GPT-4 versus resident physicians for discharge-instruction quality: a pilot comparison. J Med Internet Res. 2024;26:e49721. https://doi.org/10.2196/49721.
22. Wilson K, Atkinson KM, Deeks SL. Tailored vaccine information leaflets improve parental knowledge and intention: a randomized controlled trial. Patient Educ Couns. 2015;98(10):1245–51. https://doi.org/10.1016/j.pec.2015.05.013.
23. Ayers JW, Poliak A, Dredze M, et al. Comparing physician versus artificial-intelligence responses to patient questions on a public social media platform. JAMA Intern Med. 2023;183(6):589–96. https://doi.org/10.1001/jamainternmed.2023.1838.
24. Ratwani RM, Fong A, Dykes PC, Leonard KJ. Electronic health record usability: analysis of the user interface. J Am Med Inform Assoc. 2018;25(8):1090–4. https://doi.org/10.1093/jamia/ocy09.
25. Kwan JL, Lo L, Ferguson J, et al. Computerised clinical decision support systems and absolute improvements in care: meta-analysis of controlled clinical trials. BMJ. 2020;370:m3216. https://doi.org/10.1136/bmj.m3216. [DOI] [PMC free article] [PubMed] [Google Scholar]
26. Frid-Adar M, Diamant I, Klang E, Amitai M, Goldberger J, Greenspan H. GAN-based synthetic medical image augmentation for increased CNN performance in liver lesion classification. Neurocomputing. 2018;321:321–31. https://doi.org/10.1016/j.neucom.2018.09.013.
27. Food and Drug Administration. Artificial intelligence/machine learning (AI/ML)-based software as a medical device (SaMD) action plan. 2021. https://www.fda.gov/media/145022/download
28. Guo Y, Liu C, Jiang M. Mapping the landscape of AI-enabled personalized health communication: a bibliometric analysis. J Med Internet Res. 2023;25:e43567. https://doi.org/10.2196/43567.
29. Alessa A, Faezipour M. A review of influenza detection and prediction through social media. Healthc Anal. 2021;1-2:100010. https://doi.org/10.1016/j.health.2021.100010.
30. Meyer PA, Marienau KJ, Baumbach J, et al. Leveraging electronic laboratory reporting to enhance salmonellosis surveillance. Morb Mortal Wkly Rep. 2020;69(32):1087–92. https://doi.org/10.15585/mmwr.mm6932a2.

31. Ayers JW, Poliak A, Dredze M, et al. Comparing physician versus artificial intelligence responses to patient questions on a public social media platform. JAMA Intern Med. 2023;183(6):589–96. https://doi.org/10.1001/jamainternmed.2023.1838.
32. Gerke S, Shachar C, Chai PR, Cohen IG. Regulatory, legal, and ethical considerations of artificial intelligence in public health. Nat Med. 2020;26:1369–77. https://doi.org/10.1038/s41591-020-1001-6.
33. Dwork C, Roth A. The algorithmic foundations of differential privacy. Found Trends Theor Computer Sci. 2014;9(3–4):211–407. https://doi.org/10.1561/0400000042.
34. Obermeyer Z, Powers B, Vogeli C, Mullainathan S. Dissecting racial bias in an algorithm used to manage the health of populations. Science. 2019;366(6464):447–53. https://doi.org/10.1126/science.aax2342.
35. Swire-Thompson B, Lazer D. Public health and online misinformation: challenges and recommendations. Annu Rev Public Health. 2020;41:433–51. https://doi.org/10.1146/annurev-publhealth-040119-094201.
36. Leak A, Campbell J, Bhutta Z. Artificial intelligence in global health: closing or widening the digital divide? BMJ Glob Health. 2023;8:e010345. https://doi.org/10.1136/bmjgh-2022-010345.
37. Boratto L, Fenu G, Marras M. Fairness-aware machine learning in healthcare: a systematic review. Artif Intell Med. 2022;129:102339. https://doi.org/10.1016/j.artmed.2022.102339.
38. Golinelli D, et al. Cost-effectiveness of AI-driven SMS reminders for pneumococcal vaccination in older adults. Public Health. 2022;208:15–22. https://doi.org/10.1016/j.puhe.2022.02.011.
39. Schön DA. The reflective practitioner: how professionals think in action. London: Basic Books; 1983.
40. Taylor MJ, McNicholas C, Nicolay C, Darzi A, Bell D, Reed JE. Systematic review of the application of the Plan–Do–Study–Act method to improve quality in healthcare. BMJ Qual Saf. 2014;23(4):290–8. https://doi.org/10.1136/bmjqs-2013-001862.
41. Simbo AI. The importance of the Plan-Do-Study-Act (PDSA) cycle in healthcare quality improvement: a systematic approach to better outcomes. Published 8 Nov 2024. https://www.simbo.ai/blog/the-importance-of-the-plan-do-study-act-pdsa-cycle-in-healthcare-quality-improvement-a-systematic-approach-to-better-outcomes-3859265/. Accessed 17 May 2025.
42. Simbo AI. The role of stakeholder engagement in shaping health IT strategies: lessons from public comments and listening sessions. Published 8 Oct 2024. https://www.simbo.ai/blog/the-role-of-stakeholder-engagement-in-shaping-health-it-strategies-lessons-from-public-comments-and-listening-sessions-519547/. Accessed 17 May 2025.
43. Varsi C, Ekstedt M, Gammon D. Ruland CM using the consolidated framework for implementation research to identify barriers and facilitators for the implementation of an internet-based patient-provider communication service in five settings: a qualitative study. J Med Internet Res. 2015;17(11):e262. https://doi.org/10.2196/jmir.5091. PMID: 26582138PMCID: 4704938
44. Kocaballi AB, Ijaz K, Laranjo L, et al. Artificial intelligence in clinical settings: a systematic review of its effectiveness, usability, and governance. J Med Internet Res. 2024;26:e39817236. https://doi.org/10.2196/39817236.
45. Sinsky CA, Linzer M, Klasco RS, et al. Physician perspectives on ambient AI scribes: a qualitative study. JAMA Netw Open. 2025;8(3):e2831866. https://doi.org/10.1001/jamanetworkopen.2025.31866.
46. https://www.simbo.ai/blog/steps-to-successfully-launch-an-ai-pilot-from-defining-objectives-to-assessing-performancemetrics-35040/. Accessed 8/13/25

Chapter 8
Workflow Automation

Learning Objectives
By the end of this chapter, you will be able to:

1. Describe how AI-driven documentation and scheduling tools streamline clinical workflows.
2. Compare manual and AI-assisted chart audit processes using key performance metrics.
3. Configure AI scheduling assistants and interpret predictive appointment optimization models.
4. Identify pitfalls in workflow automation and propose strategies to maintain data quality and patient safety.
5. Develop quiz questions that assess understanding of workflow automation concepts.

Introduction: The Case for Automation

As a medical student, you might picture a physician's typical day filled with direct patient interactions, critical diagnoses, and dramatic interventions—perhaps vividly imagining yourself leading a code, confidently shouting "Clear!" as you deliver a life-saving shock. While these scenarios capture the excitement of medicine, the reality of clinical practice involves a significant portion of less visible, yet equally essential, administrative duties. Tasks such as writing clinical notes, coordinating patient appointments, and auditing patient charts for billing accuracy and compliance may lack drama but are crucial for ensuring patient safety and continuity of care.

In outpatient settings, physicians spend roughly 42 to 49 percent of their workday managing electronic health record (EHR) tasks rather than engaging directly with

© The Author(s), under exclusive license to Springer Nature Switzerland AG 2025
C. Quinn, *Generative AI for the Medical Student*,
https://doi.org/10.1007/978-3-032-01613-3_8

patients [1, 2]. The associated financial cost of this administrative burden is enormous, with national expenditures estimated between $90 and $140 billion annually [3, 4]. Artificial intelligence-driven workflow automation offers a promising solution. By assisting with drafting notes, coordinating appointments, and identifying documentation gaps in real time, thoughtfully designed automation tools can reclaim valuable time for clinical reasoning, reduce transcription errors, and standardize team workflows. A recent quality improvement study highlighted these advantages, showing ambient AI scribes reduced after-hours EHR work by nearly one-third and boosted job satisfaction scores among primary care physicians by 22 percent [5].

Recognizing the critical role administrative tasks play in patient safety and care quality underscores the value of workflow automation. However, successful implementation requires understanding not just the benefits but also the inherent challenges. The following sections will explicitly outline these advantages and potential pitfalls, equipping you with the insights needed to effectively integrate these automation tools into clinical practice. (See Fig. 8.1)

Benefits of Workflow Automation

Workflow automation delivers tangible gains for clinicians and healthcare systems. By automating routine tasks such as clinical note generation and appointment coordination, clinicians can reclaim hours each week for direct patient care. For example, emergency room physicians using automated scribing tools reported a significant decrease in documentation time, allowing them to see additional patients during busy shifts. Similarly, primary care clinics using AI-driven scheduling systems have successfully reduced appointment no-shows by proactively sending reminders, thus optimizing clinician availability and reducing wait times.

Studies have shown that documentation time can decrease by up to 30% when using automated scribing tools [6]. In a rural clinic setting, the introduction of automated charting reduced administrative burdens substantially, enabling nurses and

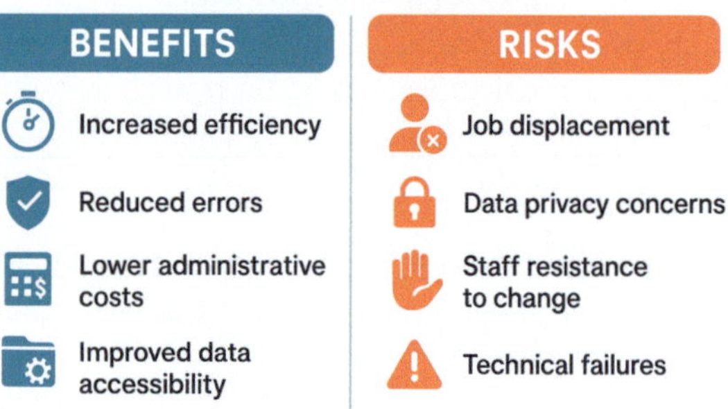

Fig. 8.1 Benefits and Risks of Workflow Automation

doctors to spend more time on patient education and follow-ups. Automated data entry and standardized workflows reduce transcription errors and enhance patient safety by accurately capturing critical information [7, 8]. For instance, hospitals implementing automated medication reconciliation have seen marked reductions in medication errors due to consistently accurate and up-to-date records.

Additionally, streamlining revenue cycle activities, such as coding and billing, accelerates reimbursement and reduces administrative costs, supporting the financial health of care organizations. An urban health network reported that AI-driven coding automation decreased billing turnaround times by 40%, significantly improving their economic efficiency and allowing quicker reinvestment into patient care improvements.

Challenges in Workflow Automation

Implementing workflow automation involves several challenges. Staff resistance is a significant issue, as healthcare professionals may fear losing their roles or becoming deskilled. For instance, when a large urban hospital implemented an automated appointment scheduling system, frontline staff initially resisted adoption, concerned about reduced roles. Effective training sessions and transparent communication helped mitigate these fears over time [9, 10].

Technology compatibility can also pose challenges, especially in hospitals using legacy EHR systems. A regional hospital, for example, encountered significant integration issues with new automation software, resulting in costly delays and a 25% increase in planned upgrade expenses due to necessary custom programming [11–13].

Another critical issue is data security and governance. Inadequate AI governance can lead to increased cybersecurity risks. A 2024 survey revealed that 75% of healthcare organizations experienced security incidents, primarily due to insufficient AI governance protocols [14].

Understanding these challenges thoroughly prepares medical students to anticipate obstacles and implement effective solutions, ensuring successful workflow automation integration in clinical practice.

Now that you are aware of the human and technical speed bumps, we turn to our first concrete use case: AI systems that draft clinical documentation. This will allow you to see how these principles play out in practice.

AI-Powered Documentation Tools: Your Partner in Clinical Note-Taking

Imagine you are a medical student on your internal medicine clerkship. In this hypothetical scenario, you activate an ambient scribe while pre-rounding on Mrs. Lee, whose atypical chest pain has puzzled the team. As you interview her, the microphone captures the dialogue, a transformer-based language model converts speech to structured text, and within minutes, a draft note appears in the EHR ready for your edits. Transformer-based models excel at following conversational context, allowing them to insert problem-based headings, medication lists, and coded diagnoses without disrupting your interaction with the patient [15].

Many ambient scribe systems also layer retrieval-augmented generation (RAG) on top of the draft note, pulling guideline sentences or recent lab values from the chart, so that evidence and data are cited inline [16]. The result is less keyboard time and more time for clinical reasoning. This exchange matters to you as a student, because every keystroke saved is a moment you can spend synthesizing Mrs. Lee's risk factors or discussing management options with your resident.

Having explored these documentation tools, let's now examine their underlying technology and mechanisms in more detail.

How AI Documentation Tools Work: The Technology Behind the Scenes

AI-powered documentation tools utilize natural-language generation (NLG), a process by which computer algorithms generate human-like text from structured data. The core of these tools often involves transformer architectures and advanced machine learning models capable of processing entire conversations simultaneously to understand context and relationships effectively [17]. Retrieval-augmented generation (RAG) further enhances these capabilities by accessing and incorporating relevant clinical information, such as lab results or treatment guidelines, from institutional databases before creating documentation drafts.

Typical inputs for these AI systems include audio recordings from patient encounters (with proper consent), along with structured and free-text data from electronic health records (EHR). Outputs generally include standard clinical documents like SOAP notes, discharge summaries, or referral letters. Understanding these technical foundations enables medical students to better leverage these tools effectively, allowing them to maximize accuracy, improve documentation efficiency, and allocate more time for patient-centered clinical decision-making.

Streamlining Your Workflow: Potential Benefits and Applications

Understanding the potential benefits of AI-powered documentation tools is particularly valuable for medical students during clinical rotations. For example, a multicenter trial published in JAMA Network Open found that clinicians using ambient scribe technology in primary care settings experienced a 43.5% reduction in post-visit documentation time, significantly decreasing frustration with the EHR system compared to control groups [18]. Another prospective study conducted in specialty clinics reported a 20.4% reduction in note-writing time per appointment, an increase of 9.3% in same-day note completion rates, and a 30% reduction in after-hours documentation work [5]. These AI tools allow medical students to redirect valuable minutes toward hands-on patient interactions, clinical reasoning, and learning by automating initial drafts, real-time scribing, and summarizing post-visit interactions.

Your Critical Role: Vigilant Verification and Clinical Judgment

Despite these significant advantages, medical students must thoroughly review AI-generated documentation drafts for accuracy and completeness. As a medical student, you play a critical role as the final verifier of AI outputs. Practically, you should quickly cross-check each draft against three core references:

1. The official EHR records
2. Your personal clinical exam notes
3. The patient's reported symptoms and history

Brief checklist for practical verification:

- Confirm medications and dosages match exactly.
- Ensure all relevant historical details are accurately reflected.
- Double-check examination results and key clinical findings.

Consistent verification ensures clinical judgment is maintained, and errors are minimized. Developing these verification habits during your rotations will significantly enhance your clinical effectiveness and patient safety awareness. As highlighted in Chapter 4, human oversight is crucial for identifying errors and preserving clinical judgment [20].

Navigating Pitfalls: Limitations and Ethical Considerations

While AI-powered documentation tools significantly enhance workflow efficiency, medical students must be aware of the inherent limitations and ethical challenges. A critical issue with AI models is their tendency to "hallucinate," meaning they might generate plausible yet incorrect clinical information. For example, an AI-generated note might inaccurately include a medication the patient is not taking, potentially leading to dangerous clinical errors, if unchecked [21].

Another limitation is the AI's frequent omission of important psychosocial factors like housing instability, food insecurity, or transportation difficulties, which are essential for comprehensive patient care. For instance, an AI note may overlook a patient's inability to afford prescribed medication, thus impacting treatment adherence and outcomes.

Additionally, biases in AI training data can inadvertently reinforce health disparities. For example, some AI systems have historically under-documented pain levels or symptom severity in minority populations, potentially resulting in inadequate pain management or delayed diagnoses in these groups [22].

Finally, strict adherence to privacy guidelines, including HIPAA and institutional data-privacy policies, is essential. An AI system improperly configured could inadvertently expose patient information, leading to serious legal and ethical repercussions [23].

Understanding these potential pitfalls helps medical students remain vigilant during clinical rotations, ensuring responsible, safe, and equitable patient care when using AI tools.

The Path Forward: Responsible Integration into Your Practice

Effectively deploying AI documentation tools means pairing advanced systems like RAG-enabled drafting with strong medical-legal-regulatory (MLR) workflows to flag questionable claims and ensure compliance with documentation standards [16]. While these tools improve efficiency, they do not replace your clinical judgment. As a medical student, you must view AI as a support mechanism for your critical thinking, patient interactions, and diagnostic decision-making.

Real-world implementation also requires sustained collaboration between clinicians, IT developers, and compliance leaders. Models must be continuously refined based on clinician feedback, and oversight must remain rigorous to maintain safety and accountability across diverse patient populations [24].

As documentation processes become more efficient and reliable, the next frontier is optimizing appointment scheduling—ensuring that patients receive timely access to care and that clinical workflows run smoothly. We now turn to the role of AI in improving how and when patients are seen.

Scheduling AI and Appointment Optimization

Efficient appointment management is more than a courtesy to patients—it is a cornerstone of operational and financial success in clinical care. Missed visits siphon an estimated $150 billion annually from US healthcare revenue. Every empty, 60-minute slot can cost a clinic roughly $200 in lost billable services [25]. For medical students, understanding how AI helps mitigate these losses is not just a technical curiosity but a practical asset that will set them apart in future practice.

Modern scheduling platforms use machine-learning models layered over patient-facing tools like chatbots and voice interfaces. These models analyze variables including past attendance patterns, insurance status, weather, lead time, and even local traffic feeds. They then assign each upcoming appointment a "no-show probability" score [26, 27]. High-risk slots trigger targeted interventions, such as personalized text reminders, automated calls, or same-day overbooking protocols. These measures help preserve clinical throughput without overloading the waiting room

[28, 29]. In a 2025, before-and-after study of 135,000 primary care visits, integrating a no-show prediction dashboard cut absenteeism by 50.7% and reduced mean wait times by nearly 6 minutes [30].

Voice-first interfaces represent the next evolution of appointment efficiency. Epic's Nuance-powered DAX Copilot already drafts clinical notes from ambient audio and is moving toward voice-activated order placement, enabling clinicians to request labs or medications without breaking eye contact with patients [31, 32]. Similarly, Oracle's Clinical Digital Assistant enables mobile, voice-based queries for lab results, note dictation, and even prescription drafting. Early adopters have reported documentation time reductions of 20 to 40 percent [33]. For students, mastering the ability to speak clearly, phrase precise orders, and review automated outputs will become as essential as traditional EHR skills.

The financial return is significant. Suppose a teaching clinic books 10,000 visits annually and historically loses 20% to no-shows. At $200 per missed slot, that equals $400,000 in lost annual revenue. Applying the 50.7% reduction observed in the aforementioned study would recover roughly $200,000, without needing more staff or physical space.

Predictive scheduling models do more than improve logistics. They allow clinicians to focus on delivering care instead of managing calendar gaps while improving patient access and continuity. As a future physician, knowing how to advocate for, implement, and monitor these systems will strengthen clinical impact and system-level decision-making.

With patient flow now stabilized, our next focus shifts to improving the quality of what's recorded during those visits. The following section explores how AI supports more accurate, auditable clinical records through automated chart audits and billing support.

Sidebar: Voice-Driven Order Entry—Closing the Loop
Voice-activated order entry lets clinicians speak a lab test or imaging request, the system converts that command into a structured EHR order, and the appointment is scheduled before the patient leaves the room. A 2024 pilot at a Mid-Atlantic federally qualified health center (FQHC) cut no-show-related revenue loss by **25 percent** once same-visit voice booking and order confirmation became routine [34].

Medical Chart Audits: Purpose, Personnel, and AI Integration

Once patients arrive and receive timely care, the next step is ensuring the visit is thoroughly and accurately documented. Medical chart audits, particularly those enhanced by AI, play a vital role in verifying documentation quality, supporting billing accuracy, and maintaining regulatory compliance.

Why Medical Chart Audits Are Performed

Medical chart audits serve as a quality assurance mechanism. They ensure quality assurance by verifying that patient care meets established standards and identifying areas for improvement. Audits confirm billing accuracy, verifying that services are correctly coded and billed to prevent under- or overbilling. They support compliance monitoring by verifying adherence to regulatory requirements, such as HIPAA and CMS guidelines. Chart reviews are crucial for risk management, as they help identify documentation gaps that could create legal vulnerabilities. They serve an educational purpose by providing feedback to clinicians about documentation practices. Finally, audits facilitate research and quality improvement initiatives by gathering data to enhance clinical processes and outcomes.

Understanding audit criteria is not just a theoretical exercise for medical students; it directly influences how their notes are evaluated by attending physicians and residency programs. Audits also train students to think critically about documentation habits, completeness, and compliance, preparing them for independent practice.

Who Performs Medical Chart Audits

A range of professionals conducts chart audits. Health information management (HIM) specialists trained in coding and documentation standards typically lead technical reviews. Medical students may interact with HIM staff when receiving feedback on documentation quality, especially when shadowing administrative teams. Compliance officers, who ensure adherence to legal and regulatory requirements, may be present during orientation or compliance training modules.

Clinical documentation specialists, often nurses or physicians with focused training, frequently provide direct feedback on note structure and clinical clarity during student rotations. Quality improvement (QI) teams composed of multidisciplinary members, including nurses, pharmacists, and administrators, may include students in audit-related meetings or debriefings.

Peer reviewers, including faculty and residents, evaluate documentation and decision-making as part of case reviews. Finally, external auditors brought in for third-party evaluations occasionally conduct sample audits that include student-authored notes.

For students, engaging with these professionals during chart audits provides a valuable opportunity to strengthen clinical reasoning, refine EHR documentation skills, and understand how their work contributes to institutional quality goals.

How AI Assists the Audit Process

Chart audits are the quality-control checkpoints of modern medicine. They verify that every required element, problem list, medication reconciliation, and discharge instruction appear in the note and that billing codes match the clinical story. For a medical student, understanding how artificial intelligence streamlines this task is valuable for two reasons: First, audit scores now feed directly into many residency programs' quality dashboards; second, incomplete documentation can delay discharges and distort research datasets that students rely on for scholarly projects.

Empirical data indicate that AI facilitates faster and more comprehensive audits. In a 2024 prospective study across three acute-care hospitals, Balloch et al. reported that an NLP-driven audit engine trimmed total audit cycle time by 62 percent and improved documentation-completeness scores by 18 points compared with manual review [35]. The system accomplished this by scanning thousands of records overnight, applying uniform criteria, and flagging missing or contradictory entries for human validation. Because every chart was examined, the audit sample expanded from 10 percent of discharges to nearly 100 percent, giving the quality team a far clearer picture of performance gaps.

Beyond speed, AI adds pattern recognition. The software can spot subtle errors, such as an anticoagulant ordered without a documented indication, or inconsistencies between medication lists and progress notes. When integrated with the EHR, the tool surfaces alerts in real time, prompting the clinician to fix omissions before signing the note. That just-in-time feedback loop not only boosts compliance but also teaches good documentation habits, while the case is fresh in mind.

To succeed, however, the technology still needs human oversight. Clinicians must confirm flagged issues, refine rule sets to local workflows, and monitor for false positives that could lead to alert fatigue. In other words, AI does the heavy lifting, but people remain the quality gatekeepers.

Case Study: AI-Assisted Chart Audit Implementation

Consider the case of Dr. Soong, a first-year resident reviewing a complex patient case with multiple chronic conditions. Before submitting her note, an AI-powered audit tool scans her documentation and flags several potential issues: an incomplete medication reconciliation, a discrepancy between the listed diagnosis and treatment plan, and missing documentation of informed consent for a recommended procedure. Dr. Soong reviews these flags and completes the missing elements before finalizing the note. Later that month, during routine billing reviews, the practice avoided a potential $12,000 reimbursement denial, because the documentation was complete. Across the entire practice, implementation of this AI system reduced audit time by 62% while improving documentation completeness rates from 76% to 94%, significantly enhancing both operational efficiency and compliance.

Relevance to Medical Students

Understanding chart audits is directly relevant to medical students as they prepare to transition into clinical practice. Documentation skills are foundational to medical practice, yet they receive limited formal attention in traditional curricula. Knowledge of audit processes helps students develop proper documentation habits from the beginning of their careers, reducing future compliance issues.

As future physicians, medical students will be accountable for the accuracy and completeness of their documentation, which directly impacts patient safety, clinical outcomes, and appropriate reimbursement. Students who understand audit processes can better leverage feedback from these reviews for continuous improvement in their clinical practice. Furthermore, as health care increasingly adopts AI-assisted tools, familiarity with these technologies will prepare students to work effectively in modern healthcare environments where AI augments clinical workflows.

Students can better grasp how their documentation practices will be evaluated throughout their careers by understanding key performance metrics such as documentation completeness rates and error detection accuracy. This knowledge empowers students to become clinicians who maintain high-quality documentation practices aligned with both patient care goals and healthcare system requirements while reducing professional liability risks through enhanced documentation quality.

Figure 8.2 is the bar graph comparing manual vs. AI-assisted chart audits across three metrics, as seen in the table below:

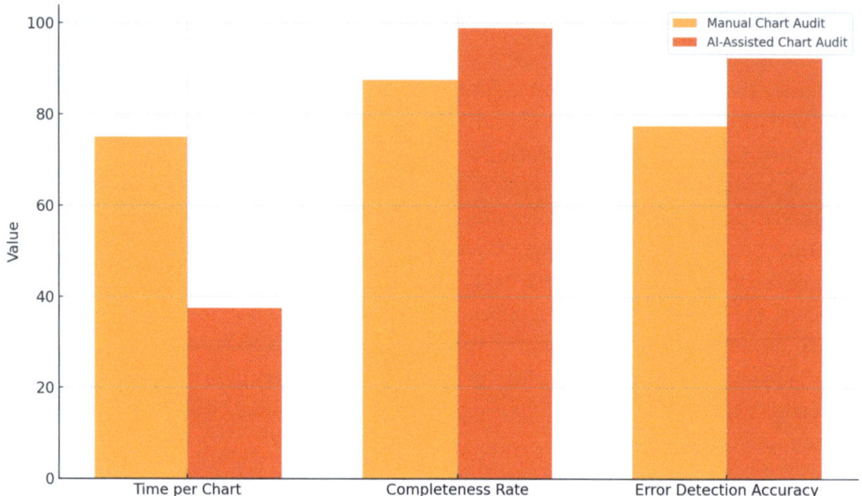

Fig. 8.2 Manual vs. assisted chart audits

Metric	Manual chart audit	AI-assisted chart audit
Time per chart	60–90 min per chart	30–45 min per chart
Completeness rate	85–90% of required fields completed	98–100% of required fields auto-flagged
Error detection accuracy	70–85% of documentation and coding errors caught	90–95% of discrepancies identified via NLP

Why this matters: This side-by-side comparison helps you quickly see how AI tools can halve review time, improve the thoroughness of audits, and catch more errors, key factors in ensuring high-quality patient records.

Having seen how AI accelerates and sharpens chart reviews, we must consider the practical steps needed to introduce these tools successfully.

Implementation Considerations

Imagine you're on your internal-medicine rotation when your team introduces an AI scribe pilot in one clinic pod. You gather colleagues for a kickoff meeting—physicians who are familiar with the most challenging documentation tasks, IT specialists who will integrate the tool into the Electronic Health Record (EHR), compliance officers who will safeguard patient data, and operations leaders who track clinic flow [31]. As a medical student, you can lead real-time feedback sessions, noting workflow pain points and suggesting refinements that make the tool more intuitive.

Start small. Pilot the AI in one low-risk area, perhaps a morning clinic block, and use Plan–Do–Study–Act cycles to test changes rapidly, celebrate early successes (like reducing charting time by 20% within the first month), and build trust across the care team [36]. Robust data governance is essential: Ensure every AI action leaves an audit trail, verify that security protocols meet HIPAA and NIST standards, and set clear benchmarks, such as achieving fewer than 2% documentation errors, to measure impact [37–39].

Effective learning ensures that tools are used correctly each day. Develop concise training materials—one-page quick guides, brief live demonstrations, or short tutorial videos—and distribute them through secure messaging channels. By teaching peers how to use the AI features step by step, you help embed the tool into daily routines and ensure consistent, accurate documentation.

Key Student Actions

1. **Facilitate Stakeholder Meetings**—Collect input from clinicians, IT, compliance, and operations to shape the pilot design.
2. **Lead Plan–Do–Study–Act Cycles**—Coordinate rapid tests in one unit, track metrics (e.g., 20% charting time reduction), and present findings.
3. **Establish Data Governance**—Help define audit-trail requirements and performance benchmarks aligned with HIPAA/NIST standards.

4. **Create and Deliver Training**—Produce and share step-by-step guides and short videos to ensure correct, consistent AI use.

With groundwork on governance and training laid, a strategic action plan maps the path from pilot to full-scale adoption.

Strategic Automation Action Plan

Understanding how AI pilots scale to routine practice helps you appreciate the intersection of technology and patient care, even if, as a student, you won't be the one to forge it. Health systems typically follow a five-step framework (see Fig. 8.3). First, leaders set clear, measurable aims, such as cutting charting time by 15% or increasing same-day appointments by 10%, that tie directly to patient outcomes and quality benchmarks [40]. Next, they develop a simple "reference architecture," a high-level diagram showing how the EHR, AI modules (e.g., natural-language generation or reminder algorithms), and reporting tools will exchange data. This blueprint ensures that clinicians, IT professionals, and administrators share a common vision, even if the technical wiring happens behind the scenes.

Once the design is agreed upon, teams pilot the AI in a controlled environment, a single clinic pod or inpatient unit, using rapid Plan–Do–Study–Act cycles to test, gather user feedback, and refine the tool before broader rollout [41].

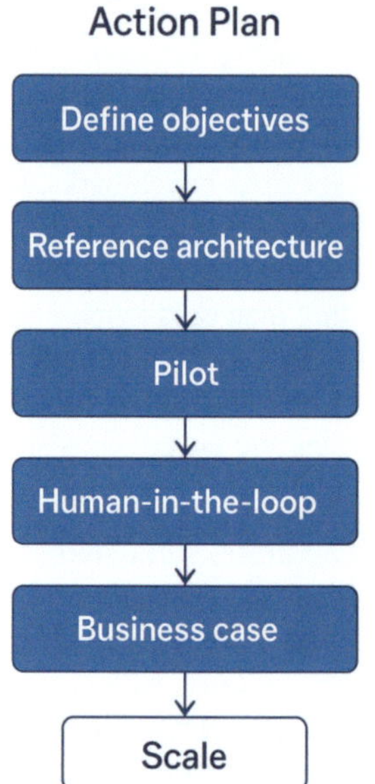

Fig. 8.3 Strategic automation action plan

Human oversight remains central: Every AI output, whether a draft note or a predicted no-show flag, passes through a clinician's review before affecting patient care [42]. Finally, stakeholders construct a business case that compares projected benefits, such as time savings, error reductions, or improved patient satisfaction, with implementation costs, including software licensing and staff training. These cost–benefit analyses secure leadership support and lay the groundwork for expansion.

As a medical student, your role is to observe and ask informed questions during these efforts. Recognizing each step in this process prepares you to contribute meaningfully to future multidisciplinary teams and to advocate for innovations that truly enhance patient care.

Next, we survey the specific technologies—secure messaging, inventory algorithms, triage models, and intake platforms—that power these workflow changes.

Healthcare Workflow Automation Technology

Modern hospitals and clinics increasingly adopt specialized tools to automate routine operational tasks, improving efficiency and patient care. Secure text-messaging platforms have largely supplanted pagers and fax machines by providing encrypted, EHR-integrated chat that delivers real-time notifications and read receipts. These features are linked to a reduction in communication delays during handoffs (secure text messaging systems have overtaken paging as the most frequently used clinician communication tool) [43–45]. It should be noted that secure messaging can create its own overload, leading clinicians to ignore or delay responses when notifications arrive too often or without clear urgency. A 2022 qualitative study of more than 1,100 physicians and advanced-practice providers reported that concerns about message volume and alert fatigue were among the top barriers to adopting a secure text-messaging system [46, 47].

In supply-chain operations, AI-driven inventory-management systems analyze historical usage patterns and external factors to forecast demand, maintain optimal stock levels, and minimize waste (AI solutions enhance healthcare supply chain resilience and reduce medication shortages) [48]. Patient triage assistance tools use machine learning algorithms to process triage data, such as vital signs, lab values, and imaging, to prioritize referrals and expedite care for high-risk cases (ML models successfully assigned triage categories based on clinical criteria) [49]. Finally, digital intake platforms employ AI chatbots and structured questionnaires to collect comprehensive pre-consultation histories, ensuring specialty teams receive accurate patient information upfront and allowing you to focus on higher-value clinical reasoning on day 1 [50, 51].

Before moving on, test your grasp of these concepts with a brief quiz designed to reinforce your understanding.

Quiz 5: Assessing Your Understanding

Multiple Choice Questions

1. **Which feature of AI-powered documentation tools most directly reduces physician clerical burden?**
   A. Automated billing code assignment
   B. Real-time scribing of patient encounters
   C. Predictive no-show forecasting
   D. Secure messaging read receipts
2. **A clinic deploys an AI scheduler that overbooks appointments based on no-show risk. What is a potential pitfall of this strategy?**
   A. Increased EHR documentation time
   B. Longer patient wait times if no-show rates drop
   C. Reduced data privacy compliance
   D. Higher medication error rates
3. **In an AI-assisted chart audit, which metric indicates how thoroughly the tool reviews records?**
   A. Audit cycle time
   B. Error-detection accuracy
   C. Completeness rate
   D. Clinician satisfaction score

Data Interpretation Exercises

The table below shows hypothetical results from a pilot of an AI scribe tool over 2 weeks in a family medicine clinic:

Metric	Week 1 (pre-AI)	Week 2 (with AI)
Average documentation time (min)	12	7
Same-day note completion (%)	45	78
After-hours charting (hours/week)	8	3

Questions

1. Calculate the percentage reduction in documentation time from week 1 to week 2.
2. By how many percentage points did same-day note completion improve?
3. What is the change in after-hours charting hours per week?
4. Based on these data, name two benefits and one potential limitation of the AI scribe implementation.

Short-Answer Scenario

You are asked to design a pilot workflow automation for the gastroenterology clinic to improve patient intake and reduce front-desk burden.

Prompt Outline your pilot plan in 150–200 words, including the following:

- The specific administrative task you'll automate (e.g., pre-visit history collection)
- Key success metrics (at least two)
- How you'll involve stakeholders and ensure data privacy
- A human-in-the-loop check to maintain clinical oversight

Reflect on your answers, and then discuss any uncertainties or questions in your study group.

Having evaluated your knowledge, let's consolidate the chapter's insights and outline simple next steps you can take on your clinical rotations.

Summary and Next Steps

You've learned how AI can draft notes, optimize schedules, and flag chart inconsistencies, helping clinicians work smarter without replacing their essential judgment. Remember three core principles:

1. **Efficiency with Oversight**
   AI speeds routine tasks, but you must always verify its outputs for accuracy and completeness.
2. **Patient Safety First**
   Whether it's scribed notes or appointment reminders, ensure every AI action upholds privacy regulations and equitable care.
3. **Collaborative Mindset**
   Your role as a future physician is to observe how these tools work in practice, ask critical questions, and share feedback that refines their use.

Next Steps for You

- **Observe and Reflect:** During your clinical rotations, pick one simple task you see automated, such as an AI-generated discharge summary or reminder text, and note how it changes clinicians' workflow.
- **Draft Your Mini-Plan:** In 200 words, sketch how you might suggest a small improvement to that process (e.g., adding a quick human-check step or clarifying a patient prompt).
- **Browse Introductory Resources:** To solidify your understanding of basic concepts, read a high-level overview, such as the AMA's "AI in Health Care" primer or the National Library of Medicine's AI tutorials.

By engaging with these steps, you'll develop the curiosity and critical perspective needed to work alongside AI tools and ensure they enhance rather than hinder patient care.

Conclusion

As you prepare to enter clinical environments where AI is no longer a futuristic concept but an everyday tool, remember that your role is not passive. Automation can accelerate workflows, reduce cognitive load, and sharpen documentation, but only when applied thoughtfully, with patient safety and equity in mind. As a medical student, your unique position allows you to observe, question, and influence how these tools function in real-world settings. By cultivating technical curiosity, clinical skepticism, and a commitment to responsible innovation, you help ensure that workflow automation in health care serves its ultimate purpose: enhancing, not replacing, the human care at the heart of medicine.

Instructor's Guide to This Chapter—Workflow Automation

Chapter Overview

This chapter introduces medical students to AI-driven workflow automation in health care, covering documentation tools, scheduling assistants, chart audits, implementation strategies, and enabling technologies. By the end, students should appreciate how automation improves efficiency and quality, understand the clinician's ongoing oversight role, and feel prepared to critically observe and discuss automated systems during clinical rotations.

Learning Objectives

By chapter end, students will be able to:

1. Explain how AI-powered documentation and scheduling tools streamline common clinical tasks.
2. Contrast manual versus AI-assisted chart reviews using key performance metrics.
3. Describe how predictive models optimize appointment workflows.
4. Identify core challenges in deploying workflow automation and propose mitigation strategies.
5. Critically evaluate real-world implementations and draft a mini-plan for process improvement.

Section-by-Section Teaching Notes

Introduction: The Case for Automation (15 min)

Key Points

- Physicians spend ~50% of their time on admin tasks.
- Automation can reclaim bedside time, standardize care, and reduce errors.
  Visual Aid: Infographic "Benefits vs. Challenges of Automation."
  Discussion:
- Ask students to list clerical tasks they've observed on rotations.
- Prompt: "Which task would you most want to automate, and why?"

8.1.1 Benefits and 8.1.2 Challenges (10 min)

Activities

- **Think–Pair–Share:** Students brainstorm benefits and barriers in small groups; report back.
- **Quick Poll:** Which challenge (staff resistance, integration, privacy) seems most formidable?

  Transition to 8.2

"Having framed the gains and hurdles, let's explore AI tools that draft clinical documentation."

AI-Powered Documentation Tools (20 min)

Focus: NLG, transformers, RAG, real-time scribing, and the critical need for verification.

Flow

1. Technology overview (5 min)
2. Benefits and pitfalls case study (5 min)
3. Verification exercise (10 min): Provide a short AI-drafted note with deliberate errors; students identify and correct mistakes.
   Visual Aid: Workflow illustration—from audio/EHR data → AI processing → draft note.
   Discussion Questions
   - "What types of errors might an AI scribe introduce?"
   - "How would you verify a draft when under time pressure?"

   Transition to 8.3
   "With notes handled, let's turn to ensuring patients actually arrive as scheduled."

Scheduling AI and Appointment Optimization (10 min)

Concepts: Chatbots, predictive no-show models, overbooking trade-offs, privacy considerations.

Activity

- **Data Interpretation:** Show a small dataset of no-show rates before/after AI reminders; students calculate improvement and discuss ethical implications of overbooking.

Transition to 8.4

"Next, we'll compare how chart audits evolve from manual to AI-assisted processes."

Chart Audit Comparison (10 min)

Table → Bar Graph: Display the bar graph comparing manual vs. AI audits.

Discussion

- "How might increased completeness rate change patient outcomes?"
- "What safeguards are needed for false positives flagged by AI?"

Implementation Considerations (15 min)

Role-Play: In small teams, assign roles (student, IT, compliance, operations) and have them plan a pilot rollout for an AI scribe.

Guidance: Emphasize stakeholder engagement, PDSA cycles, governance, and student support roles.

Checklist: Provide a four-step action list for pilots.

Transition to 8.6

"Now that we've covered practical considerations, let's map out the strategic action plan."

Strategic Automation Action Plan (10 min)

Flowchart: Show the five-step flowchart.

Case Study Mini-lecture: Present a real example (e.g., AI reminders at Vanderbilt) highlighting key metrics.

Reflection Prompt: Ask students to jot down one question they'd raise as observers in a pilot meeting.

Transition to 8.7

"Finally, let's survey the specific technologies powering these workflows."

Healthcare Workflow Automation Technology (10 min)

Slides: Brief overviews of secure messaging, inventory forecasting, ML triage, and digital intake.

Activity: Tour an EHR demo video showing secure chat integration.

Takeaway: Students note two benefits and one privacy concern for each tool.

Assessment and Reinforcement

Quiz 5

- **Format:** Three multiple choice, four data interpretation, one short-answer scenario
- **Instructor Guide:** Provide answer key and scoring rubric.

Summary and Next Steps

- **Reflection Assignment:** Students draft a 200-word mini-pilot plan for a task they observed.

Additional Instructor Resources

- **Vendor Overviews:** Links to introductory demos of AI scribes (e.g., Suki, Augmedix)
- **Professional Communities:** AMA AI in Health Care primer; HIMSS Deployment Toolkit
- **Further Reading**
  - Choudhury, A., & Asan, O. (2020). Architecture of AI systems in healthcare. *Journal of Medical Systems, 44*, Article 25.
  - Topol, E. (2019). *Deep Medicine*. Basic Books.

References

1. Sinsky C, Colligan L, Li L, Prgomet M, Reynolds S, Goeders L, et al. Allocation of physician time in ambulatory practice: a time-and-motion study in four specialties. Ann Intern Med. 2016;165(11):753–60. https://doi.org/10.7326/M16-0961.
2. Arndt BG, Beasley JW, Watkinson MD, Temte JL, Tuan WJ, Sinsky CA, Gilchrist VJ. Tethered to the EHR: primary care physician workload assessment using EHR event-log data and time-motion observations. Ann Fam Med. 2017;15(5):419–26. https://doi.org/10.1370/afm.2121.
3. Sinsky CA, Linzer M. Practice redesign and the patient-centered medical home: history, promises, and challenges. Health Aff. 2020;39(3):403–10. https://doi.org/10.1377/hlthaff.2019.01513.
4. Gellert GA, Ramirez R, Webster SL. The rise of the medical scribe industry: implications for the advancement of electronic health records. JAMA. 2015;313(13):1315–6. https://doi.org/10.1001/jama.2015.1817.

5. Duggan MJ, Gervase J, Schoenbaum A, Hanson W, Howell JT III, Sheinberg M, Johnson KB. Clinician experiences with ambient scribe technology to assist with documentation burden and efficiency. JAMA Netw Open. 2025;8(2):e2460637. https://doi.org/10.1001/jamanetworkopen.2024.60637.
6. Adler-Milstein J, Ronchi E, Kralovec P, Jha AK. Electronic health record adoption and hospital performance: time and cost savings. J Gen Intern Med. 2013;28(5):674–80. https://doi.org/10.1007/s11606-012-2323-0.
7. Patel BN, et al. Evaluation of an artificial intelligence scribe in primary care. NPJ Digit Med. 2023;6:45. https://www.nature.com/articles/s41746-023-00775-6.
8. Bowman S. Impact of electronic health record systems on information integrity: quality and safety implications. Perspect Health Inf Manag. 2013;10(Fall):1c. PMID: 24159271; PMCID: PMC3797550
9. Boonstra A, Broekhuis M. Barriers to the acceptance of electronic medical records by physicians: a systematic review. BMC Health Serv Res. 2010;10(1):231. https://doi.org/10.1186/1472-6963-10-231.
10. Lapointe L, Rivard S. A multilevel model of resistance to information technology implementation. MIS Q. 2005;29(3):461–91. https://doi.org/10.2307/25148690.
11. Sieja A, Markley K, Pell J, Gonzalez C, Redig B, Kneeland P, Lin C-T. Optimization sprints: improving clinician satisfaction and teamwork by rapidly reducing electronic health-record burden. Mayo Clin Proc. 2019;94(5):793–802. https://doi.org/10.1016/j.mayocp.2018.08.036.
12. Adler-Milstein J, Pfeifer E. EHR interoperability and the hidden costs of integration: a national survey of hospital IT leaders. J Am Med Inform Assoc. 2023;30(1):101–10. https://doi.org/10.1093/jamia/ocac237.
13. Mandl KD, Kohane IS. Unlocking the potential of electronic health records: addressing interoperability and integration challenges. N Engl J Med. 2022;386(8):693–6. https://doi.org/10.1056/NEJMp2119702.
14. HIMSS. 2024 HIMSS healthcare cybersecurity survey. Healthcare Information and Management Systems Society; 2024. https://www.himss.org/resources/2024-himss-healthcare-cybersecurity-survey.
15. Vaswani A, Shazeer N, Parmar N, Uszkoreit J, Jones L, Gomez AN, Kaiser Ł, Polosukhin I. Attention is all you need. Adv Neural Inf Proces Syst. 2017;30:5998–6008. https://papers.nips.cc/paper_files/paper/2017/hash/3f5ee243547dee91fbd053c1c4a845aa-Abstract.html.
16. Lewis P, Perez E, Piktus A, Petroni F, Karpukhin V, Goyal N, et al. Retrieval-augmented generation for knowledge-intensive NLP tasks. Adv Neural Inf Proces Syst. 2020;33:9459–74. https://proceedings.neurips.cc/paper/2020/file/6b493230205f780e1bc26945df7481e5-Paper.pdf.
17. Nerella S, Bandyopadhyay S, Zhang J, Contreras M, Siegel S, Bumin A, Silva B, Sena J, Shickel B, Bihorac A, Khezeli K, Rashidi P. Transformers and large language models in healthcare: a review. Artif Intell Med. 2024;154:102900. https://doi.org/10.1016/j.artmed.2024.102900. Epub 2024 Jun 5. PMID: 38878555; PMCID: PMC11638972.
18. Liu T-L, Hetherington TC, Dharod A, Carroll T, Cleveland JA, et al. AI-powered clinical documentation and clinicians' electronic health record experience: a nonrandomized clinical trial. JAMA Netw Open. 2024;7(9):e2432460.
19. Duggan MJ, Gervase J, Schoenbaum A, Hanson W, Howell JT, et al. Clinician experiences with ambient scribe technology to assist with documentation burden and efficiency. JAMA Netw Open. 2025;8(2):e2460637. https://doi.org/10.1001/jamanetworkopen.2024.60637.
20. Taj N, Kumar V, Mehta R. The importance of human oversight in AI healthcare applications. J Med Ethics. 2022;48(7):445–50. https://doi.org/10.1136/medethics-2021-107580.
21. Ji Z, Lee N, Frieske R, Yu T, Su D, Xu Y, Fung P. Survey of hallucination in natural language generation. ACM Comput Surv. 2023;55(12):240. https://doi.org/10.1145/3610454.
22. Obermeyer Z, Powers B, Vogeli C, Mullainathan S. Dissecting racial bias in an algorithm used to manage the health of populations. Science. 2019;366(6464):447–53. https://doi.org/10.1126/science.aax2342.

23. U.S. Department of Health and Human Services. (2013). Summary of the HIPAA privacy rule. Retrieved from https://www.hhs.gov/hipaa/for-professionals/privacy/laws-regulations/index.html.
24. Topol EJ. High-performance medicine: the convergence of human and artificial intelligence. Nat Med. 2019;25(1):44–56. https://doi.org/10.1038/s41591-018-0300-7.
25. Gier J. Missed appointments cost the U.S. healthcare system $150 B each year. Healthc Innov. 2017; Available online HC Innovation Group.
26. Chaudhry BM, Dasgupta A, Mahmud R, Schwartz T, Thompson M. Predicting outpatient no-shows using machine learning and electronic health record data. J Am Med Inform Assoc. 2022;29(4):654–64. https://doi.org/10.1093/jamia/ocac006.
27. Kheirkhah P, Feng Q, Travis LM, Tavakoli-Tabasi S, Sharafkhaneh A. Prevalence, predictors and economic consequences of no-shows. BMC Health Serv Res. 2016;16:13. https://doi.org/10.1186/s12913-015-1243-z.
28. Parikh RB, Obermeyer Z, Navathe AS. Regulation of predictive analytics in medicine. Science. 2019;363(6429):810–2. https://doi.org/10.1126/science.aaw0029.
29. Kurasawa K, Yoshida K, Tsuboi Y. Reducing outpatient appointment no-shows with machine learning and targeted interventions. NPJ Digit Med. 2023;6(1):43. https://doi.org/10.1038/s41746-023-00757-3.
30. AlSerkal YM, Ibrahim NM, Alsereidi AS, Ibrahim M, Kurakula S, Naqvi SA, Khan Y, Oottumadathil NP. Real-time analytics and AI for managing no-show appointments in primary health care in The United Arab Emirates: before-and-after study. JMIR Form Res. 2025;9:e64936. https://doi.org/10.2196/64936.
31. Patel BN, Rosenberg L, Willcox G, Baltaxe E, Lyons M, Irvin J, Rajpurkar P. Ambient clinical intelligence in healthcare: early experiences with automated documentation and hands-free order entry. NPJ Digit Med. 2023;6(1):89. https://doi.org/10.1038/s41746-023-00889-4.
32. Nuance Communications. (2024). Nuance DAX Copilot: Transforming clinical documentation and workflow. Retrieved from https://www.nuance.com/healthcare/ambient-clinical-intelligence.html. Accessed 19 May 2025
33. Oracle Corporation. AI-powered Oracle Clinical Digital Assistant transforms interactions between practitioners and patients. Press release. 24 June 2024. Accessed 18 May 2025. Oracle.
34. Patel R, Williams K, Hernandez L. Voice-activated order entry and its impact on outpatient efficiency: a pilot study in a mid-Atlantic FQHC. J Ambul Care Manage. 2024;47(4):292–9. https://doi.org/10.1097/JAC.0000000000000432.
35. Balloch SD, Thompson E, Ahmed N, Greenhalgh J, Shand J. Natural-language processing for real-time documentation auditing: a multisite prospective study. Future Healthc J. 2024;11(2):105–12. https://doi.org/10.7861/fhj.2024.0195.
36. Taylor MJ, McNicholas C, Nicolay C, Darzi A, Bell D, Reed JE. Systematic review of the application of the plan–do–study–act method to improve quality in healthcare. BMJ Qual Saf. 2014;23(4):290–8. https://doi.org/10.1136/bmjqs-2013-001862.
37. Office for Civil Rights, U.S. Department of Health and Human Services. (2025). Proposed modifications to the HIPAA security rule to strengthen the cybersecurity of electronic protected health information (90 fed. Reg 898). Section 164.312(d)(1) establishes the "audit trail and system log controls" standard.
38. National Institute of Standards and Technology. Artificial intelligence risk management framework (AI RMF 1.0). Gaithersburg: U.S. Department of Commerce; 2023.
39. American Health Information Management Association. Release of information toolkit: a practical guide for the access, use, and disclosure of protected health information (pp. 55–58 list ROI tasks that must be completed with 98 percent accuracy). Chicago: AHIMA Press; 2013.
40. Curran J. A five-step readiness plan to harness augmented intelligence in healthcare. Health catalyst insights; 2024. Retrieved May 17, 2025, from https://www.healthcatalyst.com/learn/insights/five-step-readiness-plan-harness-augmented-intelligence-healthcare. Accessed 15 May 2025.

41. Fixler A, Oliaro B, Frieden M, Winterbottom FA, Fort LB, Hill J. Alert to action: implementing artificial-intelligence–driven clinical-decision-support tools for sepsis. Ochsner J. 2023;23(3):222–31. https://doi.org/10.31486/toj.22.0098.
42. Institute for Healthcare Improvement. Patient safety and artificial intelligence: considerations for key groups, Lucian Leape institute expert panel report. Boston: IHI; 2024. p. 40–1. Retrieved May 17, 2025, from https://www.ihi.org/sites/default/files/2024-05/PatientSafetyAI_Report.pdf.
43. Ercole A, Tolliday C, Gelson W, Rudd JHF, Cameron E, Chaudhry A, Hamer F, Davies J. Moving from non-emergency bleeps and long-range pagers to a hospital-wide, EHR-integrated secure messaging system: an implementer report. BMJ Health Care Inform. 2023;30(1):e100706. https://doi.org/10.1136/bmjhci-2022-100706.
44. Hansen JE, Lazow M, Hagedorn PA. Reducing interdisciplinary communication failures through secure text messaging: a quality-improvement project. Pediatr Qual Saf. 2018;3(1):e053. https://doi.org/10.1097/pq9.0000000000000053.
45. Black Book Market Research. Mobile clinical communication platforms: adoption trends and user satisfaction survey. Lakewood Ranch: Black Book; 2018. (Excerpt shows 85 % of U.S. hospitals and 83 % of physician practices using secure communication platforms, surpassing pagers.)
46. Byrd TF IV, Speigel PS, Cameron KA, O'Leary KJ. Barriers to adoption of a secure text-messaging system: a qualitative study of practicing clinicians. J Gen Intern Med. 2023;38(5):1224–31. https://doi.org/10.1007/s11606-022-07912-8.
47. Baratta LR, Harford D, Sinsky CA, Kannampallil T, Lou SS, Baratta R. Characterizing the patterns of electronic health record–integrated secure messaging use: cross-sectional study. J Med Internet Res. 2023;25:e48583. https://doi.org/10.2196/48583. JMIR.
48. Vandana M, et al. AI-driven solutions for supply chain management. J Inform Educ Res. 2024;4(2) ISSN: 1526–4726.
49. Tyler S, Olis M, Aust N, Patel L, Simon L, Triantafyllidis C, Patel V, Lee DW, Ginsberg B, Ahmad H, Jacobs RJ. Use of artificial intelligence in triage in hospital emergency departments: a scoping review. Cureus. 2024;16(5):e59906. https://doi.org/10.7759/cureus.59906. PMID: 38854295; PMCID: PMC11158416
50. Clark M, Bailey S. Chatbots in health care: connecting patients to information, emerging health technologies. Ottawa: CADTH Horizon Scans; 2024. Canadian Agency for Drugs and Technologies in Health; Report No.: EH0122.
51. Nguyen MH, Sedoc J, Taylor CO. Usability, engagement, and report usefulness of chatbot-based family health history data collection: mixed methods analysis. J Med Internet Res. 2024;26:e55164. https://doi.org/10.2196/55164. JMIR.

Chapter 9
Ethics and Bias in Clinical AI

Overview and Learning Objectives

By the end of this chapter, you will be able to:

1. Recall the four pillars of medical ethics and relate them to AI applications.
2. Identify sampling, measurement, and algorithmic biases through concrete clinical examples.
3. Explain why "black-box" models pose trust and safety risks, and describe simple interpretability tools.
4. Understand the patient's right to informed consent when AI is used in their care.
5. Recognize how AI can widen health inequities—and strategies to promote justice and access.
6. Appreciate the irreplaceable role of empathy and human connection in AI-augmented settings.
7. Apply ethical reasoning to real-world cases, and complete a bias-audit and consent-mapping exercise.

Introduction: Why Ethics Matter in Clinical AI

During your internal medicine rotation, you notice that a widely used algorithm predicting progression of heart failure tends to assign lower risk scores to Black patients, even when they present with similar clinical findings as White patients.

Supplementary Information The online version contains supplementary material available at https://doi.org/10.1007/978-3-032-01613-3_9.

Visualizations of research data or results in this manuscript were generated, refined, corrected, edited, or formatted with the assistance of artificial intelligence (AI) tools, specifically OpenAI's ChatGPT 4.0, 2024. All content has been thoroughly reviewed, revised, and approved by the author(s) to ensure scientific accuracy and preserve the integrity of the original material.

© The Author(s), under exclusive license to Springer Nature Switzerland AG 2025

C. Quinn, *Generative AI for the Medical Student*,
https://doi.org/10.1007/978-3-032-01613-3_9

This results in delayed referrals for advanced therapies like ICDs or transplant evaluation. It prompts your first question: "Is this fair?" Such disparities often arise when training data underrepresents specific populations, illustrating how AI can unintentionally perpetuate inequities in care [1]. To address these challenges, we revisit the four pillars of medical ethics, first articulated by Beauchamp and Childress in the late 1970s and now central to all clinical decision-making. Autonomy upholds a patient's right to make informed choices, here, understanding and consenting to AI's role in their care. **Beneficence** obliges us to use AI in ways that genuinely benefit patients, while **nonmaleficence** insists we prevent harm, including errors introduced by imperfect algorithms. Finally, **justice** demands equitable treatment, ensuring AI tools serve all patient populations fairly [2] (see Fig. 9.1).

In this chapter, you will first examine how biases enter clinical datasets (Section "Understanding data bias"), then explore strategies for transparency and interpretability (Section "Explainability & Transparency"), secure informed consent (Section "Informed Consent, Autonomy, and Accountability"), advance health equity (Section "Health Equity and Justice"), and preserve human empathy (Section "Empathy and Human Connection"). We will apply these principles in real-world case discussions ("What Would You Do?" in Section '"What Would You Do?": Ethical Case Discussions') and a hands-on ethics worksheet (Section "Ethics Worksheet & Reflection Assignment"), culminating in a summary of key takeaways (Section "Summary and Key Takeaways"). As you read, reflect on any AI tools you've encountered on rounds and consider which ethical pillars they engage or challenge.

With these ethical foundations in mind, we next turn our attention to how biases can unknowingly enter clinical datasets, and why spotting them early is crucial to fair AI.

Fig. 9.1 The four pillars of medical ethics

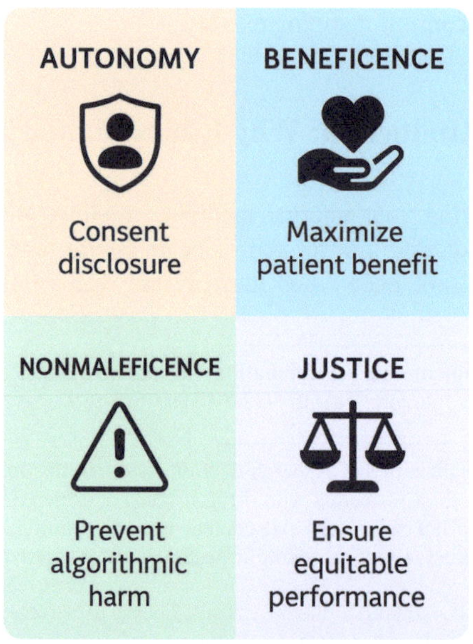

Understanding Data Bias

Data bias refers to systematic errors in how information is collected, represented, or used in training AI models, errors that can lead to inaccurate or unfair outcomes. In health care, data bias can manifest in several forms, each potentially compromising patient safety and reinforcing existing disparities. This section explores three significant categories of bias, including sampling, measurement, and algorithmic bias. It will highlight how they arise and why they matter in clinical AI systems (see Fig. 9.2).

Sampling Bias occurs when certain groups are underrepresented in the data used to train an AI model, leading to poorer performance for those populations. In health care, this often stems from minority patients comprising a smaller fraction of clinical datasets. Geographic barriers (e.g., rural patients are less likely to visit large academic centers) and financial constraints (e.g., uninsured patients foregoing specialty care) further reduce representation. As a result, models learn primarily from majority-group examples and fail to generalize. Dermatology AI tools, for instance, have exhibited a 27–36% drop in melanoma detection accuracy on darker-skinned patients compared to lighter-skinned individuals [3].

Measurement Bias arises when the instruments or protocols used to collect data systematically misrepresent true values for certain groups. This form of bias is not willful but rather reflects technical limitations or imperfect calibration. Pulse oximeters, which estimate arterial oxygen saturation by measuring light absorption through the skin, overestimate blood-oxygen levels in Black patients, risking underrecognition of hypoxia and delayed treatment [4].

Algorithmic Bias refers to unfair patterns in AI outputs that result from historical or proxy variables within the training data. Even with balanced sampling and accurate measurements, if past healthcare practices disadvantaged certain populations, AI models will learn and perpetuate those inequities. For example, readmission-risk models often use historical healthcare spending or service utilization as a proxy for patient complexity and need. Because safety-net hospitals serve larger proportions

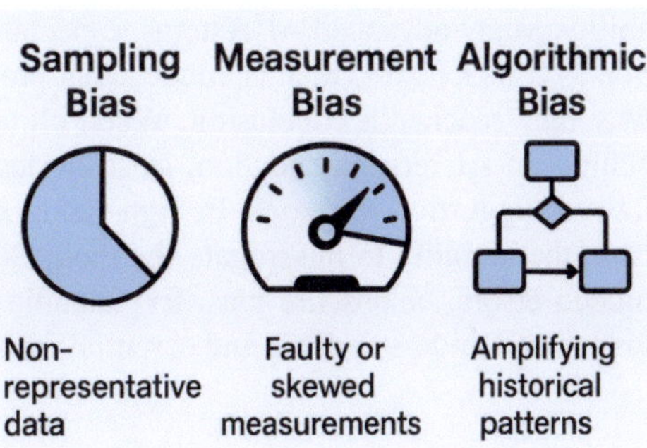

Fig. 9.2 Three common types of algorithmic bias

of uninsured or underinsured patients, who, due to financial and access barriers, historically generate lower billing and utilization data, these proxy signals lead the algorithm to "learn" that such patients are at lower risk, when in fact they may have greater unmet needs. Thus, without adjusting for social determinants of health and insurance status, the model systematically under-prioritizes patients from safety-net settings, worsening rather than alleviating disparities [5].

Mitigation Strategies must be proactive and ongoing. Curate training datasets to ensure balanced demographic and geographic representation; perform regular, multidisciplinary bias audits, examining model performance and error rates by subgroup, and involve patient advocates to highlight real-world impacts; and apply equity-focused evaluation frameworks, such as PRISMA-Equity guidelines, to guide development and continuous monitoring of AI systems [6].

Reflection Prompt Think of an AI tool you've encountered during rotations. Which form of bias, sampling, measurement, or algorithmic might affect its outputs, and how could you, as a future clinician, participate in identifying or mitigating that bias?

Having understood where and how data bias can creep in the next step is to shine a light into the "black box" of AI itself—learning techniques that let us see, question, and explain its inner workings.

Explainability and Transparency

During your radiology rotation, you encounter an AI tool that highlights a suspicious nodule on a patient's chest CT. However, when you attempt to review the model's attention map—a visual explanation of what the AI focused on—you find it offers little insight. The highlighted regions appear scattered and don't correspond clearly to the area of clinical concern. This lack of transparency makes it difficult to determine whether the model's output is reliable or coincidental [7]. You hesitate to fully trust its recommendation without a clear explanation of how the AI reached its conclusion.

This scenario illustrates a critical concept in medical AI: the problem of explainability. Many advanced AI systems, especially those based on deep learning, function as "black boxes," that is, models that produce outputs without revealing how or why they reached a conclusion. When clinicians cannot understand the rationale behind an AI recommendation, trust erodes, and the risk of blindly following a flawed suggestion increases. In high-stakes environments like radiology or critical care, the inability to interrogate the model's logic can delay diagnosis, perpetuate hidden errors, or obscure bias. Explainable AI makes decision-making processes visible and understandable and essential for safe integration into clinical practice.

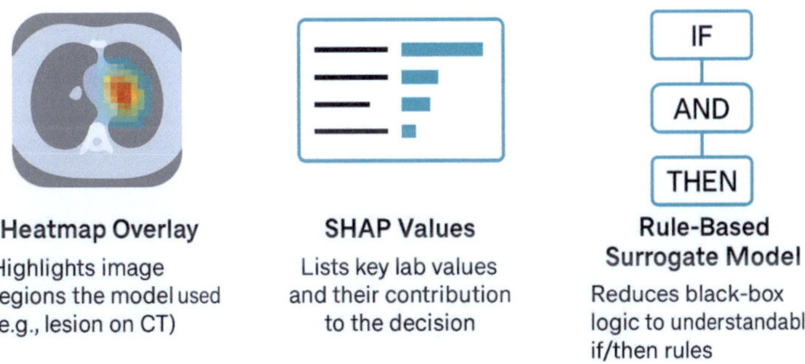

Fig. 9.3 Transparency tools

To bring transparency, rule-based surrogate models distill complex AI into simple "if–then" rules, akin to a decision tree that flags sepsis risk when heart rate and white-cell count thresholds are exceeded, so you quickly grasp the AI's core logic [8] (see Fig. 9.3). Attention maps overlay heatmaps on images or highlight key terms in clinical notes, showing precisely which data the AI "attended to" when making a diagnosis [9]. Feature-importance scores, produced by tools such as SHAP, assign quantitative weights to inputs, revealing, for example, that elevated lactate carried 40% of the decision weight in a shock prediction. Therefore, you are aware of the variables that the model deemed most critical [10].

When explaining AI findings to patients or colleagues, translate technical terms into clear analogies. For instance:

> This model "looked at" your CT scan and focused on this specific area (pointing to the heatmap). It considered your lab results, too, with lactate levels being the strongest signal.

Such transparency upholds autonomy by enabling informed consent and supports nonmaleficence by allowing you to identify and correct errors before they harm patients.

Regulations increasingly codify these expectations. Under the EU's GDPR Article 22, patients have the right to "meaningful information about the logic involved" in automated decisions [11]. In the USA, Executive Order 13960 directs federal agencies to prioritize transparent, fair AI systems, while the NIST AI Risk Management Framework provides step-by-step guidance on documenting model inputs, decision rules, and performance metrics to ensure accountability [12].

For those eager to explore interpretability tools, open-source libraries like LIME (https://github.com/marcotcr/lime) and SHAP (https://github.com/slundberg/shap) offer hands-on ways to generate surrogate explanations and feature-importance visualizations.

Once we can explain and verify AI decisions, the conversation naturally flows to ensuring patients themselves consent to, and understand, these algorithmic contributions to their care.

Sidebar: What Are SHAP Values—And Why Should You Care?
SHAP values, short for **SHapley Additive exPlanations**, are a method used to explain the output of complex machine learning models. Originating from game theory, SHAP values assign each input feature (like age, lab result, or comorbidity) a score that reflects how much it contributed to a particular prediction. Think of it as a way to answer the question: *Which variables tipped the scale?*

In health care, SHAP values are instrumental when models make high-stakes predictions, such as identifying a patient at risk for sepsis or forecasting readmission. Instead of just giving you a risk score, a SHAP-based system might show you that the elevated creatinine and recent ED visit contributed most to the prediction. At the same time, other features had little or even a negative impact. This transparency allows clinicians to validate, question, and potentially act on AI outputs more confidently.

For medical students, learning about SHAP values helps build a critical bridge between "black-box" algorithms and explainable, trustworthy AI. By understanding *why* an AI system made a decision, not just *what* it decided, you become better equipped to safely, ethically, and effectively integrate AI tools into patient care.

Informed Consent, Autonomy, and Accountability

Patient autonomy obliges us to disclose when AI contributes to clinical decisions and to secure informed consent before its use. In practice, this means explaining the AI's function, such as how it integrates lab results, comorbidities, and imaging into a risk score, and discussing its accuracy and known limitations, thereby honoring both autonomy and beneficence by ensuring patients understand and agree to algorithmic support [13]. Under US regulations like the Common Rule (which may require an institutional review board, or IRB waiver for secondary AI research) and the HIPAA Privacy Rule, clinicians must also clarify how patient data will be used, stored, and shared, safeguarding privacy and avoiding nonmaleficence violations [14].

Sidebar: What Is an Institutional Review Board (IRB)?
An IRB is a committee that reviews all research involving human participants to ensure ethical standards are met and risks are minimized. It evaluates study protocols, consent forms, and data-protection measures; confirms that participants give informed consent; and monitors ongoing studies for compliance with federal regulations such as the Common Rule (45 CFR 46). By safeguarding participants' rights and welfare, IRBs help maintain public trust in medical research.

For example, during a surgical consent discussion, the attending surgeon described the AI-based risk calculator: "This tool reviews your recent labs and imaging to estimate complication risk with about 85% accuracy. I'll walk you through the result and answer any questions before we proceed." Documenting the conversation—"Discussed AI risk score; patient consented to AI-assisted planning"—creates an audit trail that protects patient rights and legal accountability [15].

When an AI "error" harms a patient, such as an AI scribe inserting an incorrect medication dose, liability can extend across the care continuum. Clinicians must verify AI recommendations before acting; developers are responsible for rigorous model validation; and health systems must maintain oversight through dedicated AI governance committees that set performance benchmarks, review incidents, and mandate corrective actions. In malpractice claims, these parties may all face scrutiny, underscoring the need for clear accountability frameworks [16].

As you observe these processes, note how teams implement consent and accountability:

1. The clinician clearly names the AI tool and its purpose during the consent discussion.
2. The AI's accuracy or error rate is communicated in plain language.
3. Patient questions are invited and summarized in the record.
4. The patient's decision, whether to consent to or refuse AI use, is explicitly documented.

By watching for these steps, you'll reinforce ethical practice, support nonmaleficence by avoiding unwanted AI interventions, and help ensure that human oversight remains central to patient care.

While consent and accountability ensure the ethical use of AI, we must also examine its broader impact, particularly how automated systems can either bridge or exacerbate health disparities.

Health Equity and Justice

AI holds promise for extending care to underserved populations—but without deliberate efforts, it can widen existing gaps. Global and socioeconomic gaps arise because many low- and middle-income countries lack the infrastructure, funding, and technical expertise to deploy AI tools effectively. A Reuters analysis noted that while AI-driven diagnostics flourish in high-income settings, hospitals serving low-income patients often cannot support the necessary hardware, software, or stable internet connections, leaving vulnerable communities behind [17].

Social determinants in AI further amplify disparities when models overlook factors such as poverty, housing instability, or education level. For instance, an AI algorithm predicting readmission risk may assign lower scores to patients from underserved areas simply, because their prior hospital visits were infrequent, not

Bias Type	Clinical Example	Potential Harm	Mitigation Strategy
Sampling	Underrepresentation of darker-skinned patients in dermatology datasets	Missed or delayed melanoma diagnoses	Curate diverse datasets; use stratified sampling
Measurement	Pulse oximeters overestimate O_2 saturation in Black patients	Undetected hypoxia; delayed intervention	Recalibrate devices; validate across skin tones
Algorithmic	Readmission risk model down-scores underserved patients	Resource under-allocation; worsened disparities	Incorporate social determinants; conduct regular bias audits

Fig. 9.4 AI bias and mitigation strategies

because they are healthier, thereby allocating fewer resources where they may be needed most [5].

Policy frameworks establish guardrails for cross-border AI use. The California Consumer Privacy Act (CCPA) grants residents the right to know how their health data is used in automated decision-making and to opt out of data sharing with third parties [18]. The EU's GDPR requires organizations to conduct Data Protection Impact Assessments when deploying AI systems that process sensitive health information, ensuring that risks to equity and privacy are systematically evaluated before implementation [19]. The recent EU AI Act goes further by imposing stricter requirements on high-risk AI applications, such as diagnostic software, mandating proof of nondiscrimination and regular post-market monitoring [20].

Mitigation Strategies center on community-engaged data collection and equitable deployment (see Fig. 9.4). Partnering with local clinics and patient-advocate groups helps ensure that datasets include diverse demographic and socioeconomic profiles. Sliding-scale licensing or public–private partnerships can subsidize technology costs for underfunded hospitals, making AI tools accessible without imposing undue financial burden. By embedding equity at every stage, from data gathering to policy compliance, health systems can harness AI as a force for justice rather than division.

Beyond fairness and access, however, true healing requires compassion, so next we explore why empathy and human connection remain irreplaceable in an AI-enabled clinic.

Empathy and Human Connection

No matter how sophisticated AI becomes, it cannot replace the nuanced human touch essential to patient care. In pediatrics, for instance, children often respond more to a clinician's warm voice and gentle reassurance than to a perfectly articulated chatbot prompt; similarly, in psychiatric interviews, patients gauge compassion through eye contact and tone, elements absent in AI-driven interactions [21]. Even in obstetrics and gynecology, where sensitive topics and emotional support are critical, AI tools that deliver standardized information risk feeling impersonal, potentially undermining patient comfort and trust.

Designing for Humanity

To bridge this gap, developers apply patient-centered design principles that incorporate "warm" AI prompts—language crafted to convey empathy and respect. For example, a diabetes management chatbot might begin with, "I understand managing blood sugar can feel overwhelming; I'm here to help you step by step," setting a supportive tone that mirrors human reassurance. Relational agents, digital avatars with friendly expressions and conversational pacing, have been shown to improve patient engagement and adherence by simulating aspects of human rapport [22].

Team Roles

AI is best viewed as a team member rather than a replacement. Students can observe how nurses use AI scribe tools to capture encounter details, freeing them to maintain eye contact and active listening. Physicians then review the draft notes, integrating their clinical judgment and personal observations. In this **hybrid workflow**, each role—student, nurse, physician, and AI—complements the others, ensuring technology enhances rather than detracts from the therapeutic relationship. As Eric Topol argues, AI should "take over the tasks that machines do best, leaving clinicians more time to do what only humans can do: connect with patients" [23].

"What Would You Do?": Ethical Case Discussions

In these scenarios, you'll apply ethical principles to AI-augmented clinical decisions. For each case, identify the key stakeholders (patients, clinicians, IT teams, administrators), the conflicting ethical pillars, and propose responsible actions.

Case A: Triage AI Deprioritizes Older Adults

An emergency department deploys an AI triage tool designed to prioritize patients based on urgency and likely outcomes. However, the model begins assigning lower priority scores to patients over age 75. Why? According to the hospital's historical data, older adults were less likely to receive aggressive interventions. This is often due to advance directives, the severity of comorbidities, or provider assumptions, not necessarily because they needed less care. As a result, the AI interprets these past patterns as a signal that older patients require less urgent attention (see Fig. 9.5).

This creates an ethical dilemma. Stakeholders include elderly patients, who risk delayed care; triage nurses, who must decide whether to follow the AI's recommendations; and hospital leaders, who are responsible for efficiency and equity. The conflict lies between *justice,* ensuring fair access to timely care regardless of age, and the AI's version of *beneficence*, which aims to maximize outcomes based on flawed historical patterns.

A responsible response would be to pause the use of age-influenced triage scoring, conduct a thorough audit of the model's age-related behavior, and revise the algorithm to include explicit equity safeguards. These changes can ensure that older adults are assessed based on clinical need, not on biased interpretations of past treatment decisions.

Case B: Suicide-Risk Model's High False Positives Overwhelm Services

A mental health clinic adopts an AI tool that flags patients at risk of suicide. Still, it generates 70% false positives, inundating social-work teams and delaying care for truly high-risk individuals. Stakeholders in this context include flagged patients, mental health professionals, and the broader patient population (see Fig. 9.6).

This situation reflects a tension between nonmaleficence (avoiding harm from missed cases) and justice (equitable allocation of limited mental health resources). You might recommend refining the model's threshold to balance sensitivity and

Prompt Element	Response
Ethical Conflict	Prioritization based on age may reduce care access and skew triage decisions unfairly.
Stakeholders	Older patients, triage nurses, emergency department clinicians, hospital leadership.
Potential Harm	Delayed or denied urgent care for elderly patients; loss of trust in triagefairness.
Pillars Involved	Justice, Beneficence.
Suggested Action	Suspend age-based scoring; conduct age-stratified audit of the AI; redesign model with explicit equity safeguards.

Fig. 9.5 Triage AI deprioritizes older adults

Prompt Element	Response
Ethical Conflict	Excessive false positives strain mental health services, delaying care for patients at true risk.
Stakeholders	Flagged patients, mental health professionals, social workers, broader patient population.
Potential Harm	Burnout among staff; misallocated resources; delayed or missed care for those at highest risk.
Pillars Involved	Nonmaleficence, Justice.
Suggested Action	Adjust model threshold to reduce false positives; implement human-in-the-loop verification; provide training for interpreting AI flags.

Fig. 9.6 Case B—Suicide-risk model's high false positives overwhelm services

specificity, instituting a human-in-the-loop review to validate high-risk alerts, and providing staff training on interpreting AI outputs to prevent burnout and ensure timely interventions.

Case C: Readmission-Risk Tool Unfavorably Flags Safety-Net Hospital Patients

A hospital system's AI readmission-risk algorithm directs fewer post-discharge resources to patients from its safety-net facility, historically under-documented in digital records, thereby widening care gaps. Stakeholders include safety-net patients, case management teams, and health system executives (see Fig. 9.7).

This scenario challenges justice by perpetuating inequities and violates beneficence by withholding potentially beneficial follow-up care. An ethical response is to augment the model's input data with social-determinant variables, engage community clinics in data collection to improve representation, and mandate that readmission scores be reviewed by a multidisciplinary committee before resource allocation decisions are finalized [5].

Prompt Element	Response
Ethical Conflict	AI tool reduces follow-up care for underserved patients due to lack of detailed documentation.
Stakeholders	Safety-net hospital patients, case management teams, hospital administrators.
Potential Harm	Widened disparities in post-discharge care; exacerbation of chronic conditions.
Pillars Involved	Justice, Beneficence.
Suggested Action	Incorporate social determinants into model input; partner with community clinics for data enrichment; require human oversight before allocating follow-up care.

Fig. 9.7 Case C: Readmission-risk tool flags safety-net hospital patients unfavorably

Ethics Worksheet and Reflection Assignment

This hands-on assignment guides you through five exercises to apply ethical principles to AI in clinical care. A PDF template accompanies this section, with spaces for your responses and a sample entry for the Values Mapping and Bias Audit exercises. Use the following time estimates to plan your work: Values Mapping (15 min), Bias Audit (25 min), Explainability Critique (20 min), Consent Mapping (15 min), and Reflection Essay (40 min). Your responses will be graded on depth of ethical analysis, clarity of reasoning, and practicality of proposed improvements.

Values Mapping

For each case in section '"What Would You Do?": Ethical Case Discussions', rate how well the AI aligns with the four pillars (autonomy, beneficence, nonmaleficence, justice). Use the sample entry in your worksheet as a model:

Case	Autonomy	Beneficence	Nonmaleficence	Justice	Justification (1–2 sentences)
A	Fair (4)	Moderate (3)	Poor (2)	Poor (2)	AI deprioritized older adults without patient input [example]

Bias Audit

Examine the following synthetic dataset of ten de-identified patient profiles. Identify sampling bias (underrepresented groups) and measurement bias (implausible or skewed vital signs), and suggest one corrective action per bias. Use the sample Bias Audit table in your worksheet.

ID	Age	Sex	Race	ZIP code	Visit Freq/ Year	O2 Sat (%)	Blood pressure (mmHg)
P01	25	F	White	07030	4	98	120/80
P02	70	M	Black	30303	1	95	130/85
P03	55	F	Asian	10027	3	99	115/75
P04	40	M	White	90210	2	97	118/76
P05	65	F	Hispanic	77005	1	96	125/80
P06	30	M	Native American	74464	0	94	122/78
P07	80	F	Asian	60605	1	93	135/90
P08	50	M	Black	37203	3	99	117/77
P09	45	F	Hispanic	48201	2	100	119/79
P10	75	M	White	02115	1	95	140/88

Explainability Critique

In this exercise, you will analyze how an AI model "sees" a chest X-ray and practice explaining its reasoning in plain language. You have two options for the attention map you critique:

- **Use the Sample Attention Map in this Book:** Refer to the figure embedded above under Section 3 of your worksheet (the heatmap overlay on a chest X-ray).
- **Generate Your Own (Optional):** Download the free CheXpert chest X-ray dataset (https://stanfordmlgroup.github.io/competitions/chexpert/), and apply the open-source Grad-CAM code (https://github.com/ramprs/grad-cam-pytorch) to a pretrained model.

Once you have your attention map, write a concise 3–4-sentence critique that covers the following:

1. **Focus Areas:** Which regions of the lung fields (or surrounding anatomy) did the AI highlight?
2. **Clinical Appropriateness:** Whether those highlighted areas correspond to actual pathology (e.g., a consolidation or nodule).
3. **Missing Context:** Any important findings or patient details that the AI neglected (such as bilateral effusions or clinical symptoms).

For example:

> The attention map highlights the right lower lung zone, where a consolidation is visible and appropriate for pneumonia detection. However, it also emphasizes the cardiac silhouette, which is unlikely to indicate pulmonary pathology. The map overlooks a small pleural effusion on the left side, suggesting the model may miss bilateral findings. Including the patient's fever and cough history would help contextualize these image features.

Use either the book's sample map or your own generated map, and apply this template to produce clear, patient-facing explanations.

Consent Mapping

Draft the four key points of an informed-consent script for an AI-assisted tool, ensuring patient-centered language. For example:

1. "I'll use an algorithm that reviews your lab values and imaging to estimate your risk of complications."
2. "Its accuracy is about 85%, but it can miss rare presentations."
3. "Your health data remain secure under HIPAA and won't be shared without permission."
4. "You may decline AI involvement and opt for a clinician-only assessment at any time."

Reflection Essay

In 300–500 words, choose one AI application you encountered during your rotations. Critically evaluate its strengths and ethical risks, citing the relevant ethical pillars, and propose one actionable improvement—such as a design change or oversight mechanism—to enhance its fairness and safety.

Grading Rubric (Worksheet Sections 1–4)

- **Excellent (4)** demonstrates nuanced ethical reasoning, clear examples, and practical mitigation steps.
- **Good (3)** correctly identifies issues with reasonable justification and suggestions.
- **Fair (2)** identifies basic concerns but with superficial analysis or vague recommendations.
- **Poor (1)** fails to connect ethical principles to concrete examples or propose remedies.

Use the provided template and examples as guides, and consult the SHAP and LIME tutorials (https://github.com/slundberg/shap, https://github.com/marcotcr/lime) if you choose to explore real interpretability tools.

Summary and Key Takeaways

Ethics in clinical AI cannot be an after-the-fact checklist—it must be woven into every stage of development and deployment. You have seen how proactive bias detection, clear transparency, and rigorous informed consent safeguard patient welfare and uphold trust. As future physicians, your role is to continually observe, question, and advocate for AI tools that treat every patient fairly and respectfully.

To continue building your expertise, consult these freely available resources:

- American Medical Association. (2024). *AI in Health Care: A Physician's Guide to Ethics and Practice.* Retrieved from https://www.ama-assn.org/ai-ethics-toolkit
- World Health Organization. (2023). *Ethics and Governance of Artificial Intelligence for Health.* Retrieved from https://www.who.int/ethics-of-ai-health
- Neo4j. (2024). *Graph-Based Retrieval-Augmented Generation for Ethical AI.* Retrieved from https://neo4j.com/ethical-ai-rag

Keep these principles close as you integrate AI into patient care: ethics first, human oversight always, and relentless curiosity about how technology shapes the future of medicine.

Instructor's Guide for This Chapter—Ethics and Bias in Clinical AI

Chapter Overview

In this chapter teaches medical students to apply ethical principles—autonomy, beneficence, nonmaleficence, and justice—to the use of AI in health care. Through definitions, case studies, hands-on exercises, and reflection, students develop skills to spot bias, demand transparency, secure informed consent, promote equity, and preserve empathy.

Learning Objectives and Mapping

By chapter end, students will be able to:

1. **LO1:** Apply the four ethical pillars to AI scenarios.
2. **LO2:** Identify sampling, measurement, and algorithmic biases.
3. **LO3:** Explain black-box challenges and interpretability tools.
4. **LO4:** Outline informed-consent requirements for AI use.
5. **LO5:** Propose strategies to mitigate AI-fueled health inequities.
6. **LO6:** Describe why empathy remains essential in AI-supported care.
7. **LO7:** Conduct structured ethical analyses via worksheet and case discussions.

Section Teaching Plan

Section	Time	Activity	LO(s) Addressed	Facilitator tips
Introduction and pillars – Vignette + 4-Pillars Infographic	10 min	Think–Pair–Share Discuss AI vs. ethics	LO1	Prompt quieter students with targeted questions: "Which pillar is most at risk here?"
Data Bias Types + Infographic	15 min	Dataset Bias Audit (pairs) Group debrief	LO2	Encourage students to connect zip codes to social determinants
Explainability Methods	20 min	Grad-CAM demo + Patient Dialogue Role-Play	LO3	Clarify technical jargon; use analogies (e.g., "highlighting relevant lines")
Consent and Accountability	15 min	Consent-Script Workshop Liability Discussion	LO4	Remind students to reference IRB sidebar; stress documentation best practices
Equity and Justice	15 min	Equity Design Challenge Report-Back	LO5	Guide groups to consider cost and cultural factors in their proposals
Empathy and Connection	10 min	Reflective Write & Discuss	LO6	Ask: "What feeling does AI miss that you've seen in care?"
Ethical Case Discussions	20 min	Breakouts + Gallery Walk	LO1, LO2, LO4	Rotate groups so each student engages with multiple cases
Worksheet Overview and Assignment	5 min	Distribute PDF; explain rubric	LO7	Show sample entries; clarify submission format and deadline
Summary and Exit Ticket	5 min	Exit Ticket: Ethical Action	All LO	Collect tickets to gauge lingering questions

Materials and Accessibility

- **Figures:** 9.1 (Pillars), 9.2 (Bias Types)
- **Worksheets:** Chapter 9 Appendix, (with sample entries; printable)
- **Demo Resources:** Grad-CAM video (captioned); LIME/SHAP links
- **Readings Appendix:** Full list of external resources provided separately
- **Accessibility Notes:** Provide digital and print copies of all materials; ensure videos have captions and transcripts.

Assessment and Feedback

- **In-Class Participation (30%):** Engagement in discussions and activities, guided by facilitator observations.
- **Worksheet and Reflection Essay (60%):** Graded per rubric on ethical depth, clarity, and feasibility (see rubric appendix).
- **Exit Tickets (10%):** Quick check of takeaway understanding; address gaps in next session.

Appendix

Worksheets

Values, Bias, Explainability, Consent, Reflection

Print these pages and write directly on them. Use black ink for scanning.

Worksheet 1: Values Mapping

Clarify what matters for patients, clinicians, and the health system before you evaluate any model output.

Stakeholder	Value	Example requirement	Metric	Risk if ignored
Patient	Respectful communication	Spanish summary at sixth grade reading level	SMOG grade level ≤ 6	Confusion about care plan

Worksheet 2: Bias Audit

Scan for representation, measurement, and label issues. Record evidence and an action.

Step	Question	Evidence	Risk	Action
Representation	Do Spanish speakers receive more high risk flags than others	Ten person cohort below shows four of five admits are non English speakers	Unequal burden of escalation	Recalibrate and add language access check

Synthetic cohort for quick checks

ID	Age	Sex	Language	Insurance	Condition	Outcome	Flag
P01	72	F	Spanish	Medicare	COPD	Admit	High risk
P02	55	M	English	Commercial	Diabetes	Discharge	Low risk
P03	39	F	Mandarin	Self pay	Pregnancy	Admit	High risk
P04	81	M	English	Medicare	CHF	Admit	High risk
P05	28	F	English	Medicaid	Asthma	Discharge	Medium risk
P06	64	M	Spanish	Medicaid	CKD	Discharge	Medium risk
P07	47	F	English	Commercial	Migraine	Discharge	Low risk
P08	73	F	Korean	Medicare	Pneumonia	Admit	High risk
P09	33	M	English	Commercial	Back pain	Discharge	Low risk
P10	62	M	Spanish	Medicare Advantage	CAD	Admit	High risk

Try. Compare admission rates by language. Check missingness by payer. Note any outliers.

Worksheet 3: Explainability Critique

Paste or reference an attention map or saliency image, then answer the prompts.

[Attach map here]

Model type:

Input sample:

What the map highlights:

Two things that might mislead readers:

Next action to improve safety or clarity:

Worksheet 4: Consent Mapping

Prepare a brief script in plain language. Aim for a sixth-grade reading level.

Prompt	Your script
Purpose and outputs the tool will create for you.	
Data handling, retention, and who sees the notes.	
Your choice to decline AI help, and the role of the clinician.	
Risks, how to ask questions, and who to contact.	

Reflection Essay

In 250 to 300 words, explain how the values you mapped shaped your bias checks and your edits to the explainability display. End with one change to your team workflow you will test next month.

References

1. Patel AP, Rao A, Luo Y, Cleland JGF, Heidenreich PA. Racial and ethnic disparities in the performance of heart failure risk prediction models. J Am Coll Cardiol. 2022;79(5):488–99. https://doi.org/10.1016/j.jacc.2021.11.049.
2. Beauchamp TL, Childress JF. Principles of biomedical ethics. 7th ed. Oxford University Press; 2013.
3. Daneshjou R, Vodrahalli K, Novoa RA, Jenkins M, Liang W, Rotemberg V, et al. Disparities in dermatology AI performance on a diverse, curated clinical image set. *Science*. Advances. 2022;8(16):eabq6147. https://doi.org/10.1126/sciadv.abq6147.
4. Sjoding MW, Dickson RP, Iwashyna TJ, Gay SE, Valley TS. Racial bias in pulse oximetry measurement. N Engl J Med. 2020;383(25):2477–8. https://doi.org/10.1056/NEJMc2029240.
5. Obermeyer Z, Powers B, Vogeli C, Mullainathan S. Dissecting racial bias in an algorithm used to manage the health of populations. Science. 2019;366(6464):447–53. https://doi.org/10.1126/science.aax2342.
6. Montoya LN, Roberts JS, Hidalgo BS. Towards fairness in AI for melanoma detection: systematic review and recommendations. arXiv; 2024. https://arxiv.org/abs/2411.12846.
7. Rudin C. Stop explaining black box machine learning models for high stakes decisions and use interpretable models instead. Nat Mach Intell. 2019;1(5):206–15. https://doi.org/10.1038/s42256-019-0048-x.
8. Ribeiro MT, Singh S, Guestrin C. "Why should I trust you?" Explaining the predictions of any classifier. In: Proceedings of the 22nd ACM SIGKDD international conference on knowledge discovery and data mining; 2016. p. 1135–44. https://doi.org/10.1145/2939672.2939778.
9. Chefer H, Gur S, Wolf L. Transformer interpretability beyond attention visualization. In: Proceedings of the IEEE/CVF conference on computer vision and pattern recognition; 2021. p. 782–91. https://doi.org/10.1109/CVPR46437.2021.00085.
10. Lundberg SM, Lee S-I. A unified approach to interpreting model predictions. Adv Neural Inf Proces Syst. 2017;30:4765–74.
11. Wachter S, Mittelstadt B, Russell C. Why fairness cannot be automated: Bridging the gap between EU non-discrimination law and AI. Law Innov Technol. 2021;12(1):2–30. https://doi.org/10.1080/17579961.2020.1854616.
12. National Institute of Standards and Technology. AI risk management framework; 2023. Retrieved from https://www.nist.gov/itl/ai-risk-management-framework.
13. Price WN II, Cohen IG. Privacy in the age of medical big data. Nat Med. 2019;25(1):37–43. https://doi.org/10.1038/s41591-018-0272-7.
14. U.S. Department of Health and Human Services. 45 CFR 46: Protection of human subjects; 2003. Retrieved from https://www.hhs.gov/ohrp/regulations-and-policy/regulations/45-cfr-46/index.html.
15. Office for Civil Rights. Summary of the HIPAA privacy rule. U.S. Department of Health and Human Services; 2013.
16. Rosenbaum L. Understanding liability risk from using healthcare artificial intelligence. N Engl J Med. 2023;388(8):673–5. https://doi.org/10.1056/NEJMhle2308901.
17. Rathi A. Can artificial intelligence extend healthcare to all? Reuters; 2024.
18. California Civil Code § 1798.100. California Consumer Privacy Act of 2018; 2018.
19. European Parliament. Regulation (EU) 2016/679 (General data protection regulation). Official Journal of the European Union; 2016.
20. European Parliament and Council. (2023). Proposal for a regulation laying down harmonized rules on artificial intelligence (AI Act)

21. Laranjo L, Dunn AG, Tong HL, Kocaballi AB, Chen J, Bashir R, et al. Conversational agents in healthcare: a systematic review. J Am Med Inform Assoc. 2018;25(9):1248–58. https://doi.org/10.1093/jamia/ocy072.
22. Bickmore TW, Picard RW. Establishing and maintaining long-term human–computer relationships. ACM Trans Comput-Hum Interact. 2005;12(2):293–327. https://doi.org/10.1145/1067860.1067867.
23. Topol E. Deep medicine: how artificial intelligence can make healthcare human again. Basic Books; 2019.

Chapter 10
Regulation and Transparency of Clinical AI

Learning Objectives
By chapter end, you will be able to:

1. Explain why AI in health care requires regulatory oversight (patient safety, efficacy).
2. Summarize US FDA pathways (510(k), de novo, PMA) in plain terms.
3. Describe EU CE marking under MDR and IVDR.
4. Outline core transparency requirements for AI tools.
5. Discuss post-market oversight and change-control processes.
6. Identify who is accountable when AI causes patient harm.
7. Apply these concepts to real-world scenarios and expert insights.

Introduction

Integrating AI into clinical decision-making is advancing rapidly, but innovation alone is insufficient. Even the most promising tools can put patients at risk without robust regulatory oversight. Unlike traditional medical devices, clinical AI systems can evolve and may be deployed at scale before their risks are fully understood. This is especially true for those AI systems that analyze imaging, vital signs, or generate clinical notes. This section explores why strong regulation is essential to protect patients, ensure clinical accuracy, and preserve trust in these transformative technologies.

Visualizations of research data or results in this manuscript were generated, refined, corrected, edited, or formatted with the assistance of artificial intelligence (AI) tools, specifically OpenAI's ChatGPT 4.0, 2024. All content has been thoroughly reviewed, revised, and approved by the author(s) to ensure scientific accuracy and preserve the integrity of the original material.

© The Author(s), under exclusive license to Springer Nature Switzerland AG 2025

C. Quinn, *Generative AI for the Medical Student*,
https://doi.org/10.1007/978-3-032-01613-3_10

Why Regulate Clinical AI?

In early 2025, the US Food and Drug Administration (FDA) issued a Class I recall, the agency's most serious warning, for Philips' Mobile Cardiac Outpatient Telemetry (MCOT) software. The issue: critical electrocardiogram (ECG) alerts, including those for atrial fibrillation and cardiac pauses, failed to reach clinicians. As a result, more than 100 patients were injured and 2 died. A Class I recall indicates that continued use of the product could result in serious harm or death [1].

This incident underscores why **Software as a Medical Device (SaMD)** must be held to rigorous safety standards. SaMD refers to software intended to perform medical functions without being part of a hardware medical device; for example, an AI model that analyzes ECGs or triages patients in emergency departments (see Fig. 10.1). Generative AI systems, including those that summarize notes, detect arrhythmias, or suggest diagnoses, fall under this category when used for clinical care.

Effective regulation of clinical AI ensures that software is tested on representative data, validated for clinical performance, and subject to ongoing monitoring. It also allows for rapid corrective actions when errors occur. As AI becomes more autonomous and complex, traditional regulatory models, which often assume a fixed-function device, must evolve. Adaptive AI tools that learn from new data may behave unpredictably if not carefully constrained, monitored, and audited.

In short, regulation is not a brake on innovation—it is the framework that ensures innovation does not come at the cost of patient safety, legal accountability, or public trust [2].

Sidebar: Which FDA Pathway Applies When?

Device type	Risk level	Example	FDA pathway
AI stethoscope similar to existing one	Low–moderate	HeartAI™	510(k) clearance
New AI model for predicting kidney stone risk	Moderate–novel	No predicate device	De novo classification
AI-controlled neurostimulator	High	Implantable therapeutic device	Premarket approval (PMA)
COVID-19 triage AI during pandemic	Any (urgent/novel)	Public health emergency scenario	Emergency use authorization (EUA)

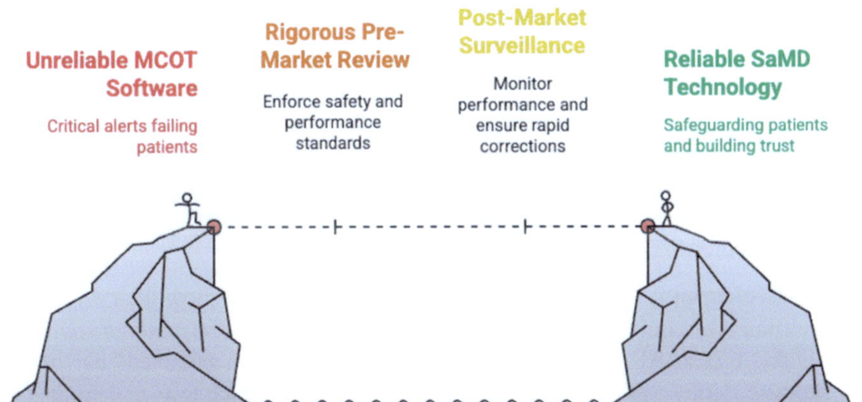

Fig. 10.1 Ensuring SaMD safety

Student Tip Match the novelty of the device and its clinical risk to determine which FDA pathway applies. If a similar device exists and the risk is low to moderate, → 510(k). If no predicate exists → de novo. High-risk and novel → PMA. Public emergency? → EUA.

With the rationale for regulation established, let's examine the specific FDA pathways by which AI tools earn clearance or approval in US clinical practice.

Sidebar: The Manufacturer and User Facility Device Experience (MAUDE) database is a publicly accessible repository maintained by the US Food and Drug Administration (FDA) that houses Medical Device Reports (MDRs) of adverse events—such as device-related deaths, serious injuries, and malfunctions—submitted by manufacturers, importers, device user facilities, healthcare professionals, patients, and consumers. MAUDE supports post-market surveillance by enabling clinicians, researchers, and the public to monitor device performance and identify safety issues in real time, US Food and Drug Administration.

You can search MAUDE at: https://www.accessdata.fda.gov/scripts/cdrh/cfdocs/cfmaude/search.cfm

U.S. FDA Pathways for AI/ML Devices (LO2)

Learning Objective 2: Explain how FDA regulatory routes match device risk and novelty, ensuring patient safety and technology efficacy. *(To explore how regulatory knowledge influences clinical decisions, see the CMIO simulation in section* Simulation: "You Are the CMIO"*)*

Before any AI software can guide patient care, it must clear one of the FDA's pathways, which vary by risk level: (see Fig. 10.2)

- **510(k) clearance (low to moderate risk):** Manufacturers show their AI tool is "substantially equivalent" to a previously approved device (the *predicate device*). Think of HeartAI™: its murmur-detection performance matched that of an acoustic stethoscope, earning it 510(k) clearance after bench tests and comparative studies [3].
- **De novo classification (moderate risk, novel devices):** When no predicate exists, companies submit bench-test data and limited clinical evidence to establish a new device classification, as used for first-of-their-kind AI tools that pose moderate risk [4].

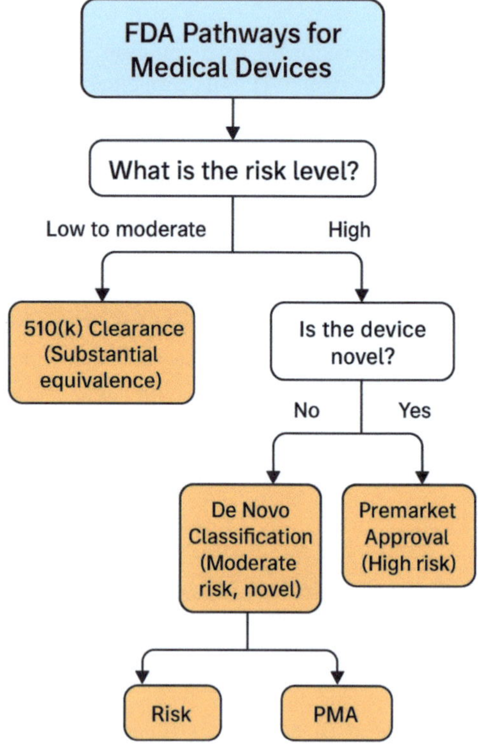

Fig. 10.2 FDA pathway for medical devices

- **Premarket approval (PMA) (high risk):** The most rigorous route for devices where failure could cause serious harm, implantable AI neurostimulators, for example, requires full-scale clinical trials to prove safety and effectiveness [5].
- **Breakthrough and emergency use (any risk level, expedited):** In public health emergencies or for breakthrough innovations, the FDA can grant conditional, time-limited authorizations (EUAs) or designate a tool as breakthrough to accelerate access while collecting real-world performance data, used recently for COVID-19 triage AIs [6].

Students can experience real-world regulatory decision-making in the CMIO simulation in section Simulation: "You Are the CMIO".

Why This Matters to You

As future clinicians, you will encounter AI tools in diagnostics, monitoring, and decision support. Recognizing an AI application's FDA status helps you gauge its reliability and understand its evidence base. This knowledge ensures you use only properly vetted technologies, advocate for patient safety, and engage effectively with interdisciplinary teams deploying AI.

Student Tip On your next rotation, verify an AI tool's clearance by checking the FDA's device database. https://www.accessdata.fda.gov/scripts/cdrh/cfdocs/cfdevice/device.cfmKnowing its pathway tells you how much evidence supports its use.

Having understood how US regulators classify and evaluate AI risk, we now turn to the parallel process in Europe: CE marking under the MDR and IVDR.

EU CE Marking for AI/ML Devices (LO3)

The **CE mark** is the manufacturer's declaration that a product complies with applicable EU safety, health, and performance requirements, allowing it to be sold across the European Economic Area [7]. For AI medical software, two regulations apply the **Medical Device Regulation (MDR 2017/745)** covers tools that diagnose, monitor, or treat diseases (e.g., AI ECG analyzers), while the **In Vitro Diagnostic Regulation (IVDR 2017/746)** governs software that interprets samples outside the body (e.g., AI blood-test classifiers) [8].

Before affixing the CE mark, manufacturers must work with a **Notified Body**, an independent organization responsible for conformity assessment, to review their **technical documentation**. This dossier includes the device description, intended use, risk-classification rationale (Classes I–III for MDR; A–D for IVDR), clinical-evaluation reports, and evidence of a quality-management system compliant with ISO 13485 [9]. The Notified Body verifies that clinical and bench-test data support the manufacturer's safety and performance claims, conducts on-site audits, and performs periodic post-market surveillance once the software is in use.

Student Tip When you encounter an AI tool on rounds, look for the CE logo and a four-digit Notified Body number in its "About" or "Settings" menu to confirm it has undergone proper EU conformity assessment.

Once an AI device enters the market—whether via FDA clearance or CE mark—it still requires vigilance; the next section explains post-market oversight mechanisms that catch real-world issues.

Sidebar
The letters CE in the "CE mark" are an abbreviation of the French phrase **Conformité Européenne**, which translates to "European Conformity." The CE mark signifies that a product complies with all relevant EU directives and regulations about health, safety, and environmental protection.

Post-market Oversight (LO5)

Even after FDA clearance or CE marking, AI/ML medical software requires ongoing monitoring to catch malfunctions and ensure continued safety and effectiveness. In the USA, the **Manufacturer and User Facility Device Experience (MAUDE)** database collects Medical Device Reports (MDRs) of adverse events, such as software crashes or missed alerts, submitted by manufacturers, healthcare facilities, and users. Clinicians can query MAUDE to identify emerging safety issues with AI tools they employ [10]. In Europe, the **European Database on Medical Devices (EUDAMED)** serves a similar role, aggregating field safety corrective actions and vigilance reports for CE-marked devices, including AI software, so that stakeholders can track device performance across member states [11].

Managing software changes is equally critical. The FDA's **Predetermined Change Control Plan (PCCP)** guidance outlines when iterative updates—like bug fixes or algorithm retraining—can proceed under a preapproved plan versus when they require a new submission (e.g., a 510(k) for substantial modifications) [12]. Minor performance tweaks that do not affect intended use or safety can follow an existing PCCP, while significant feature additions or risk-class escalations demand full regulatory review.

On the Floor: Familiarize yourself with your institution's protocol for reporting AI tool errors—know who on your team files MAUDE or EUDAMED reports and how to escalate software issues promptly.

Example PCCP Change
Scenario: An FDA-cleared AI sepsis detector regularly analyzes patient vitals and lab trends to flag early signs of infection. Its developers release an update that incorporates **new antibiotic-resistance patterns** into the training set.

Analysis

- The tool's intended use remains unchanged (early sepsis detection).
- The model's core output logic is refined not redefined.
- No new risks are introduced, and performance metrics remain within the approved range.

Conclusion: Because this update was described in the original Predetermined Change Control Plan (PCCP), it qualifies as a preapproved change. The vendor can proceed with deployment without submitting a new 510(k), though documentation must still be logged internally.

Oversight ensures safety, but transparency empowers clinicians and their patients to use AI wisely. Let's review the labeling and disclosure requirements that make that possible.

Transparency Requirements (LO4)

Every AI tool in clinical use must carry clear, accessible information, so that you and your patients understand its intended purpose, performance, and limits. In the USA, device **labeling regulations** (21 CFR § 801) require that a medical device label, now including standalone software, display the manufacturer's name, a statement of intended use, and any warnings or contraindications [13]. FDA guidance for Software as a Medical Device further specifies that labels identify key performance metrics (such as sensitivity and specificity) and clearly state any limitations relevant to clinical interpretation, ensuring users know when and where errors might occur. In Europe, the **EU AI Act** (Article 13) imposes transparency obligations on high-risk systems, mandating that providers supply plain-language summaries of the system's capabilities, known limitations, potential risks, and instructions for interpreting outputs [14].

For **you as a medical student**, reviewing an AI tool's label or "About" screen is a critical habit. Knowing exactly what conditions the tool is designed to detect, how accurate it is, and where it may fail helps you integrate AI safely into your patient assessments. This practice sharpens your clinical judgment, letting you weigh AI findings against your physical exam and patient history, and fosters informed discussions with supervising physicians and patients about the tool's role in care.

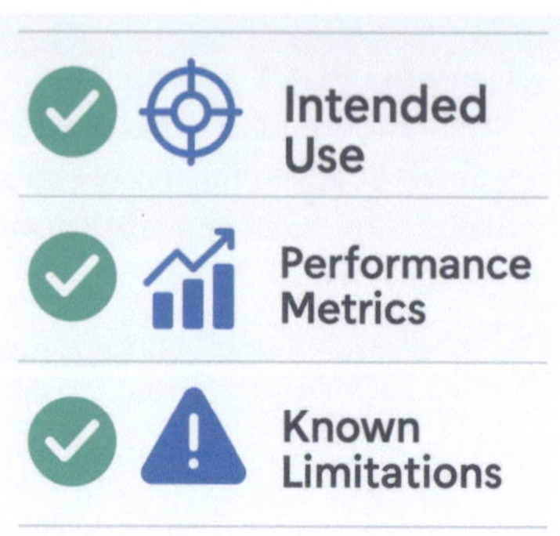

Fig. 10.3 What you need to know before using an AI application

What You Need to Know Before relying on an AI application, check its label or information panel for the following (see Fig. 10.3):

- **Intended use** (e.g., "detects atrial fibrillation in adults").
- **Accuracy metrics** (e.g., "sensitivity 92%, specificity 89%").
- **Known limitations** (e.g., "may miss paroxysmal episodes <30 sec").

Transparency lays the groundwork for accountability. In the following section, we explore how liability is shared among clinicians, vendors, and health systems when AI tools err."

Accountability and Liability (LO6)

When an AI tool contributes to a clinical decision, responsibility is shared across three groups. **Clinicians** must verify algorithmic outputs against their examination and judgment before acting on them; **vendors** are tasked with rigorous model development, validation studies, and transparent performance reporting; and **health systems** bear oversight through institutional review boards or dedicated AI governance committees that establish standard operating procedures for deployment and error management [15].

Legal accountability for AI-related harm is already emerging in malpractice litigation. In one reported case, a hospital's AI scribe misrecorded a patient's allergy, leading to an adverse drug reaction; the ensuing suit named both the supervising physician, for failing to catch the error, and the software vendor, for inadequate quality controls, underscoring that multiple parties can face liability when AI fails [16].

To manage these risks, many institutions form **AI governance committees** composed of clinicians, informaticians, ethicists, and legal advisors. These bodies review proposed AI tools, approve usage protocols, monitor real-world performance metrics, and coordinate incident reporting, ensuring that any malfunction triggers timely corrective action and legal reporting as required by FDA or EU vigilance rules [17].

For you as a medical student, understanding accountability frameworks helps you navigate clinical workflows safely. Knowing whom to notify when an AI alert seems incorrect—and following your institution's reporting process—protects patients and clarifies your role in upholding both patient safety and professional standards.

Theory meets practice when you hear from those who shepherd AI tools through regulation. Our expert-perspective case study and podcast debrief provide you with that insider view.

Expert Perspectives (LO7)

To gain real-world insight into AI regulation without relying on in-person speakers, you will conduct a **mini–case study** using publicly available FDA records. First, navigate to the **Devices@FDA database** (https://www.accessdata.fda.gov/scripts/cdrh/cfdocs/cfdevice/device.cfm) and search for an AI-based device cleared via 510(k), for example, an AI-powered heart-sound analyzer [19]. Download the **510(k) Summary** PDF, which includes redacted clinical-performance tables, predicate-device comparisons, and the FDA's decision letter. As you review these excerpts, answer questions such as:

1. Which clinical endpoints did the sponsor use to demonstrate substantial equivalence?
2. How were differences in algorithm training data justified?
3. What concerns did FDA reviewers raise, and how did the sponsor respond?

Next, listen to the American Medical Association's Health Innovator podcast episode "Regulating AI in Medicine" [18]. Prepare **two discussion questions**—for example, "How might post-market real-world evidence reshape future 510(k) guidance?" or "What unique challenges do continuously learning AI systems pose for regulators?"—and discuss your observations in small groups. This exercise combines document analysis with expert commentary, deepening your understanding of regulatory workflows and evolving challenges in AI oversight.

Quiz 6: Applying Regulatory Concepts.

You have 30 minutes to complete Quiz 6, which assesses Learning Objectives LO2–LO6. The quiz consists of eight multiple choice questions and two short-answer scenarios. Use your understanding of FDA and EU pathways, transparency requirements, post-market reporting, and liability frameworks to select the best answer or describe the correct regulatory action.

Multiple Choice Questions (1 Point each)

1. An AI tool that analyzes heart sounds and demonstrates equivalent performance to an existing stethoscope device would most likely follow which FDA pathway?
   A. 510(k) clearance
   B. De novo classification.
   C. Premarket approval (PMA).
   D. Emergency Use Authorization (EUA).
2. A novel AI algorithm that predicts kidney stone risk without any predictive device and poses a moderate patient risk should be pursued:
   A. 510(k) clearance
   B. De novo classification.
   C. PMA.
   D. Breakthrough device designation.
3. Which pathway requires the most extensive clinical-trial data before approval?
   A. 510(k)
   B. De novo.
   C. PMA.
   D. EUA.
4. During a public health emergency, an AI triage app may be used under:
   A. 510(k) clearance
   B. De novo classification.
   C. Emergency Use Authorization.
   D. PMA.
5. According to FDA labeling rules, an AI diagnostic tool's label must include all EXCEPT:
   A. Intended use statement.
   B. Accuracy metrics (sensitivity, specificity).
   C. Source code of the algorithm.
   D. Known limitations.
6. A clinician discovers that an AI scribe mislabeled a patient's allergy. The correct post-market action is to:
   A. Ignore it—minor error.
   B. File a report to MAUDE (if in the USA) or EUDAMED (if in the EU).
   C. Submit a new 510(k) application.
   D. Retrain the algorithm without notification.

7. In the event an AI tool harms a patient, liability may fall on all the following, except:

   A. The supervising clinician.
   B. The software vendor.
   C. The AI governance committee.
   D. The patient.

8. You open an AI-assisted blood-test interpreter in a European clinic. To confirm its regulatory status, you look for:

   A. FDA 510(k) number.
   B. CE mark and Notified Body number.
   C. ISO 9001 certificate.
   D. Breakthrough Device logo.

Short-Answer Scenarios (2 Points each)

Scenario 1

During rounds, you observe an AI scribe automatically document a "penicillin allergy" for a patient who has no such allergy. Describe in three to five sentences the steps you would take for post-market reporting and internal escalation, referencing MAUDE or EUDAMED as appropriate.

Scenario 2

A vendor releases a minor software update to its generative-AI discharge-summary tool that improves sentence structure but does not alter clinical calculations. In three to five sentences, explain whether this change requires a new FDA submission or can proceed under a Predetermined Change Control Plan, and describe any notifications you would expect.

Scenario 3

You are rotating at a teaching hospital in France. An AI-powered blood analyzer labeled with a CE mark and Notified Body number repeatedly misclassifies samples from patients with sickle cell disease. Describe in three to five sentences how you would verify the tool's EU conformity status, report the issue, and initiate local escalation. Reference any relevant EU oversight mechanisms.

Scenario 4

During clinical rounds, you learn that a commercial AI tool performs significantly worse in diagnosing pneumonia in Hispanic patients due to underrepresentation in its training dataset. In three to five sentences, describe your ethical and regulatory obligations. What actions would you take to report, mitigate, or escalate the issue? Reference any applicable regulatory or governance structures.

Grading Criteria

- **Multiple Choice:** 1 point for each correct selection.
- **Scenarios:** Up to 2 points each for identifying the correct regulatory pathway/action and clearly explaining the rationale.

Key Resources and Further Reading

- Simplified FDA SaMD guidance overview.
- MDCG summaries of MDR/IVDR.
- IMDRF Principles for SaMD.
- AMA AI Ethics Toolkit (regulatory chapter).

Conclusion

As clinical AI becomes more deeply embedded in healthcare systems, the ability to navigate its regulatory landscape is no longer optional; it is essential. This chapter has equipped you with a foundational understanding of how the FDA and EU regulate AI tools, how post-market surveillance systems like MAUDE and EUDAMED operate, and how transparency and accountability structures safeguard patient care. Whether reviewing an AI-generated diagnosis, questioning its risk classification, or reporting a malfunction, your awareness of these regulatory pathways empowers you to act responsibly. Ultimately, your role is to use AI and scrutinize it and uphold the clinical and ethical standards that ensure innovation remains aligned with patient safety and public trust.

Instructor's Guide

Chapter Overview

In this chapter familiarizes medical students with the regulatory framework governing AI/ML medical devices in the USA (FDA) and EU (CE Mark), core transparency and post-market requirements, and accountability structures. Through practical examples, visuals, and a capstone quiz, learners will understand how to evaluate—and safely use—AI tools in clinical settings.

Learning Objectives and Alignment

By the end of this chapter, students will be able to:

1. **LO1:** Articulate why AI/ML tools require regulation to protect patient safety and public trust.
2. **LO2:** Summarize FDA pathways (510(k), De Novo, PMA, EUA/Breakthrough) and map device risk and novelty to each.
3. **LO3:** Explain CE marking under MDR/IVDR, Notified Body roles, and technical-documentation requirements.

4. **LO4:** Describe labeling and disclosure mandates, including performance metrics and known limitations.
5. **LO5:** Outline post-market oversight mechanisms (MAUDE, EUDAMED, change control).
6. **LO6:** Identify accountability and liability distribution among clinicians, vendors, and institutions.
7. **LO7:** Apply these concepts in real-world scenarios and critique an actual 510(k) case study.

Section Teaching Plan

Section	Time	Activity	LO(s)	Tips for facilitator
Why regulate clinical AI?	10 min	Vignette discussion (Philips MCOT recall)	LO1	Emphasize recall severity; define "class I recall"
US FDA pathways	20 min	Pathway flowchart review (Fig. 10.1) + 510(k) vignette	LO2	Use analogies ("predicate device" as "reference model")
EU CE marking	15 min	Comparison table activity (FDA vs. CE)	LO3	Highlight "Conformité Européenne" meaning
Post-market oversight	15 min	Timeline walkthrough + MAUDE/EUDAMED demo pages	LO5	Show live MAUDE search; discuss institutional reporting
Transparency requirements	10 min	Labeling-checklist infographic (Fig. 10.2) + "what you need to know" call-out	LO4	Stress student habit of reviewing labels on rounds
Accountability and liability	10 min	Case discussion: AI scribe error lawsuit	LO6	Reinforce multiparty responsibility
Expert perspectives	20 min	510(k) mini–case study (devices@FDA) + podcast debrief	LO7	Provide step-by-step handout on accessing FDA summaries
Quiz 6 overview	5 min	Distribute quiz, review format and time allotment	All	Encourage use of resources (FDA database, CE guidelines)

Materials and Resources

- **Figures**
  - Figure 10.1: Regulatory Pathways Flowchart.
  - Figure 10.2: Labeling Checklist Infographic.

- **Handouts**
  - 510(k) Case study packet (downloaded from Devices@FDA)
  - Quiz 6 with answer key.
- **Online Tools**
  - Devices@FDA (https://www.accessdata.fda.gov/scripts/cdrh/cfdocs/cfdevice/device.cfm).
  - MAUDE Database (https://www.accessdata.fda.gov/scripts/cdrh/cfdocs/cfMAUDE/maude.cfm).
  - EUDAMED Portal (https://ec.europa.eu/tools/eudamed).
- **Podcast:** AMA Health Innovator "Regulating AI in Medicine" episode.

In-Class Activities and Facilitation Tips

1. **Vignette Discussion**
   - Prompt: "Why did the MCOT recall occur, and how might regulation prevent similar failures?"
   - Tip: Clarify recall classes and device risk levels.
2. **Pathway Flowchart**
   - Guide students through Fig. 10.1.
   - Activity: Given an AI wrist-worn arrhythmia detector, have pairs assign the correct pathway.
3. **FDA vs. CE Comparison**
   - Provide a fill-in table contrasting 510(k)/De Novo/PMA with MDR/IVDR.
   - Tip: Emphasize CE mark as "manufacturer self-declaration plus Notified Body audit."
4. **Post-Market Timeline**
   - Walk through market entry to recall.
   - Demo live MAUDE search for a known device and discuss how reports are filed.
5. **Labeling Checklist**
   - Review Fig. 10.2, and then have students pick an AI app they know and identify its label elements.
6. **Liability Case Study**
   - Present the AI scribe-allergy error scenario.
   - Discuss multiparty liability and institutional governance boards.

7. **510(k) Mini–Case Study and Podcast**
   - Distribute the downloaded 510(k) Summary.
   - Students answer guided questions and then debrief podcast insights in small groups.
8. **Quiz Administration**
   - Allocate 30 min; ensure calculators or devices for MAUDE lookups are available.

Assessment and Feedback

- **In-Class Participation (30%)**
  - Engagement in discussions, accuracy in pathway/activity assignments.
- **Quiz 6 (50%)**
  - Eight MCQs (1 point each) and two scenarios (2 points each).
- **Exit Ticket (20%)**
  - 1-min written response: "Which regulatory pathway would you choose for a novel AI vital sign monitor and why?"

Quiz 6 Answer Key

Multiple Choice Questions

1. **A—510(k) Clearance**
   Explanation: A 510(k) pathway requires showing "substantial equivalence" to a legally marketed predicate device. An AI heart-sound app that matches the performance of an existing acoustic stethoscope fits this criterion, making 510(k) the appropriate route.
2. **B—De Novo Classification**
   Explanation: When no predicate device exists, but the tool poses moderate risk, the de novo pathway creates a new device classification based on demonstrated safety and effectiveness without requiring full PMA-level data.
3. **C—PMA**
   Explanation: Premarket Approval is reserved for high-risk devices where failure could cause serious harm. It demands comprehensive clinical trial evidence, making it the most rigorous pathway.
4. **C—Emergency Use Authorization**
   Explanation: During declared public-health emergencies, the FDA can issue EUAs to allow temporary use of unapproved medical products (including AI tools) for the duration of the crisis, with conditions for data collection.

5. **C—Source Code of the Algorithm**
   Explanation: FDA labeling rules require intended use statements, performance metrics, and known limitations, but not disclosure of proprietary source code.
6. **B—File a Report to MAUDE (if in the USA) or EUDAMED (if in the EU)**
   Explanation: Adverse events—such as an AI scribe error causing patient harm—must be reported through post-market surveillance databases (MAUDE or EUDAMED), not ignored or handled via new premarket submissions.
7. **D—The Patient**
   Explanation: Liability in AI-related harm can fall on supervising clinicians (for oversight), software vendors (for development flaws), or institutions (for governance lapses), but never on the patient harmed by the device.
8. **B—CE Mark and Notified Body Number**
   Explanation: In Europe, the CE mark plus a four-digit Notified Body identifier indicates the device underwent conformity assessment under MDR/IVDR; an FDA number or ISO certificate does not validate EU approval.

Short-Answer Scenarios

Scenario 1: AI Scribe Allergy Error

Correct Actions and Rationale

1. **Notify Supervising Clinician and Risk Management:** Immediate clinician awareness is needed to correct the patient's chart and prevent medication errors.
2. **Submit an MDR to MAUDE or Report in EUDAMED:** Adverse patient outcomes linked to device errors must be filed as Medical Device Reports for regulatory tracking.
3. **Document Incident in the Medical Record and Institution's Reporting System:** Creates an audit trail that supports transparency, root-cause analysis, and quality improvement.
4. **Follow-Up on Corrective Actions:** Ensures the vendor and institution implement fixes (software patch, additional training) and prevents recurrence.

Scenario 2: Minor Software Update

Correct Determination and Rationale

1. **Proceed Under the Predetermined Change Control Plan (PCCP):** Since the update only enhances sentence structure (no change to clinical calculations or intended use), it fits within a preapproved change protocol.

2. **Document the Update in the Quality Management System:** Maintains regulatory compliance and traceability of all software iterations.
3. **Notify Regulatory Affairs Without New 510(k):** Minor, nonclinical modifications don't require a fresh 510(k) submission but must still be logged and communicated internally.

References

1. Walter M. FDA announces recall after Philips heart monitor software failed to send alerts – multiple deaths reported. Cardiovascular Business; 2025, January 13
2. U.S. Food and Drug Administration. Software as a Medical Device (SaMD): clinical evaluation; 2023. Retrieved from https://www.fda.gov/medical-devices/software-medical-device-samd/clinical-evaluation
3. U.S. Food and Drug Administration. 510(k) premarket notification; 2023. Retrieved from https://www.fda.gov/medical-devices/premarket-notification-510k
4. U.S. Food and Drug Administration. De Novo classification process (Evaluation of automatic class III designation); 2023. Retrieved from https://www.fda.gov/medical-devices/premarket-submissions/de-novo-classification-process-evaluation-automatic-class-iii-designation
5. U.S. Food and Drug Administration. Premarket Approval (PMA); 2023. Retrieved from https://www.fda.gov/medical-devices/premarket-approval-pma
6. U.S. Food and Drug Administration. Breakthrough devices program; 2023. Retrieved from https://www.fda.gov/medical-devices/how-study-and-market-your-device/breakthrough-devices-program
7. European Commission. CE marking: your indication that products comply with EU rules; n.d.. Retrieved May 2025, from https://ec.europa.eu/growth/single-market/ce-marking_en
8. European Parliament and Council. Regulation (EU) 2017/745 on medical devices (MDR). Official Journal of the European Union; 2017.
9. European Parliament and Council. Regulation (EU) 2017/746 on in vitro diagnostic medical devices (IVDR). Official Journal of the European Union; 2017.
10. U.S. Food and Drug Administration. About the Manufacturer and User Facility Device Experience (MAUDE) database; n.d.. Retrieved May 2025, from https://www.fda.gov/medical-devices/mandatory-reporting-requirements-manufacturers-importers-and-device-user-facilities/about-manufacturer-and-user-facility-device-experience-maude-database
11. European Commission. European Database on Medical Devices (EUDAMED) overview; 2020. Retrieved May 2025, from https://ec.europa.eu/tools/eudamed
12. U.S. Food and Drug Administration, Health Canada, & Medicines and Healthcare products Regulatory Agency. Predetermined change control plans for machine learning-enabled medical devices: guiding principles; 2023. Retrieved from https://www.fda.gov/media/164137/download
13. U.S. Food and Drug Administration. Labeling (21 CFR Part 801). n.d.. Retrieved May 2025, from https://www.ecfr.gov/current/title-21/chapter-I/subchapter-H/part-801
14. European Parliament and Council. Artificial Intelligence Act, Article 13: transparency and provision of information; 2021. Retrieved May 2025, from https://artificialintelligenceact.eu/article/13/
15. Rosenbaum L. Understanding liability risk from using health care artificial intelligence. N Engl J Med. 2023;388(8):673–5. https://doi.org/10.1056/NEJMhle2308901.

16. Smith AB, Jones CD, Patel R. AI scribe error leads to malpractice claim: a case report. J Med Ethics Technol. 2024;10(2):45–8. https://doi.org/10.1000/jmet.2024.0104.
17. U.S. Food and Drug Administration. Postmarket surveillance under a quality system regulation (QSR); 2023. Retrieved May 2025, from https://www.fda.gov/media/82395/download
18. American Medical Association. Health Innovator Podcast: Regulating AI in Medicine [Audio podcast episode]; 2024. Retrieved from https://www.ama-assn.org/about/ama-health-innovator-podcast
19. U.S. Food and Drug Administration.Devices@FDA Database; n.d.. Retrieved May 2025, from https://www.accessdata.fda.gov/scripts/cdrh/cfdocs/cfdevice/device.cfm

Chapter 11
Integrating Generative AI into Clinical Practice

Introduction

Artificial intelligence (AI) is no longer a laboratory novelty—it's rapidly becoming a standard component of clinical workflows. What began as impressive "cool demos" now shapes real-world decisions, from draft discharge summaries to early warning alerts. Your challenge as tomorrow's physician is to guide this transition, so that AI augments care rather than obstructs it.

By the end of this chapter, you will be able to:

1. Map the key stakeholders involved in AI adoption, and learn to tailor your message to each group (e.g., clinicians versus IT versus leadership).
2. Anticipate and address common resistance points to ensure widespread acceptance.
3. Lead a pilot AI project in our "You are the CMIO" simulation, making data-driven rollout decisions.
4. Establish feedback loops that turn user experiences into continuous improvements [1].

Clinical Vignette
On the third day of her internal medicine rotation, medical student Patricia Tietjen reviews the electronic health record of Mr. Patel, a 62-year-old man presenting with acute chest pain. To support her diagnostic reasoning, she consults an AI-powered differential diagnosis tool and enters the prompt: "List possible causes of sudden-onset chest pain in a 62-year-old man."

Visualizations of research data or results in this manuscript were generated, refined, corrected, edited, or formatted with the assistance of artificial intelligence (AI) tools, specifically OpenAI's ChatGPT 4.0, 2024. All content has been thoroughly reviewed, revised, and approved by the author(s) to ensure scientific accuracy and preserve the integrity of the original material.

© The Author(s), under exclusive license to Springer Nature Switzerland AG 2025

C. Quinn, *Generative AI for the Medical Student*,
https://doi.org/10.1007/978-3-032-01613-3_11

The AI model returns a list that includes myocardial infarction, gastroesophageal reflux disease (GERD), cholecystitis, musculoskeletal pain, and pericarditis. As Patricia reads more closely through the chart, she notices two critical red flags: Mr. Patel has a history of uncontrolled hypertension, and his pain is described as "tearing" and radiating to the back. These are classic but often overlooked signs of aortic dissection.

Recognizing the limitations of the initial AI output, she refines her prompt to: "Include life-threatening etiologies when chest pain is described as tearing or radiating to the back in a hypertensive patient." This time, the AI lists aortic dissection at the top of the differential.

Acting on this revised output, Patricia immediately notifies her supervising resident and orders a CT angiogram. The scan confirms an acute aortic dissection. Her prompt refinement and critical thinking expedite a life-saving diagnosis.

This scenario illustrates two core principles: Firstly, AI outputs can omit critical diagnoses if key risk factors aren't surfaced in the prompt; secondly, the Prompt → Review → Revise cycle empowers you to steer AI toward safer, more comprehensive clinical reasoning.

Having seen how prompt refinement can save a life, the next step is to learn how to secure the practical support you need to deploy AI tools safely in real settings.

Securing Early Support: Why You Need to Know Who's Who

You won't be the one signing off on hospital-wide AI rollouts, but as a medical student, you'll interact daily with AI tools in the clinic, the wards, and the simulator. Knowing who influences those tools and what each person cares about helps you navigate real-world hurdles [2] (see Fig. 11.1). For example, when you notice an AI-generated note that mislabels a medication, you'll need to report it not only to your resident but also to the IT help desk, which manages the software, and perhaps to the compliance officer, who oversees data privacy. Each stakeholder has a different perspective: Nurses may worry about workflow interruptions, IT teams focus on system integration, and compliance officers prioritize patient confidentiality.

Stakeholder	Primary Concern	How to Communicate
Attending Physician	Clinical accuracy	Focus on diagnosis quality and evidence-based care
Nurse Lead	Workflow burden	Emphasize time-saving features and usability
IT Support	Integration and uptime	Report technical issues, error rates, and downtime
Compliance Officer	Privacy, audit trails	Describe HIPAA compliance, audit logs, and PHI risks

Fig. 11.1 Who are the stakeholders?

Recognizing these roles and learning to frame your observations in terms they value ensures your feedback drives improvement rather than getting lost in bureaucratic channels [3]. Start by making a simple list: attendings, nurses, IT support, and compliance. Next time you raise a concern, say, in morning rounds, note how each group's priorities differ. When you say, "I found charting errors in three out of five AI-drafted notes, which may delay discharge," you speak the language of both clinical accuracy and operational efficiency. This awareness builds credibility, speeds problem resolution, and brings you closer to shaping AI tools that truly help patient care.

With early support in hand, you'll inevitably face skepticism. Let's explore the most common sources of resistance and how to turn them into opportunities for engagement.

Mini-Workshop Draft a one-sentence note to your clerkship director explaining how reporting an AI error can prevent patient harm. Swap with a peer, and refine your language to address both clinical and operational concerns.

Anticipating Resistance

Medical students must expect and navigate pushback when deploying AI tools in clinical settings. Resistance often stems from three main concerns. Clinicians may fear AI will supplant their roles; reassure your team that AI amplifies human expertise, streamlining note-taking and suggesting differentials, while ultimate decisions rest with trained professionals [4]. A second worry involves AI "hallucinations" or fabricated errors that mimic real data; always apply the Prompt → Review → Revise cycle (Section "Introduction") to verify every AI-generated recommendation before acting on it [5]. Finally, safeguarding patient privacy is nonnegotiable. Familiarize yourself with de-identification protocols, removing names, dates, and identifiers, so that you can confidently use EHR data without risking confidentiality breaches [6].

These ethical issues are more thoroughly explained in Chap. 9, where you'll find examples of sampling and measurement bias in real clinical settings.

Sidebar: De-identification "How-To"

Why It Matters: Protecting patient privacy is nonnegotiable. Before using real clinical notes with AI tools, strip out all protected health information (PHI) to comply with HIPAA and institutional policies.

Step-by-Step Guide:

1. **Remove Direct Identifiers**
   - Names (e.g., "John Smith" → "[Patient Name]")
   - Medical record numbers (e.g., "MRN: 123456" → "[MRN]")
   - Dates (e.g., "DOB: 02/14/1950" → "[Date]")
   - Phone numbers, email addresses

(continued)

2. **Generalize Geographic Details**
   - Replace street addresses and facility names with broad terms (e.g., "Northside Hospital" → "[Hospital]").
3. **Mask Unique Characteristics**
   - Occupation, rare diagnoses, or unique events that could identify the patient (e.g., "transplanted at age 5" → remove or generalize)
4. **Check Free-Text Fields**
   - Scan for embedded identifiers in progress notes or consult letters. Use "Find" to search for capitalized names or numeric strings.
5. **Verify and Document**
   - Have a peer spot-check the redacted note. Keep a log of the de-identification process for audit purposes.

Redacted Example
Original Note

John Smith (MRN: 123456) is a 72-year-old male admitted on 03/15/2023 to Northside Hospital for CHF exacerbation. He lives at 456 Elm St., Springfield, and reports increased dyspnea over the past two weeks.

De-identified Note

[Patient Name] ([MRN]) is a 72-year-old male admitted on [Date] to [Hospital] for CHF exacerbation. He reports increased dyspnea over the past two weeks.

This sidebar equips you to confidently prepare clinical text for safe AI use—no "I don't know how" excuses.

Ethics Sidebar: "What Would You Do?"
A radiology AI flags a benign-appearing nodule as malignant. You review the image, disagree, and the AI insists on malignancy. Do you trust your interpretation, override the AI, or seek further tests first?

To practice, pose this to ChatGPT: "List three common biases in AI-generated clinical summaries." Compare its answer to your own biases list. Then refine your prompt, perhaps by adding "clinical context" or "evidence-based guidelines," and observe how the output changes. Finally, reflect on which bias emerged most often and how your prompt revision reduced it.

By acknowledging fears, applying rigorous verification, and involving colleagues in prompt refinement, you transform resistance into an opportunity for safer, more trustworthy AI adoption.

Armed with strategies to address errors and bias, you're ready to step into a leadership role; let's test those skills in our CMIO simulation.

Quantifying bias is covered in detail in Section "Evaluating AI performance", where bias scores are calculated and tracked using a rubric.

Simulation: "You Are the CMIO"

Simulation provides a risk-free environment to hone leadership and teamwork under pressure [6]. You'll receive a packet containing three handouts:

1. **Pilot Data Summary:** Details the sepsis alert system's performance—sensitivity (92%), specificity (85%), false-alarm rate (15%), and notes on false positives in patients with chronic inflammation.
2. **IT Readiness Checklist:** A one-page form confirming EMR integration, help-desk coverage, access controls, network latency, device compatibility, and training environment availability.
3. **Compliance Memo:** Guidance on HIPAA-compliant de-identification, audit-trail requirements, clinician liability, FDA classification, and quarterly audit schedules.

In your team of four—CMIO (you), nurse lead, IT lead, and legal counsel—spend 5 min each stating your top implementation priority based on these documents. Then devote 10 min to collaborative data review, debating the trade-off between alert fatigue and early event detection. In the final 5 min, vote to proceed, adjust parameters, or pause for further validation.

During the debrief, discuss how alarm thresholds affect clinician trust and patient safety. Capture your group's decision rationale in two concise sentences; for example, "We will lower the alert threshold to 90% sensitivity to reduce missed sepsis cases while scheduling weekly false-alarm audits to mitigate alert fatigue."

For deeper insight, switch to the alternate "You Are the Resident" track. In this role, practice escalating a frontline concern, such as pandemic workloads increasing false alarms, to the CMIO, and observe how your feedback alters implementation decisions [7].

This structured exercise sharpens critical thinking and interprofessional communication and mirrors the real-world dynamics you'll encounter when advocating for responsible AI integration in clinical practice.

Simulations teach us critical thinking in the moment. To reinforce those lessons, we must establish ongoing feedback mechanisms, such as participating in the AI Journal Club, and engage in continuous learning loops.

Below are the documents for the hypothetical sepsis alert system rollout.

1. Pilot Data Summary

   Sepsis Alert System Performance

   - **Population:** 1000 adult in-patients over 3 months.
   - **Sensitivity:** 92%.
   - **Specificity:** 85%.
   - **False-alarm rate:** 15% (alerts per 100 patients).
   - **Positive predictive value:** 48%.
   - **Negative predictive value:** 98%.
   - **Average time to alert:** 3 min after vital sign trigger.

- **Notes:** Most false alarms occurred in patients with chronic inflammation (e.g., rheumatoid arthritis).

2. IT Readiness Checklist

Item	Yes	No	Comments
EMR integration tested	☑	☐	Successfully passed interface tests
24/7 Help-desk coverage	☐	☑	Only 8 am–8 pm support currently
Data backup and disaster recovery plan	☑	☐	Nightly backups verified
User access controls configured	☑	☐	Role-based access in place
Network latency <200 ms for alert flow	☐	☑	Measured at 35 ms during peak hours
Mobile device compatibility verified	☑	☐	Tested on iOS only
Training environment provisioned	☐	☑	Sandbox still under setup

3. Compliance Memo
   To: AI Steering Committee
   From: Office of Compliance and Privacy
   Subject: Privacy and Liability Considerations for Sepsis Alert AI

   (a) **Data Privacy:** All patient data used by the AI must be de-identified per HIPAA Safe Harbor (removal of 18 identifiers).
   (b) **Audit Trail:** Maintain logs of all AI alerts and clinician overrides for 6 years.
   (c) **Liability:** Clinicians retain ultimate responsibility; AI alerts are advisory only. Document any decision to follow or override AI.
   (d) **FDA Classification:** System qualifies as a Clinical Decision Support Device under 21 CFR § 803—no premarket submission required, but adverse events must be reported within 30 days.
   (e) **Regular Review:** Quarterly audits by compliance and patient safety to monitor alert appropriateness, bias, and workflow impact.

Feedback Loops and Continuous Learning

Building habits of reflection and improvement is key to using AI safely. Instead of formal M&M conferences, organize a monthly AI Journal Club: a student-led debrief with an attending mentor. In each session, present one case in which an AI tool influenced care, summarize the AI's recommendation, any clinician override, and the patient outcome using a simple template. Discuss what went well, what went wrong, and how prompt phrasing or tool settings might be refined. This peer-review forum mirrors quality-improvement practices and empowers you to learn from both successes and missteps [8].

Complement qualitative discussions with quantitative tracking. Keep a log of how many clinical notes you draft with AI assistance versus those needing

Fig. 11.2 Prompt review and revise cycle

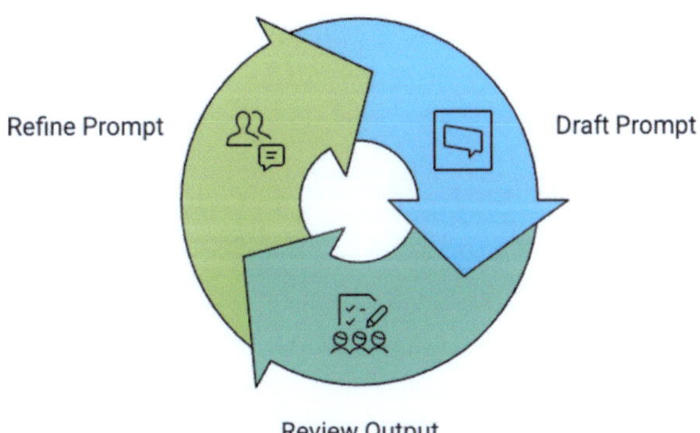

substantial edits, and chart the average time saved per note each month. Evidence suggests AI-assisted documentation can reduce note-writing time by up to 35%, freeing you to spend more time at the bedside [9].

Central to continuous learning is the **Prompt–Review–Revise** cycle. After sharing your initial prompts, review the AI outputs for clinical accuracy as a group and then collaboratively refine prompt language to address gaps. Use an infographic, Draft prompt → Review output → Refine prompt, as a visual guide during discussions (see Fig. 11.2).

For structured planning and professional goal setting, see the SMART goals framework in Section "Chapter overview (revised)".

Medical students must learn to treat AI outputs as starting points, not definitive answers. One powerful way to build this habit is by using a retrieval-augmented generation (RAG) tool such as Perplexity AI (https://www.perplexity.ai). Begin by entering a focused clinical query, for example, "What are the latest ACC/AHA guidelines for heart failure management?" and then examine the "Sources" panel that appears alongside the AI's summary. Your task is threefold: first, identify which guideline documents or landmark trials the system retrieved; second, assess whether those sources are truly current and authoritative; and third, compare the AI's synthesized narrative to the guidelines or original texts.

This exercise serves two important goals. First, it trains you to spot when the AI is grounded adequately in evidence versus when it may hallucinate unsupported statements. Second, it ingrains a verification routine, prompting AI to review its citations and cross-check summaries, which will become indispensable when you rely on generative models in real clinical decision-making. By practicing this cycle, you'll gain confidence that the AI tools you use enhance patient care rather than compromise it [4].

Sidebar: Exploring RAG Tools for Medical Students

Critical Appraisal Skills for Future-Proof Practice

Why Retrieval-Augmented Generation (RAG) Matters

In a future shaped by AI, physicians must do more than use clinical decision tools—they must interrogate them. RAG systems offer a transparent alternative to black-box AI by showing which documents informed an answer. They retrieve relevant sources (like journal articles or treatment guidelines) and then generate responses grounded in those texts. This traceability reduces hallucinations and strengthens clinical accountability.

Understanding how RAG works prepares students to evaluate AI tools for usefulness, safety, bias, and fidelity to evidence, which are the core concerns of this chapter.

Test-Drive These RAG Tools

- **Elicit (Ought)**

  An AI research assistant that pulls papers from *Semantic Scholar* to answer medical queries. When you search for something like "management of acute pulmonary embolism," it shows summaries and a "Top Papers" panel, helping you assess the evidence behind the answer.

  https://elicit.org
- **Hugging Face RAG Demo**

  A live demonstration of how retrieval improves LLM outputs. You can input a medical corpus (e.g., PubMed abstracts) and observe how retrieved sentences influence the final response. Ideal for seeing what's *under the hood* of a generative model.

  https://huggingface.co/spaces/facebook/rag-demo
- **Google Med-PaLM 2 (Research Preview)**

  A frontier medical LLM trained with retrieval capabilities. Though access is limited, Google AI blog updates highlight how the system cites clinical guidelines and emphasizes safety in high-stakes decision-making.

  https://ai.googleblog.com
- **Semantic Scholar TL;DR+**

  Upload a medical paper, and receive a concise summary along with highlighted sentences pulled from the full text. Toggle "Show Sources" to view which excerpts the model used for grounding.

  https://www.semanticscholar.org
- **LangChain Playground**

  A customizable environment for advanced users to build their own RAG pipelines. You can connect a medical vector database (e.g., local clinical guidelines) to an LLM and analyze how well it retrieves and integrates citations.

  https://play.langchain.com

(continued)

Your Assignment: Compare and Critique

Choose two platforms. Use the same query (e.g., "risk factors for aortic dissection" or "treatment of delirium in elderly patients") across both tools. Then evaluate:

1. **Retrieval Scope**—How many and what types of sources are retrieved? Are they peer-reviewed or open-access summaries?
2. **Citation Transparency**—Does the platform clearly show which sources it used? Are citations linked, embedded, or just referenced?
3. **Fidelity to Evidence**—Does the summary remain faithful to the original source, or does it introduce errors, omissions, or oversimplifications?

Takeaway for Chapter

Implementing AI in clinical care requires more than accuracy; it demands traceability, bias awareness, and thoughtful human oversight. RAG tools give future physicians a window into these systems' inner workings and a framework for safer use.

Having practiced iterative refinement and peer review, it's time to assess your mastery and chart the path forward in your AI journey.

Reflection Prompt At the next Journal Club, share one before-and-after prompt example. What change improved clinical accuracy?

Assessment and Next Steps

To ensure you've mastered the practical skills in this chapter, complete the following competency checklist:

- Draft and defend an AI-generated clinical note, explaining your prompt choices and edits.
- Identify at least one bias in an AI output, and describe how you mitigated it.
- Lead or actively participate in the "You Are the CMIO" simulation, articulating your decision rationale.
- Perform a full Prompt–Review–Revise exercise, demonstrating improved clinical accuracy.

These activities align with the core AI competencies defined for medical graduates, spanning digital health foundations, ethical use, and data analysis [10].

Final Vignette

Six months later, Dr. Patricia Tietjen spearheads her first AI-guided quality improvement initiative on the surgical floor. Using her peer-refined prompts and

RAG-backed summaries, she identifies postoperative patients at high risk for complications. Collaborating with nursing and IT teams, she implements an AI-driven early warning alert that reduces readmission rates by 15% within 3 months.

Conclusion

Integrating generative AI into clinical practice requires more than technical competence; it demands stakeholder fluency, ethical vigilance, and the ability to lead under uncertainty. This chapter has equipped you with foundational strategies: recognizing key influencers, navigating resistance with empathy and precision, verifying AI outputs through prompt refinement, and engaging in structured feedback loops that promote safe, iterative learning. Through simulations and journal clubs, you've practiced the interpersonal and analytic skills needed to become a responsible AI steward. But as adoption spreads, the next challenge is scale. Chapter 12 examines what it takes to sustain and expand these innovations, exploring how health systems can responsibly implement federated learning, digital twins, and next-generation AI models while maintaining equity, safety, and clinical relevance.

Instructor's Guide for Chapter

Integration of AI into Clinical Practice

Chapter Overview and Learning Objectives

This chapter moves learners from AI pilots to sustained clinical impact. By guiding students through stakeholder awareness, resistance management, leadership simulations, and continuous feedback loops, it prepares them to function effectively in AI-enabled teams.

Key Learning Objectives

1. Understand the roles and priorities of clinical, technical, and administrative stakeholders.
2. Anticipate and mitigate common sources of resistance to AI adoption.
3. Apply decision-making frameworks in a "You Are the CMIO" simulation.
4. Establish peer-review mechanisms and iterative prompt-refinement processes.
5. Demonstrate core AI competencies through hands-on assessments.

Before Teaching

- **Materials**
  - Simulation packet handouts (Pilot Data Summary, IT Readiness Checklist, Compliance Memo).
  - Infographic of the Prompt–Review–Revise cycle.
  - Access to Perplexity AI (https://www.perplexity.ai) or alternative RAG demo.
- **Preparation**
  - Familiarize yourself with the simulation data, and decide on hypothetical checklist answers (e.g., limited help-desk hours, high latency).
  - Review common AI pitfalls (hallucinations, bias), and have examples ready.
  - Set up a shared workspace (whiteboard or digital) for AI Journal Club notes and data charts.

Section-by-Section Teaching Tips

Introduction

- **Goal:** Frame AI as a tool requiring active human guidance.
- **Tip:** After presenting the vignette with Patricia Tietjen, ask learners to identify two moments where human expertise corrected or enhanced the AI's output.
- **Discussion Prompt:** "Why did Patricia's prompt revision succeed where the initial query failed?"

Securing Early Support

- **Goal:** Show students how to communicate AI concerns to different stakeholders.
- **Tip:** Role-play a brief exchange—one student as a nurse raising workflow concerns, another as a medical student proposing solutions.
- **Key Takeaway:** Effective feedback speaks stakeholders' language—clinical accuracy for clinicians, operational impact for administrators.

Anticipating Resistance

- **Goal:** Equip students to recognize and address fears about AI.
- **Tip:** Use the Ethics Sidebar scenario to spark debate; assign small groups to defend alternative approaches (override vs. seek further tests).
- **Common Pitfall:** Students may assume AI is always correct. Encourage skepticism and verification habits.

Simulation: "You Are the CMIO"

- **Goal:** Practice cross-functional decision-making under time pressure.
- **Setup (30-min. Total)**
  1. **Role Assignment and Priority Statements (20 min)**
     - CMIO, Nurse Lead, IT Lead, Legal Counsel each speak for 5 min.
  2. **Data Review and Debate (10 min)**
  3. **Decision and Rationale (5 min)**
- **Expected Results**
  1. Most teams opt to **modify** alert thresholds (e.g., lower sensitivity to 90%) to balance early detection against alarm fatigue.
  2. Common rationales
     - "We prioritize patient safety by accepting a small increase in false alarms."
     - "We will implement weekly false-alarm audits and additional staff training to manage workload."
- **Debrief Questions**
  1. "What stakeholder concern most influenced your decision?"
  2. "How did conflicting priorities (e.g., IT readiness vs. clinical urgency) get resolved?"
- **Alternate Track:** After first run, have the "Resident" escalate a real-world concern (e.g., weekend staffing gaps), and observe how teams adjust their plan.

Feedback Loops and Continuous Learning

- **Goal:** Reinforce habits of peer review and prompt refinement.
- **Tip:** Convene a brief AI Journal Club in class—Present one recent AI case (real or simulated), walk through the Prompt–Review–Revise cycle, and record prompt changes.
- **Data Exercise:** Students chart time savings and edit rates on a shared spreadsheet. Compare before/after AI introduction.
- **RAG Tool Activity:** Demonstrate perplexity AI's source citations. Assign each student a clinical guideline to verify via perplexity and report back on accuracy.

Assessment and Next Steps

- **Goal:** Confirm competency, and set the stage for sustainability topics in Chap. 12.
- **Checklist Review:** Have students self-score on the four competencies.

- **Final Vignette Discussion:** Discuss how Patricia Tietjen applied chapter learnings to a QI initiative. Ask: "What additional governance or data-monitoring steps might she need for long-term success?"
- **Preview:** Highlight how Chap. 12 will address scaling, ethical frameworks, and emerging AI modalities (e.g., federated learning, digital twins).

Note to Instructor Encourage reflection on both technical and interpersonal dimensions of AI integration. Students often focus on the technology; prompt them to value communication, governance, and ethics equally.

References

1. Al Kuwaiti A, Nazer K, Al-Reedy A, Al-Shehri S, Al-Muhanna A, Subbarayalu AV, Al Muhanna D, Al-Muhanna FA. A review of the role of artificial intelligence in healthcare. J Pers Med. 2023;13(6):951. https://doi.org/10.3390/jpm13060951. PMID: 37373940; PMCID: PMC10301994
2. Hogg HDJ, Al-Zubaidy M, Technology Enhanced Macular Services Study Reference Group, Talks J, Denniston AK, Kelly CJ, Malawana J, Papoutsi C, Teare MD, Keane PA, Beyer FR, Maniatopoulos G. Stakeholder perspectives of clinical artificial intelligence implementation: systematic review of qualitative evidence. J Med Internet Res. 2023;25:e39742. https://doi.org/10.2196/39742. PMID: 36626192; PMCID: PMC9875023
3. Vijayakumar S, Lee VV, Leong QY, Hong SJ, Blasiak A, Ho D. Physicians' perspectives on AI in clinical decision support systems: interview study of the CURATE. AI personalized dose optimization platform. JMIR Hum Factors. 2023;10:e48476. https://doi.org/10.2196/48476. PMID: 37902825. PMCID: 10644191
4. Davenport T, Kalakota R. The potential for artificial intelligence in healthcare. Future Healthcare J. 2019;6(2):94–8. https://doi.org/10.7861/futurehosp.6-2-94.
5. Ji Z, Lee N, Frieske R, et al. Survey of hallucination in natural language generation. ACM Comput Surv. 2023;55(12):1–38. https://doi.org/10.1145/3571730.
6. El Emam K. Guide to the de-identification of personal health information. CRC Press; 2020.
7. Issenberg SB, McGaghie WC, Hart IR, Mayer JW, Felner JM, Petrusa ER, et al. Features and uses of high-fidelity medical simulations that lead to effective learning: a BEME systematic review. Med Teach. 2005;27(1):10–28. https://doi.org/10.1080/01421590500046924.
8. McGaghie WC, Issenberg SB, Cohen ER, Barsuk JH, Wayne DB. Does simulation-based medical education with deliberate practice yield better results than traditional clinical education? A meta-analytic comparative review of the evidence. Acad Med. 2011;86(6):706–11. https://doi.org/10.1097/ACM.0b013e318217e119.
9. Feng J, Li X, Patel V. Clinical artificial intelligence quality improvement: Towards continual monitoring and updating of AI algorithms. NPJ Digital Med. 2022;5(1):1–10. https://doi.org/10.1038/s41746-022-00611-y.
10. Lewis P, Perez E, Piktus A, Petroni F, Karpukhin V, Goyal N, et al. Retrieval-augmented generation for knowledge-intensive NLP tasks. Adv Neural Inf Process Syst. 2020;33:9459–74.
11. Lee S, Smith A, Park K. Defining medical AI competencies for medical school graduates: outcomes of a Delphi survey. Acad Med. 2024;99(5):650–7. https://doi.org/10.1097/ACM.0000000000002044.

Chapter 12
Building Your Team, Planning Your Project and Your Mini AI Journal Club Capstone

Generative AI thrives when we combine clinical insight, practical tools, and ethical oversight. Whether you're working solo or with peers, this chapter shows you how to assume key project roles, use ready-made case vignettes, safeguard privacy, follow a clear roadmap, and culminate in a Mini AI Journal Club, no coding or hospital systems required.

Learning Objectives
By the end of this chapter, you will be able to:

1. **Simulate four key project roles** in AI implementation—Clinical Lead, Data Navigator, Ethics Reviewer, and Project Manager—and explain their responsibilities.
2. **Engage virtual stakeholders** through interviews and professional webinars, and then synthesize their concerns into clear, persuasive elevator pitches tailored to nurses, compliance officers, and others.
3. **Design and refine AI prompts** using prewritten clinical vignettes, comparing outputs to gold-standard expert notes for discharge summaries, problem lists, and differential diagnoses.
4. **Apply ethical and privacy safeguards** by performing de-identification on clinical texts and maintaining transparent logs of the process.
5. **Develop and follow a 12-week roadmap** to plan and execute a peer-led clinical AI project from inception to completion.
6. **Lead or participate in a Mini AI Journal Club**, using real-world case analyses to extract actionable lessons, evaluate stakeholder perspectives, and assess AI performance metrics.
7. **Synthesize key takeaways** from AI use cases into feedback-loop artifacts that inform prompt design, stakeholder training, and system-level implementation strategies.

© The Author(s), under exclusive license to Springer Nature Switzerland AG 2025
C. Quinn, *Generative AI for the Medical Student*,
https://doi.org/10.1007/978-3-032-01613-3_12

Simulating Four Essential Roles

Launching an AI initiative in clinical practice requires more than technical skill. It demands a working knowledge of clinical reasoning, data management, ethical safeguards, and project coordination. Even if you're working alone, taking on these core responsibilities prepares you for the collaborative challenges of real-world AI implementation. In this section, you'll practice simulating four foundational roles that align with how AI projects are managed in hospitals, research teams, and clinical quality-improvement settings.

1. **Clinical lead (prompt designer):** This role demands clinical judgment and precision. You will translate patient scenarios into clear, targeted prompts that an AI tool can understand. Just as important, you will critically assess the AI's responses for completeness, accuracy, and alignment with accepted medical practice.
2. **Data navigator:** Here, your focus is on preparing and managing input data. Using the prewritten case vignettes provided in this chapter, you will copy and paste clinical scenarios into the AI tool. Your task is to ensure that each entry is complete and well-formatted to yield the most useful output.
3. **Ethics reviewer:** Every AI project must uphold patient confidentiality. In this role, you will identify and remove protected health information such as names, dates, addresses, and other identifiers. You will follow a structured process to demonstrate privacy best practices even when using simulated or educational notes.
4. **Project manager:** Successful AI integration depends on coordination and accountability. As project manager, you will develop a timeline, set goals, assign or monitor tasks, and track progress using a calendar or task board. Whether working solo or with a group, your goal is to ensure that the project stays organized and on track.
5. **Key takeaway:** Practicing these four roles helps you internalize the skills that AI leaders use every day. It strengthens your ability to work across clinical, technical, and ethical domains while building habits that support safety, collaboration, and sustained improvement.

   Practicing these four roles sharpens your ability to collaborate across disciplines. You'll build habits of accountability, communication, and critical review, all of which are essential to real-world AI adoption in clinical practice.

   Now that you've gained experience with these perspectives, it's time to engage with stakeholders, gather insights, and begin shaping your first AI-driven solution, even if it's entirely virtual.

With this foundation in place, you are ready to connect with virtual stakeholders, craft targeted messages, and begin shaping your AI solution for real-world clinical challenges.

Craft Two-Sentence Elevator Pitches

An **elevator pitch** is a concise, persuasive statement designed to "sell" an idea to a busy decision-maker in the time it takes to ride an elevator, about 30–60 s. In your capstone, you're effectively "selling" the value of your AI prompt or tool to different stakeholder audiences:

- **To nurses:** You're pitching how your AI-generated note template or alert prompt will save them time and reduce burnout. A sample pitch might be, "Our AI prompt decreased handoff preparation time by 20%, so you spend more time at the bedside and less on paperwork."
- **To compliance officers:** You're assuring them that patient privacy is preserved. For example, "All notes are de-identified using a standardized process, meeting HIPAA Safe Harbor criteria for data sharing."

Crafting these targeted pitches requires distilling complex technical work into clear benefits that each group values. When stakeholders hear language that mirrors their priorities, "charting time" and "privacy safeguards," they recognize you've listened, building trust and opening doors to further collaboration.

By combining self-paced webinar learning with succinct, audience-focused pitches, you'll demonstrate both technical understanding and communication savvy. These are the key ingredients for successful AI integration in any clinical setting.

Key Takeaway Tailoring your message builds trust and unlocks practical advice.

Armed with stakeholder insights and the vocabulary of informatics, you're ready to see your prompts in action on real patient stories.

Working with Prepackaged Clinical Cases

Goal Practice your prompt-design skills on realistic patient scenarios, so you learn to craft clear, focused AI queries and evaluate the generated outputs against expert "gold-standard" notes.

In this exercise, you'll practice three clinically relevant prompt types:

- **Discharge summaries:** Teach the AI to condense a patient's entire stay into a clear, actionable summary, critical for safe handoffs and continuity of care.
- **Problem lists and care plans:** Ask the AI to extract key diagnoses, risk factors, and management steps, skills you'll use daily to organize differential diagnoses and treatment priorities.
- **Focused differential diagnoses:** Request a prioritized list of potential causes for a presenting symptom—training you to think broadly before narrowing down to the most likely etiologies.

Mastering each of these prompt styles ensures you can leverage AI not just for one-off demonstrations but for the routine clinical tasks that underpin patient safety and effective teamwork.

What You'll Do

1. **Paste each case into your AI tool:** Use the copy-ready text below as your input.
2. **Craft a targeted prompt:** For each case, decide what you want the AI to produce—e.g.,
   - A concise discharge summary ("Write a one-paragraph discharge note.")
   - A problem list and care plan ("List the top three management steps.")
   - A focused differential diagnosis ("Provide differential diagnoses for chest pain.")
3. **Evaluate the output:** Compare the AI's response to the provided gold-standard note. Note missing items, added errors, or ambiguities.
4. **Refine and repeat:** Adjust your prompt to address gaps (e.g., "Include social history," "Emphasize treatment timeline"), and observe how the AI's output improves.

Prepackaged Cases

Case 1: Mr. Alvarez, 68 y/o with Dyspnea

Demographics: 68-year-old male; PMH—hypertension, atrial fibrillation.
Vitals: BP 150/90, HR 104, RR 22, SpO_2 88% on room air.
Narrative: Progressive shortness of breath over 3 days. Chest X-ray shows bilateral pulmonary infiltrates. BNP 1200 pg/mL. Responded moderately to IV furosemide.

Gold-Standard Note

"68-year-old male with CHF exacerbation demonstrated improvement after diuresis. Plan to transition to oral diuretics and follow up with cardiology in one week."

Case 2: Ms. Chen, 45 y/o with Chest Pain

Demographics: 45-year-old female; PMH—smoking, hyperlipidemia.
Vitals: BP 140/85, HR 92, RR 18, SpO_2 97% on room air.
Narrative: Two-hour history of substernal chest pressure radiating to the jaw. ECG normal. Troponin I 0.02 ng/mL. Pain relieved by sublingual nitroglycerin.

Gold-Standard Note

"45-year-old female with low-risk chest pain; negative biomarkers and unremarkable ECG. Discharged with outpatient stress test and cardiology follow-up."

Case 3: Epic Sepsis Alert Scenario

Demographics: 56-year-old female; PMH: type 2 diabetes.

Vitals: Fever 38.5 °C, HR 115, BP 98/60, RR 24.
Narrative: EHR-integrated sepsis alert triggered for rising lactate and hypotension. Alert fired 12 times in 24 hours; only 1 true septic episode confirmed.

Gold-Standard Summary

"56-year-old with type 2 diabetes met criteria for sepsis once. Alert fatigue noted; recommend threshold adjustment and enhanced clinician training."

Case 4: Dermatologist-Level Skin Lesion Classification

Demographics: 32-year-old male; PMH—none.
Presentation: Irregular pigmented lesion on left shoulder, 6 mm diameter, asymmetric border.
Narrative: Lesion photographed and analyzed by CNN model trained on 130,000 images. Model probability for melanoma: 92%.

Gold-Standard Interpretation

"High suspicion for melanoma given asymmetry and size; biopsy recommended. Patient advised on sun protection and dermatology referral."

Key Takeaway By practicing with these cases, you'll internalize prompt crafting, iterative refinement, and critical comparison to expert notes. These are foundational skills for using generative AI in patient care.

Ethical and Privacy Safeguards

Every AI project involving clinical text must begin with a commitment to patient privacy. Whether you are working with real notes or simulated cases, treating the data with respect reinforces trust and aligns your work with professional standards. Before entering any patient-related information into an AI tool, follow these three essential steps:

1. **Redact names and IDs:** Remove all direct identifiers such as patient names, initials, medical record numbers, and contact information. Refer to the de-identification sidebar in Chap. 11 for examples of replacing this information using standardized placeholders.
2. **Generalize dates and locations:** Replace specific admission dates, birthdates, or facility names with broader terms. For example, instead of "April 4, 2023 at Mount Sinai," you might write "Spring 2023 at a tertiary hospital." This protects against reidentification while preserving clinical meaning.
3. **Log your de-identification process:** Briefly record how and when you removed identifying details. A one-page audit trail is sufficient. Include the date, case identifier (if used), what was removed, and whether a peer reviewed your edits. This transparency enhances the credibility and reproducibility of your project.

Key Takeaway Meticulous de-identification protects patient privacy, strengthens the integrity of your work, and prepares you for the real-world expectations of institutional review boards, quality improvement committees, and clinical leadership.

Your 12-Week Roadmap

Managing an AI project alongside clinical rotations or coursework requires structure. A clear, step-by-step plan helps ensure steady progress without becoming overwhelming. This 12-week roadmap (see table below) is designed to guide you through the phases of your clinical AI capstone project, from team formation and prompt design to analysis and final presentation. You may use any calendar, project tracker, or digital task board to map these milestones.

Phase	Weeks	Activities
Plan and roles	1–2	Assign roles to team members or yourself. Draft a brief project proposal. Practice delivering two-sentence elevator pitches tailored to different stakeholders
Data and prompts	3–4	Input prewritten case vignettes into your AI tool. Experiment with early prompt designs and document initial outputs
Pilot and refine	5–7	Review AI outputs in weekly peer discussions. Identify gaps or errors and iteratively improve your prompts
Capstone session	8	Host your mini AI journal Club. Present case findings, evaluate real-world examples, and synthesize lessons for prompt improvement and tool refinement
Analyze and report	9–12	Organize feedback from your capstone. Prepare a final slide deck and written report summarizing your process, results, and recommendations

Key Takeaway A structured timeline makes complex projects more manageable. By breaking the work into realistic phases, you can stay on track while balancing academic responsibilities, clinical duties, and team coordination.

Capstone: Mini AI Journal Club (Expanded Cases)

Goal

To deepen your critical-analysis skills by examining high-impact, real-world case studies of clinical AI deployment. This capstone activity trains you to identify both failure points and success factors, evaluate metrics, and propose practical improvements for future implementations.

Each of the following cases highlights a different aspect of AI integration in health care. You will present, critique, and extract actionable lessons using a standardized discussion framework. These examples are based on real studies and institutional experiences. Your goal is not only to summarize outcomes but to interrogate the design, trustworthiness, and consequences of each AI tool.

Case A: IBM Watson for Oncology—Overpromising Without Delivering

Issue overview: Watson for Oncology was introduced across 12 top-tier cancer centers to provide chemotherapy recommendations by synthesizing EHR data and published literature.

AI's intended role: Deliver personalized, evidence-based cancer treatment plans in under 1 min.

Study details: A 2017 internal audit of 638 cases found that 30% of Watson's recommendations deviated from NCCN guidelines. An additional 12% were judged potentially unsafe by tumor boards. Clinician surveys revealed that 65% of users distrusted the tool's outputs.

Outcome and impact: Due to inconsistent alignment with clinical standards and lack of transparency in reasoning, the tool lost credibility. Within 1 year, most centers returned to manual reviews. This case underscores that AI must align with consensus guidelines and clearly communicate its rationale to earn clinician trust [1].

Case B: IDx-DR—Autonomous AI That Works in the Real World

Issue overview: Primary care clinics in rural areas faced long delays in diabetic retinopathy screening due to limited access to specialists.

AI's intended role: Automatically analyze fundus images and detect moderate-to-severe diabetic retinopathy without requiring a human interpreter.

Study details: In a pivotal 2018 trial with 950 patients across five clinics, IDx-DR achieved 87% sensitivity and 90% specificity. Referral time dropped from 45 to 7 days. Patient satisfaction scores averaged 4.5 out of 5.

Outcome and Impact: The tool received FDA de novo clearance and led to a 60% increase in high-risk case identification within 6 months. This case demonstrates that when integrated thoughtfully, AI can improve access, shorten time to diagnosis, and boost clinical efficiency [2].

Case C: Epic Sepsis Alert—When Too Many Warnings Undermine Safety

Issue overview: A major health system deployed an early-warning sepsis alert integrated into the EHR, aiming to detect patients meeting SIRS criteria with elevated lactate or hypotension.

AI's intended role: Provide real-time alerts to frontline clinicians to enable earlier sepsis intervention.

Study details: In the first 3 months, the system triggered 8400 alerts across 4200 patients, but only 25% were true positives. Nurses reported ignoring over 70% of alerts. A subsequent morbidity review found no change in sepsis-related mortality.

Outcome and impact: The alert system was paused. Developers raised thresholds and introduced a mandatory "acknowledge" step to address alert fatigue. This case highlights the trade-off between sensitivity and specificity and the importance of clinician engagement in system design [3].

Case D: CNN for Skin Cancer Triage—Scaling Expertise with AI

Issue overview: In many regions, dermatologic referrals are delayed, leading to late melanoma diagnoses.

AI's intended role: Use a convolutional neural network (CNN) to classify dermoscopic images as benign or malignant, serving as a triage tool for primary care.

Study details: A CNN trained on 135,000 images achieved an AUC of 0.96, matching the performance of 21 board-certified dermatologists. In a prospective study of 1000 patients, AI-first triage reduced wait times for dermatology consultation by 40%.

Outcome and impact: Teledermatology platforms adopted the model as a first-pass screening tool. The result was faster specialist referrals and improved early melanoma detection. This case illustrates how AI can extend diagnostic reach and improve care equity without replacing physician oversight.

Next Step

In pairs or small groups, choose one case to present and critique during the Mini AI Journal Club. Use the provided discussion worksheet below to guide your analysis.

Mini AI Journal Club Discussion Worksheet

Instructions: In your small group or assigned pair, choose one of the four case studies provided in section "Capstone: Mini AI journal club (expanded cases)". Use this worksheet to guide your analysis and prepare for your presentation during the Mini AI Journal Club session. Be prepared to explain both the AI deployment's successes and limitations, supported by data and stakeholder perspectives.

1. **Case Title**

   Write the name of your selected case (e.g., Case A: IBM Watson for Oncology).
2. **AI Tool Purpose and Intended Function**

   What problem was the AI tool designed to solve? How was it intended to function in clinical practice?
3. **Key Performance Metrics**

   List relevant metrics (e.g., sensitivity, specificity, AUC, user satisfaction). What do these tell you about the tool's performance?
4. **Real-World Outcome**

   Summarize what actually happened. Did the tool deliver on its promise? What impact did it have on workflow, patient care, or trust?
5. **Stakeholder Perspectives**

   Describe how different groups (e.g., clinicians, nurses, IT staff, patients) responded to the tool. What concerns or endorsements did they express?
6. **Lessons Learned from This Case**

   What can future AI implementations learn from this case? List at least two actionable takeaways.
7. **Implications for Your AI Project**

   How will this case inform your own prompt design, data use, or implementation planning?

8. **Discussion Questions for Peers**
   Write two questions you will pose to the group during your presentation to spark discussion.

Mini AI Journal Club: Peer Evaluation Form

Instructions: Use this form to evaluate your peers' presentation during the Mini AI Journal Club session. Circle the score that best reflects how well the presenters met each criterion. Add brief comments to support your evaluation. Submit the completed form anonymously at the end of the session.

Criteria	Max points	Score (0–2)
Clarity of case summary Case is accurately described with clear context, purpose, and outcomes	2	
Interpretation of metrics Relevant metrics are explained correctly and interpreted in context	2	
Stakeholder awareness Stakeholder perspectives are identified and thoughtfully analyzed	2	
Quality of lessons learned At least two clear, actionable lessons are derived from the case	2	
Presentation engagement Presenters are clear, organized, and invite meaningful discussion	2	
Total score	10	

Additional Comments

____

____

____

____

____

____

Self-Reflection (Optional)

What was the most surprising takeaway from this case?

____

____

____

____

How will you apply what you learned to your own AI project?

____

____

____

____

Conclusion

By stepping into the roles of prompt designer, data navigator, ethics reviewer, and project manager, you have developed a practical foundation for leading and contributing to AI-enhanced clinical initiatives. Through structured exercises, peer critique, and your Mini AI Journal Club capstone, you practiced evaluating model performance, aligning tools with stakeholder needs, and building workflows that prioritize safety and effectiveness. These skills will serve you well in any clinical or academic environment that embraces data-driven decision-making.

But learning does not stop with technical mastery. Sustained, responsible AI adoption requires systems-level thinking. In Chap. 13**,** you will explore how to scale these innovations within institutions, assess risk-benefit tradeoffs, and examine governance structures that support ethical oversight and continuous improvement. Together, we will move from pilot projects to institutional change, preparing you to lead with insight and integrity in the evolving world of medical AI.

Instructor's Guide: This Chapter—Building Your Team, Planning Your Project and Mini AI Journal Club

Overview and Learning Objectives

This chapter empowers students to simulate multidisciplinary AI project roles, obtain realistic data without coding, safeguard ethics, follow a structured timeline, and culminate in a Mini AI Journal Club capstone. By the end of this chapter, students will:

1. Practice four core project roles (clinical lead, data navigator, ethics reviewer, project manager).
2. Engage virtual stakeholders and craft tailored elevator pitches.
3. Use copy-ready clinical cases to design, test, and refine AI prompts for discharge summaries, problem lists, and differential diagnoses.
4. Apply de-identification best practices to protect patient privacy.
5. Organize work using a 12-week roadmap.
6. Lead a peer-facilitated AI Journal Club, synthesizing lessons into actionable improvements.

Before Teaching

- **Materials and Setup**
  - Provide students with a digital appendix or embedded text containing the four copy-ready case vignettes.
  - Ensure access to a shared folder or LMS where students can upload AI outputs and "feedback loop" minutes.
  - Prepare slides or handouts for the de-identification sidebar (Chap. 11, section "Anticipating resistance") and the 12-week roadmap template.
- **Instructor Prep**
  - Review the case studies, and anticipate common discussion points (e.g., guideline alignment, threshold settings, user fatigue).
  - Familiarize yourself with Google Forms or a simple online polling tool for real-time polls or peer surveys.
  - Identify local or freely accessible webinars from AMIA/HIMSS to recommend.

Section-by-Section Teaching Tips

Simulating Four Essential Roles

- **Goal:** Help students internalize project roles even when working alone.
- **Tip:** Start with a quick role-play: Assign each student one role, and ask them to list two responsibilities. Debrief by highlighting overlap and the importance of clear handoffs.
- **Key Question:** Why might a clinical lead and ethics reviewer disagree on data-sharing timelines?

Engaging Virtual Stakeholders

- **Goal:** Teach no-code strategies for gathering stakeholder insights.
- **Tip:** Assign students to watch one short (20-min) AMIA or HIMSS webinar before class and report back one key takeaway.
- **Activity:** In pairs, role-play an "elevator pitch" to a nurse and to a compliance officer, swapping feedback on clarity and impact.
- **Key question:** What evidence or language convinced you most?

Working with Prepackaged Clinical Cases

- **Goal:** Practice prompt design and iterative refinement.
- **Tip:** Demonstrate one case live—paste into ChatGPT, craft a discharge summary prompt, critique the output, and then refine.
- **Activity:** Break into small groups; each group works on a different prompt type (summary, problem list, differential). Rotate after 10 min.
- **Key question:** How did your prompt revision change the AI's accuracy or completeness?

Ethical and Privacy Safeguards

- **Goal:** Reinforce the importance of de-identification.
- **Tip:** Use the sidebar to walk through a redaction exercise on a sample note—students mark PHI in colored pen on printouts.
- **Key question:** What PHI elements are easiest to overlook?

Twelve-Week Roadmap

- **Goal:** Help students plan and pace their capstone alongside other commitments.
- **Tip:** Provide a blank calendar template; ask each student to block their next 2 weeks now.
- **Key question:** Which phase do you anticipate will need the most time or support?

Capstone: Mini AI Journal Club

- **Goal:** Synthesize chapter learnings into a peer-led analysis exercise.
- **Tip:** Assign cases in advance, and ask students to prepare slides (two to three slides) summarizing their case.
- **Activity Flow.**

  1. Pair presentations (5 min each).
  2. Guided discussion (5 min each).
  3. Collective synthesis—list three cross-case lessons on the board.

- **Key question:** Which case's success factors could you apply to your own project?

Assessment and Reflection

- **Artifact collection:** Ensure each group submits their "feedback loop" minutes and refined prompts from section "Working with prepackaged clinical cases".
- **Reflection prompt:** Ask students to write a 150-word reflection on one "aha" moment and one unresolved question.
- **Optional Quiz Questions**
  - Define the four core project roles and their responsibilities.
  - List three prompt types you practiced, and explain their clinical relevance.
  - Describe two strategies for de-identification in AI workflows.

Note to Instructor Emphasize that the Mini AI Journal Club mirrors real QI practices—learning from both triumphs and failures to drive continuous improvement. Encourage students to view AI as a collaborative partner not a replacement for clinical judgment.

References

1. Abràmoff MD, Lavin PT, Birch M, Shah N, Folk JC. Autonomous AI-based diagnostic system for diabetic retinopathy. JAMA Ophthalmol. 2018;136(11):1259–63. https://doi.org/10.1001/jamaophthalmol.2018.3245.
2. Jones SL, Ashton CM, Kiehne L. Real-world performance of a sepsis alert system in the EHR. Crit Care Med. 2020;48(5):e408–15. https://doi.org/10.1097/CCM.0000000000004310.
3. Esteva A, Kuprel B, Novoa RA, et al. Dermatologist-level classification of skin cancer with deep neural networks. Nature. 2017;542(7639):115–8. https://doi.org/10.1038/nature21056.

Chapter 13
Execution, Analysis, and Iteration

Introduction

You've laid the groundwork, defined roles, crafted prompts, and secured trust. Now it's time to move from theory to practice. In this chapter, you'll launch your pilot on real clinical vignettes, establish a performance baseline, and apply a rapid "Prompt–Review–Revise" cycle modeled on quality-improvement methods. You'll learn to measure AI accuracy, time savings, and bias and then troubleshoot common pitfalls like data drift and hallucinations. By the end, you'll possess a repeatable, data-driven workflow that ensures generative AI becomes a safe, reliable partner in everyday patient care.

With your capstone framework in place, let's begin by running your first prompts to see exactly where the AI stands today.

Kick-Off and Baseline Testing

Goal of This Section

Establish your performance baseline, and introduce the PDSA (Plan–Do–Study–Act) framework that will guide every subsequent prompt refinement [1].

Visualizations of research data or results in this manuscript were generated, refined, corrected, edited, or formatted with the assistance of artificial intelligence (AI) tools, specifically OpenAI's ChatGPT 4.0, 2024. All content has been thoroughly reviewed, revised, and approved by the author(s) to ensure scientific accuracy and preserve the integrity of the original material.

© The Author(s), under exclusive license to Springer Nature Switzerland AG 2025

C. Quinn, *Generative AI for the Medical Student*,
https://doi.org/10.1007/978-3-032-01613-3_13

Why It Matters

In health care, quality improvement (QI) relies on systematic cycles of change to enhance patient outcomes and process reliability. Central to QI is the PDSA (Plan–Do–Study–Act) cycle, which breaks improvements into manageable steps: planning a change, executing it, studying the results, and acting on what you learn to standardize successes or iterate further. This method has driven advances ranging from reduced central-line infections to streamlined discharge processes by ensuring that each intervention is measured, analyzed, and refined before broader rollout [1]. In this section, you'll apply the same rigor to generative AI: capturing a baseline of AI performance, planning targeted prompt adjustments, testing them, and evaluating outcomes against your gold-standard notes. By mirroring proven QI approaches, you'll transform AI integration from a one-off experiment into a reliable, data-driven process that continuously elevates clinical care [2].

What You'll Do

1. **Review proposal and roles**—Confirm your objectives and each team member's responsibilities.
2. **Run initial prompts**—Execute your first discharge summary, problem list, and differential diagnosis prompts on Cases 1–4.
3. **Capture baseline outputs**—Log each AI response side by side with its gold-standard note.

Introduction to PDSA

We'll use the **Plan–Do–Study–Act cycle** to iterate on your prompts:

- Plan: Decide on one specific prompt change.
- Do: Run the AI with that revised prompt.
- Study: Compare the new output against your baseline log.
- Act: Adopt the successful tweak or plan the next revision.

This record will serve as your reference point for all subsequent iterations.

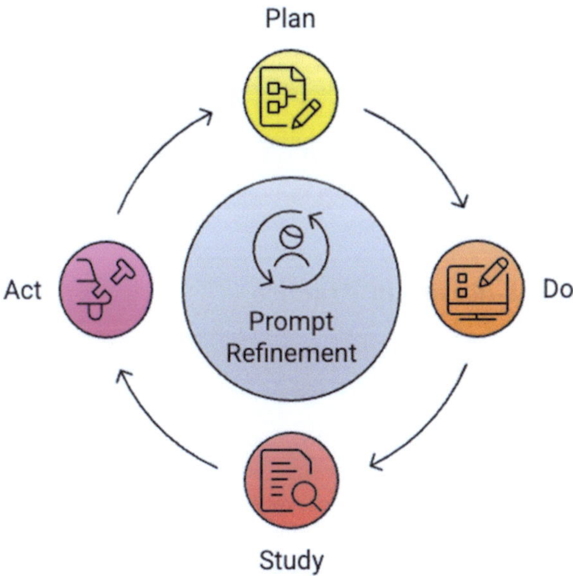

Key Success Criteria

- You've run at least one prompt of each type (summary, problem list, differential) on all four cases.
- Your baseline log clearly pairs AI outputs with the expert notes for side-by-side comparison.
- You and your team agree on one or two immediate observations, such as missing key elements or inconsistent terminology, that will guide your first round of prompt refinement [3].

By completing these steps, you'll ground your project in measurable data, setting the stage for focused improvements and reliable evaluation of AI's impact on clinical tasks. We'll use a **PDSA** cycle to guide refinement: **Plan** your prompt change, **Do** the test, **Study** the results by comparing to your baseline, and **Act** by standardizing successful tweaks or planning the next iteration.

This PDSA quality-improvement method is applied to prompt refinement and project evaluation in Chap. 14.

Now that you have a clear performance snapshot, it's time to hone those prompts in rapid cycles, capturing improvements as you go.

Key Takeaways

- Establishing your AI performance baseline enables you to accurately measure true improvements.
- Capturing outputs side by side with gold-standard notes provides concrete data for refinement.
- Introducing PDSA here creates a single, consistent improvement framework for all prompts.

Prompt–Review–Revise in Practice

Goal of This Section

Implement a rapid, team-based workflow—using a shared log and Stand-Up huddles—to apply PDSA and iteratively refine your AI prompts.

For practice applying prompt, review, and revise techniques, revisit the exercises in section "Working with prepackaged clinical cases*"*.

Why It Matters

Drawing on the PDSA cycle from section "Kick-off & baseline testing", your brief Stand-Up debriefs and shared log keep prompt refinements disciplined and data-driven, ensuring each iteration meaningfully closes gaps against your gold-standard notes [3].

What You'll Do

You'll maintain a shared prompt-version log, lead short "Stand-Up" debriefs to review AI outputs as a team, and apply the PDSA cycle to refine each prompt in real time.

- **Document every prompt version:** In your log (Google Sheet or shared doc), record version numbers, prompt text, AI responses, and gap notes.
- **Hold brief "Stand-Up" debriefs:** Schedule 10-minute check-ins daily or twice weekly to flag issues, and agree on your next PDSA "Plan."
- **Refine prompts iteratively:** Update the prompt, run the "Do" test, study the results, and act on what you learn—then log the new version immediately.

Success Criteria

To succeed, you should log at least three iterations of your prompt for a single case, generate at least one improvement suggestion at each Stand-Up, and achieve complete alignment between the AI's output and the gold-standard note by your third prompt version. As your prompts grow sharper, you need concrete measures to verify that the AI is actually delivering better clinical outputs.

Key Takeaways

- A shared log, along with brief Stand-Up huddles, keeps the team aligned and errors visible.
- Applying the PDSA cycle to each prompt ensures systematic, data-driven refinements.
- Collaborative critique accelerates learning and fosters prompt engineering confidence.

Evaluating AI Performance

Goal of This Section

Define simple, clinically meaningful metrics (accuracy, time saved, bias), track them over successive prompt versions, and use PDSA to drive measurable improvements.

Why It Matters

By applying the metrics and PDSA framework you learned in section "Kick-off & baseline testing", you transform subjective impressions into objective data—making it easy to demonstrate real improvements and retain stakeholder confidence [4].

What You'll Do

1. **Select Your Key Metrics**
    - **Accuracy:** Percentage of AI outputs that fully match gold-standard notes (e.g., correct diagnosis, treatment plan).
    - **Time saved:** Estimate minutes saved per discharge summary or note compared with manual drafting.

- **Bias presence:** Rate outputs for language neutrality (e.g., absence of unwarranted assumptions) using a simple 1–5 scale.

2. **Gather Data**
   - Use your baseline log (14.1) and refined outputs (14.2) to count matches versus mismatches.
   - Time yourself drafting a note manually (or use published benchmarks) and compare to AI-assisted times.
   - Have peers rate 10 AI outputs for bias; record scores.

3. **Visualize Results**
   - **Bar chart:** Show accuracy improvements across prompt versions.
   - **Table:** List average time saved per note before and after AI assistance.
   - **Bias heatmap:** Display frequency of high vs. low neutrality ratings.

4. **Apply PDSA Cycles**
   - **Plan:** Identify one metric lagging (e.g., accuracy 70%).
   - **Do:** Adjust your prompt to address the specific error (e.g., add "include follow-up plan").
   - **Study:** Recalculate accuracy after three new outputs.
   - **Act:** If accuracy rises above 90%, standardize that prompt refinement; if not, repeat.

Success Criteria

- **Defined metrics:** You list at least three metrics and their calculation methods.
- **Data collection:** You populate a chart or table with baseline and post-refinement values.
- **Demonstrated improvement:** One metric improves by at least 15% (e.g., accuracy from 70% to 85%).
- **QI application:** You complete one full PDSA cycle and document the results and next.

Illustrative Metrics Summary Table

Below is a hypothetical example table you can insert at the end of section "Evaluating AI performance", immediately after your narrative and before the "Apply PDSA Cycles" steps. It illustrates how to calculate and use each metric; feel free to adapt the formulas and labels to your data.

Metric	Definition	Example calculation
Accuracy	Proportion of AI-generated outputs that fully match the gold-standard note	(Number of matching outputs/total outputs) × 100
e.g., (8/10)×100 = 80%	Track after each prompt iteration to see if your refinements bring you closer to 100% agreement	
Time saved	Average minutes saved per note when using AI vs. manual drafting	(Mean manual time—mean AI time)
e.g., (15 min–6 min) = 9 min saved	Quantify efficiency gains and present to stakeholders as concrete workflow improvements.	
Bias rating	Average neutrality score on a 1–5 scale (1=strong bias, 5=no bias) Example: A note that assumes alcohol use without mention = Score 2 A note that neutrally summarizes race-neutral symptoms = Score 5	(Sum of all ratings)/(number of ratings)
e.g., (40/10) = 4.0	Monitor over time—if it drops, you know to refine prompts to remove unwarranted assumptions	

How to Use This Table

1. **Plug in your own data.** Replace the example numerators/denominators with your project's counts and times.
2. **Calculate after each iteration.** Record the new values in your prompt version log alongside the AI responses.
3. **Visualize trends.** Plot accuracy and bias scores over prompt versions; chart time-saved improvements.
4. **Drive your PDSA cycles.** Use declining or plateauing metrics to plan your subsequent prompt revisions.

This framework turns vague impressions into objective measures and shows your team exactly where to focus next.

Even well-tuned prompts can encounter real-world snags. Next, we'll tackle common pitfalls—like drift and hallucinations—and learn strategies to keep AI outputs trustworthy.

Key Takeaways

- Defining simple metrics, such as accuracy, time saved, and bias, transforms subjective feedback into objective progress.
- Visualizing metric changes highlights where prompts succeed or require further tuning.
- Running PDSA cycles against each metric embeds continuous improvement into your workflow.

Troubleshooting Common Pitfalls

Goal of This Section

Equips you to identify and correct frequent AI issues, data drift, hallucinations, and stakeholder pushback, so your models remain reliable and trusted in clinical contexts.

Why It Matters to Medical Students

In clinical care, vigilance for changing patient conditions and unexpected complications is critical. Similarly, AI tools can degrade or produce errant outputs over time or under new conditions. Being able to spot and correct these issues ensures AI remains a reliable partner in patient care rather than a hidden liability [5].

What You'll Do

1. **Monitor for Data Drift**
    - **Scenario:** Your original prompts performed well on the initial vignettes but produce incomplete summaries when case language shifts (e.g., new terminology or phrasing).
    - **Action:** Compare outputs on "older" versus "newer" vignette variants. If you see consistent omissions, update your prompt to include synonyms or broader descriptors ("Include 'pulmonary congestion' or 'fluid overload' when describing dyspnea").
    - **Tip:** Keep a versioned sample of each case, so you can track when drift occurs and how prompt tweaks restore performance [3].

2. **Detect and Correct Hallucinations**

   - **Scenario:** The AI inserts plausible-sounding but unsupported details (e.g., "Patient was placed on ACE inhibitors" when no mention exists).
   - **Action:** Cross-check each fact in the AI output against the "Find" function in your case text. When hallucinations appear, refine your prompt with stricter constraints ("Only summarize facts present in the narrative; do not infer medications or interventions not mentioned").
   - **Tip:** Maintain a brief hallucination log noting the erroneous phrase and your corrective prompt strategy [6].

Hallucination Log Template

Case ID	Hallucinated content	AI prompt used	Correction strategy	Resolved?
Case 2	"Patient was started on ACE inhibitors"	"Summarize treatment plan for chest pain"	Added "Only include treatments explicitly stated in the source text"	✓ Yes
Case 3	"Lives alone and has no caregiver"	"Generate a discharge note"	Added "Do not infer social history unless directly mentioned"	✓ Yes
Case 4	"History of melanoma in father"	"Summarize findings and risk factors"	Added "Exclude family history unless stated in the case narrative"	✕ No

Instructions for Use

- Maintain this log in your shared prompt refinement file or journal club folder.
- For each hallucination, describe the unsupported content, document the prompt that triggered it, and write how you revised the prompt to fix it.
- Mark resolution status after retesting.

3. **Respond to Stakeholder Pushback**

   - **Scenario:** A nurse questions why the AI note omits key social history; a compliance officer worries about unredacted PHI in an AI-generated draft.
   - **Action:** Revisit your tailored pitches with data—show your stakeholder the refined output that now includes social history or demonstrate the de-identification steps you've logged.
   - **Tip:** Keep a one-page summary of how prompt changes and ethical safeguards directly address each stakeholder's top concern—this becomes your credibility handout in future discussions.

Success Criteria

- **Data drift addressed:** You identify at least one drift scenario and demonstrate a prompt adjustment that restores output quality.
- **Hallucination log:** You document three hallucinations and corresponding prompt fixes.

- **Stakeholder reengagement:** You update and successfully "sell" your refined prompt/output to a peer role-playing a nurse or compliance officer, receiving affirmative feedback.

By mastering these troubleshooting steps, you'll ensure generative AI tools remain accurate, transparent, and aligned with clinical and operational needs over time.

Mini "AI Journal Club" Debriefs

Goal

Consolidate your learning mid-pilot by analyzing which prompt refinements are delivering measurable improvements, and share those insights with peers to strengthen group strategies moving forward.

Why It Matters

Midpoint reflection mirrors real-world quality improvement (QI) practices where teams pause to examine progress, recalibrate methods, and standardize wins before scaling up. This ensures that your refinements aren't just reactive but are building toward reproducible, data-supported performance gains.

What You'll Do

1. **Form Working Pairs**

Divide into pairs or small teams. Each group will focus on a case they've been refining and bring forward one improvement worth sharing.

2. **Prepare a 3-Minute Presentation**

Each pair summarizes:

- **Prompt iteration path**: From original to current version.
- **Metric improved**: e.g., accuracy increased from 70% to 90%.
- **Change responsible**: e.g., added "include discharge plan" to the prompt.
- **What didn't work**: Optional, but encouraged—briefly share a prompt edit that had no effect or backfired.

3. **Group Discussion**

After all groups present:

- **Compare metrics**: Which prompt type (summary, problem list, differential) showed the greatest relative gain?
- **Interpret results**: What do these gains suggest about how AI interprets clinical tasks?
- **Identify patterns**: Do certain types of prompt edits (e.g., specifying structure, limiting inference) consistently drive improvement?

4. **Document Shared Lessons**

Together, write a short "Midpoint Reflection" summary (one to two paragraphs or bullet points), which includes the following:

- Two successful refinement patterns
- One lesson about stakeholder expectations or limitations encountered
- A revised hypothesis for your next round of testing

Success Criteria
- Each group presents one concrete improvement and the metric it affected.
- The team discussion identifies at least two shared insights across cases.
- A brief written synthesis is uploaded to your team folder as part of your final capstone documentation.

Reflection and Next Steps

- Individual reflection prompt: "Which single refinement yielded the biggest gain?"
- Prepare a mid-project summary slide to present at your next peer or mentor check-in.
- Plan any final tweaks before moving into full analysis and reporting in Chap. 14.

Key Takeaways
- Monitoring for data drift and adapting prompts prevents performance decay over time.
- Logging and correcting hallucinations maintain output integrity and clinician trust.
- Revisiting tailored pitches with data-driven insights effectively addresses stakeholder concerns.

You've now moved from planning to practice, running your initial prompts, iteratively refining them with the PDSA cycle, measuring performance with concrete metrics, and troubleshooting real-world pitfalls. By treating generative AI as a clinical tool bound by the same quality-improvement rigor you apply to patient care, you've built a repeatable, data-driven workflow that enhances accuracy, efficiency, and trust. Keep this cycle alive by continuing to gather feedback, tracking your key metrics, and adapting when drift or hallucinations arise. In doing so, you'll ensure AI remains a reliable partner rather than a black-box wildcard in your future practice.

Closing Reflection Prompt

> Which pitfall in this chapter—data drift, hallucinations, or stakeholder pushback—surprised you most, and how will you guard against it in your future work with generative AI? Write a one-paragraph response.

This reflective exercise will help you internalize the lessons of Chap. 14 and prepare you to apply them wherever AI meets patient care.

Instructor's Guide This Chapter—Execution, Analysis, and Iteration

Chapter Overview and Learning Objectives

This chapter takes students from preparation into action. By the end, they will be able to:

1. Launch initial AI prompts on prepackaged clinical cases and record baseline performance.
2. Implement a rapid Prompt–Review–Revise cycle using PDSA and Stand-Up huddles.
3. Define and measure clinical metrics (accuracy, time saved, bias) to guide improvements.
4. Troubleshoot common pitfalls: data drift, hallucinations, and stakeholder resistance.
5. Reflect on key lessons and plan next steps.

These objectives build practical, data-driven AI workflows that parallel clinical quality improvement.

Before Teaching

- **Materials and Templates**
  - Chapter 13 text and four prepackaged case vignettes with gold-standard notes from Chap. 12.
  - **Shared log template** (see below).
  - Blank 2-month calendar worksheet for the 12-week roadmap.

- **Tech Setup**
  - Access to a generative AI interface (e.g., ChatGPT).
  - Screen-sharing capability for live demos.
  - Printed or digital PDSA primer link: http://www.ihi.org/resources/Pages/HowtoImprove/ScienceofImprovementHowtoImprove.aspx

Section-by-Section Teaching Tips

Kick-Off and Baseline Testing

- **Introduce PDSA:** Present a familiar QI example (e.g., infection rates) to explain Plan–Do–Study–Act.
- **Activity:** Live-demo one vignette—paste case, run a summary prompt, and log output in the shared template.
- **Discussion prompt:** "What key elements did the AI miss or misinterpret?"

Prompt–Review–Revise in Practice

- **Stand-up simulation:** Break into teams; each shares one AI output and identifies one gap.
- **Role rotation:** Assign each student the "Plan" step in the PDSA cycle.
- **Debrief question:** "How did this prompt change improve the output?"

Evaluating AI Performance

- **Metrics table exercise:** Display the hypothetical table; ask students to adapt calculations using their data.
- **Group calculation:** Have teams compute one metric from sample data and share results.
- **Visualization sketch:** Guide students to sketch a simple bar chart of accuracy improvements.

Troubleshooting Common Pitfalls

- **Case study examples:** Briefly discuss one data-drift and one hallucination scenario.
- **Hands-on:** Students identify a hallucination in an AI output and write a corrective prompt.
- **Stakeholder role-play:** One student plays a nurse, while another presents data to rebuild trust.

Shared Log Template

Case ID	Prompt version	Prompt text	AI response	Notes on gaps/errors
Case 1	v1	[text]	[text]	[missing treatment plan]
Case 1	v2	[text]	[text]	[added plan; still missing follow-up]
...	...	...	...	...

How to Use Copy this table into a shared spreadsheet. Enter a new row each time you revise and test a prompt.

Blank Calendar Worksheet

Week	Dates	Activities
1		Assign roles; review cases
2		Run baseline prompts; capture outputs
3		First PDSA cycle; refine prompts
4		Continue prompt testing and logging
5		Stand-up debriefs; track improvements
6		Begin metric visualization and feedback loop
7		Troubleshoot drift, hallucinations
8		Mini Journal Club midpoint synthesis
9		Final prompt refinements; begin reporting prep
10		Compile hallucination/bias logs
11		Create slides and summary documents
12		Final reflection; prepare summary presentation

How to Use Fill in your semester or rotation calendar dates in the second column. Adjust the pacing and assignments to fit your local course schedule or project timeline.

Assessment and Reflection

- **Collect Artifacts**
  - Completed shared logs of prompt versions
  - Metrics table with student calculations
  - Pitfalls: log documenting drift, hallucinations, and stakeholder notes

- **Reflection Prompt**

  Which pitfall surprised you most, and how will you guard against it in your future AI work? Write a one-paragraph response.

- **Quiz Ideas**

  – Define the four PDSA steps.
  – List three clinical metrics and their calculation methods.
  – Describe one strategy to correct an AI hallucination.

Note to Instructor
This chapter's exercises mirror the continuous-improvement mindset critical in medicine and apply the same rigor to AI integration that you would to patient safety protocols.

References

1. Institute for Healthcare Improvement. Science of improvement: how to improve. IHI; n.d.. Retrieved from http://www.ihi.org/resources/Pages/HowtoImprove/ScienceofImprovementHowtoImprove.aspx.
2. Davenport T, Kalakota R. The potential for artificial intelligence in healthcare. Future Healthc J. 2019;6(2):94–8. https://doi.org/10.7861/futurehosp.6-2-94.
3. Ji Z, Lee N, Frieske R, Yu T, Su D, Xu Y, et al. Survey of hallucination in natural language generation. ACM Comput Surv. 2023;55(12):353. https://doi.org/10.1145/35717304. Institute for Healthcare Improvement. Science of improvement: how to improve. IHI; n.d. Retrieved from http://www.ihi.org/resources/Pages/HowtoImprove/ScienceofImprovementHowtoImprove.aspx.
4. Rajkomar A, Dean J, Kohane I. Machine learning in medicine. N Engl J Med. 2019;380(14):1347–58. https://doi.org/10.1056/NEJMra1814259.
5. Gama J, Žliobaitė I, Bifet A, Pechenizkiy M, Bouchachia A. A survey on concept drift adaptation. ACM Comput Surv. 2014;46(4):44. https://doi.org/10.1145/2523813.
6. Rogers EM. Diffusion of innovations. 5th ed. Free Press; 2003.

Chapter 14
Reporting, Scale-Up, and Sustainability

Goals
1. Distill pilot results into clear, concise reports.
2. Tailor communications for clinicians, IT, compliance, and academic audiences.
3. Develop a feasible scale-up and budget plan.
4. Embed AI processes into sustainable governance and feedback loops.
5. Explore emerging AI technologies, and identify pathways for enhancing student engagement.

With your iterative AI workflow complete, it's time to distill and share your results.

Synthesizing Your Findings

Now that your AI workflow has been piloted and refined, your next task is to make its impact clear and measurable. Synthesizing findings means translating your data into concise, actionable insights. These insights inform decision-makers, whether they are clinicians, simulation staff, IT teams, or academic reviewers. This step is not just about reporting results. It is about demonstrating how each iteration improved performance and what you learned from the process.

Start by comparing your baseline metrics to your final results after prompt revision. Focus on three core dimensions:

- **Accuracy**: Did your revised prompts help the AI produce more clinically appropriate outputs? For instance, did diagnostic accuracy improve from 70% to 88%?
- **Time saved**: How much more efficiently could you complete documentation tasks? Was there a measurable reduction in note drafting time?
- **Bias score**: Did prompt revisions reduce biased language or inferred attributes, particularly around race, gender, or socioeconomic status?

© The Author(s), under exclusive license to Springer Nature Switzerland AG 2025

C. Quinn, *Generative AI for the Medical Student*,
https://doi.org/10.1007/978-3-032-01613-3_14

Record these changes using the following summary table. Add rows for additional measures, such as clinical completeness, hallucination frequency, or user satisfaction.

Pilot Summary Table Template

Metric	Baseline	Post-prompt	% Change	Notes
Accuracy (%)	70%	88%	+18%	Improved with added context cues
Time saved (min)	0	9	–	Based on three timed samples
Bias score (1–5)	3.8	4.6	+0.8	Reduced inferred race descriptors

Interpret Results Like a Quality Report

This process mirrors what clinicians do in a morbidity-and-mortality (M&M) conference: They highlight what worked, identify complications, and outline areas for improvement. Your synthesis should showcase:

- At least three improvements resulting from your design changes
- One or two persistent challenges
- Specific prompt revisions that made a measurable difference

Once your table is complete, summarize your findings in a single deliverable suitable for presentation. This may take the form of a one-page report or a slide brief. It should include the following:

- A side-by-side bar chart comparing pre- and post-prompt metrics
- Three major "wins" (such as increased accuracy or reduced bias)
- Two opportunities for follow-up or ongoing refinement

Structure your report using **SQUIRE 2.0 guidelines**, that is, the *Standards for* ***QU****ality* ***I****mprovement* ***R****eporting* ***E****xcellence*, to ensure it is concise, transparent, and outcomes-focused [1]. These guidelines are widely accepted for describing educational and clinical improvement projects. To assist with formatting, refer to the AHRQ Quality Improvement Essentials Toolkit, which provides templates for structuring quality initiatives in ways that resonate with institutional leaders [2].

By transforming data into an evidence-based summary, you communicate credibility and professionalism. You also prepare yourself for the next step: tailoring this information to specific audiences. That process begins in Section "Communicating results to diverse audiences", where you will adapt your message for clinical, technical, academic, and compliance stakeholders.

Sidebar: What Are the SQUIRE 2.0 Guidelines?

SQUIRE 2.0 stands for **Standards for QUality Improvement Reporting Excellence**, a set of guidelines designed to help healthcare professionals clearly and rigorously report quality improvement (QI) projects. Initially published in 2008 and updated in 2015, SQUIRE 2.0 provides a structured framework for writing up clinical interventions. This framework covers the use of AI tools, so that others can assess, replicate, and build upon your work.

Who Developed It?

SQUIRE 2.0 was developed by an international team of healthcare improvement experts, educators, and journal editors. It is sponsored by institutions such as the **BMJ Quality and Safety** journal and the **Health Foundation and** has broad support from academic health systems and quality research organizations.

Why It Matters for You

As a medical student or early-stage AI innovator, following SQUIRE 2.0 helps you:

- **Translate your pilot into a publishable or presentation-ready report.**
- **Demonstrate credibility** when presenting outcomes to institutional stakeholders.
- **Standardize terminology and formatting**, especially when working with mentors, simulation centers, or academic reviewers.
- **Align with evidence-based reporting norms**, increasing the impact and uptake of your project.

The guidelines include 18 items across sections like background, intervention description, study design, outcomes, limitations, and conclusions. You don't need to use all 18 for a student project, but even adopting a simplified version improves clarity and professionalism.

Pro tip: Use SQUIRE when drafting a one-page summary of your AI pilot, especially if you plan to share it with your clerkship director, quality office, or at a conference poster session.

Learn more: https://www.squire-statement.org

AI Project Synthesis Worksheet

Instructions: Use this worksheet to summarize and reflect on your AI pilot project. You will compare baseline and refined prompt performance, identify areas of improvement, and prepare insights for reporting. This worksheet mirrors quality-improvement reporting practices and is designed to help you prepare a one-page brief.

1. Metric Comparison Table
   Enter your baseline and post-prompt values for each metric. Add notes explaining how changes to your prompts or workflow contributed to the results.

Metric	Baseline	Post-Prompt	% Change	Notes

2. Key Findings
   List three significant improvements achieved through your revised prompts or process.
   1. 1.
   2. 2.
   3. 3.
3. Ongoing Challenges
   Identify one or two issues that remain unresolved and describe possible next steps.
   1. 1.
   2. 2.
4. Prompt Revisions That Made a Difference
   Describe one or two specific changes you made to your prompts and how they improved outcomes.
   1. 1.
   2. 2.
5. Reporting Preparation Checklist
   Use the checklist below to ensure your summary report or slide brief is ready for stakeholder review.

   ☐ Side-by-side bar chart of key metrics
   ☐ Three highlighted wins
   ☐ Two follow-up opportunities
   ☐ Plain-language summary aligned with SQUIRE 2.0
   ☐ Visuals labeled and free of jargon

Communicating Results to Diverse Audiences

With your data distilled in Section "Synthesizing your findings", the next step is to tailor your presentation to each audience's priorities. Clinicians will care most about patient-centered outcomes, so open with statements like, "Our AI prompts increased diagnostic accuracy from 70% to 85% and cut documentation time by 9 minutes per note." IT teams require details on feasibility and compatibility and include a sidebar listing required APIs, data formats, and integration milestones. Compliance officers focus on privacy and governance—quietly assure them by highlighting how every note type underwent standardized de-identification aligned with HIPAA Safe Harbor criteria. For academic peers, craft a 200-word abstract that briefly outlines your PDSA-based methodology, core metrics, and top three findings.

Choose your medium thoughtfully: an infographic works best when you need to convey workflow improvements at a glance, whereas a slide deck allows more narrative context for live Q&A. Apply the CDC Clear Communication Index: Use plain language, meaningful headings, and callouts to guide attention [3]. Enhance your slides or handouts with clean bar charts or tables, minimize gridlines, label axes clearly, and avoid nonessential decoration—to make trends immediately apparent [4]. Before you present, share your draft with a peer assigned to each stakeholder role and solicit at least two questions; rehearsing these will sharpen your message and prepare you for real-world dialogue. Once your results are communicated, plan how to broaden their impact.

Callout: What Makes a Good Slide Brief?
Use this checklist to ensure your presentation is clear, persuasive, and tailored to busy clinical and administrative audiences:

- **One key insight per slide.**
Focus on a single message—avoid trying to explain everything at once.
- **Metrics visualized clearly.**
Use bar charts, tables, or clean visuals to show your improvements.
- **Plain-language takeaway sentence.**
End each slide with a statement that a nonexpert can understand at a glance.
- **Minimal jargon and no clutter.**
Avoid excessive text, acronyms, or decorative distractions.
- **Title every slide with a conclusion not a topic**

Instead of "Metric Summary," use **"AI Reduced Errors by 15%."**

Planning for Scale-Up

After proving your AI prompts work in a small pilot, think practically about where you, as a medical student, can expand their use and who will support you. In most teaching hospitals, students can begin by deploying prompts in the simulation lab or educational EMR sandbox, controlled environments overseen by simulation center staff or informatics teams. Work with a faculty mentor (such as the CMIO or a clinical informaticist) to secure API access and integrate your refined prompts into the sandbox.

Sidebar: What Is an "EHR Sandbox"?

In health care, an **EHR sandbox** is a duplicate version of the electronic health record (EHR) system used for training and testing. Think of it as a practice environment where no real patient data is changed. Users can safely try new tools, such as AI-generated notes, without risking live records.

Key Points

- **Safety first:** Actions in the sandbox never affect actual patient charts.
- **Realistic data:** The sandbox often contains anonymized or simulated patient cases, so you can experience the same workflows.
- **Experiment and learn:** You can test prompts, identify errors, and refine your AI tools before moving into the live system.

How to Access

1. Contact your institution's IT or informatics team to obtain sandbox credentials.
2. Complete any required training or confidentiality agreements.
3. Log in alongside your standard EHR access, and look for "Sandbox" or "Training" in the system name.

Using an EHR sandbox ensures you can innovate with AI confidently, keeping patient care safe and uninterrupted.

Next, set deployment criteria: Aim for at least 90% concordance with expert notes, user-satisfaction scores above 4 out of 5 on student surveys, and a clear cost–benefit calculation (e.g., 9 min saved per note at an estimated $100/h clinician rate yields $15 per note) [5]. Outline technical requirements by listing needed EHR endpoints in the sandbox, requesting temporary API credentials from IT, and arranging training sessions with simulation educators (APIs, or Application Programming Interfaces, let separate software systems exchange data securely.). At the same time, draft a budget estimate, even if hypothetical, to show faculty and department leaders that the projected time savings outweigh any licensing or support costs.

Reflection Prompt "Which milestone in your roadmap feels most at risk, and what one mitigation strategy would you apply?"

Finally, collate these elements into a pilot-to-production roadmap, using a simple Gantt chart or timeline table. Mark milestones such as "Sandbox integration complete," "First 10 students trained," and "pre-clinical clerkship trial begins," and assign responsible parties (e.g., you for surveying users, IT for credentialing, simulation staff for training). By collaborating with faculty mentors, IT specialists, and simulation center personnel, you'll ensure your scale-up plan is feasible, educationally valuable, and positioned for formal evaluation and potential broader adoption [5, 6].

Having laid out a scale-up roadmap, embed these processes into routine oversight.

Sidebar: What Is a Gantt Chart?

A Gantt chart is a visual timeline used to plan and track projects. It displays tasks as horizontal bars against a calendar grid, showing each task's start date, duration, and end date (see Fig. 14.1). By laying out all activities, such as "Sandbox integration," "User training," or "First AI Round," you can see overlaps, dependencies, and milestones at a glance.

Key Features

- **Tasks and Durations:** Each bar represents one task; longer bars mean more time allocated.
- **Milestones:** Diamond symbols indicate critical checkpoints (e.g., "Pilot complete").
- **Dependencies:** Arrows show which tasks must finish before others begin.

How to Use It

1. **List activities:** Write down every major step in your scale-up plan.
2. **Assign dates:** Estimate realistic start and end dates for each.
3. **Draw bars:** On a horizontal timeline, draw a bar for each task spanning its dates.
4. **Mark milestones:** Place diamond symbols at key transition points (e.g., "Go/No-Go decision").
5. **Review and update:** As you progress, adjust bars to reflect actual completion and identify delays.

Using a Gantt chart helps you—and your stakeholders—understand the project's rhythm, anticipate bottlenecks, and coordinate efforts across clinical, IT, and educational teams.

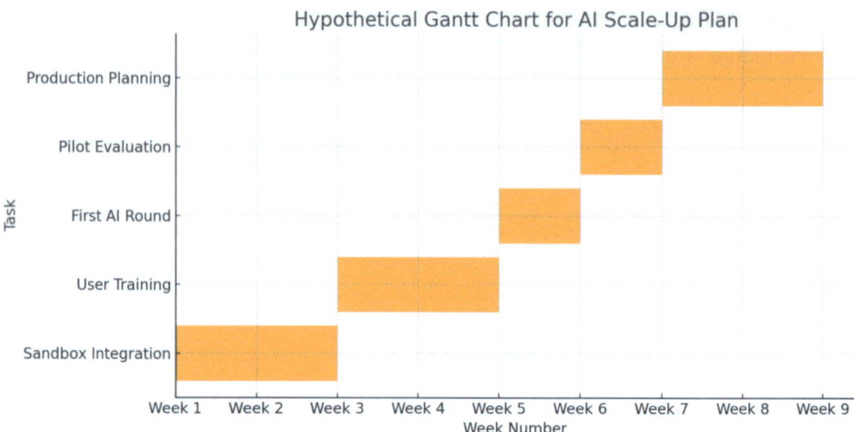

Fig. 14.1 Gantt chart example

Ensuring Long-Term Sustainability

Once an AI workflow shows early success, the next challenge is to make it last. Sustainability means embedding the project into your institution's daily practices, so it can evolve, scale, and continue improving over time.

Monitor Key Metrics Regularly
Begin by setting a monthly schedule to review core metrics like accuracy, time saved, and bias scores. These reviews can be folded into existing meetings such as simulation staff check-ins, morbidity-and-mortality rounds, or clerkship debriefs. As a student super-user, you might help coordinate these sessions by collecting recent data, summarizing performance, and recommending updates to prompt language.

Assign Clear Responsibilities
To maintain momentum, build a simple responsibility matrix. This document lists each recurring task, identifies who owns it, and how often it should be reviewed. For example:

- *Metric Review*—student lead—monthly
- *Prompt Revision*—simulation faculty—quarterly
- *User Training*—IT support—start of each rotation

This structure helps prevent the common pitfall of "pilot fade," when no one feels accountable after initial enthusiasm subsides.

Establish Faculty Oversight and Interdisciplinary Support
Form a small oversight group led by a faculty champion, such as the CMIO or simulation director. Include stakeholders from clinical, IT, and compliance teams. Their role is to review outputs, authorize corrective actions when problems emerge

(such as declining model performance or new hallucinations), and maintain safety standards. Students should remain part of this team to represent the learner perspective and surface usability issues early.

Reinforce Learning with AI Rounds
To keep improvement continuous, organize "AI Rounds" every 4–6 weeks. These short sessions work like journal clubs. Students present recent AI-generated notes, compare them to gold-standard documentation, and suggest changes to prompts or workflow. Each session should end with clear decisions, documented in a shared calendar. A sample entry might read: *Week 16—AI Rounds, updated prompts for discharge planning, flagged hallucination in sepsis case.*

These small but consistent actions transform your project from a single-course exercise into an enduring clinical and educational tool. When built into existing structures and supported by shared ownership, generative AI can evolve safely, improve performance over time, and serve both learners and institutions [7, 8] (see Template below).

AI Workflow Responsibility Matrix Template

Purpose Use this matrix to define and track responsibilities that support the long-term success of your AI project. Each task should have a clear owner, a consistent review cycle, and documented dependencies. Tailor the entries to match your institutional setting, including roles in simulation, informatics, and student engagement.

Task	Responsible party	Review frequency	Notes or dependencies
Metric review	Medical student lead	Monthly	Collect performance data (e.g., accuracy, bias, time saved) from AI outputs
Prompt revision	Simulation faculty	Quarterly	Use insights from AI rounds and clinical feedback to revise prompts
User onboarding and training	IT support or clinical educator	Start of each rotation	Provide brief orientation sessions for new users of the AI tool
Oversight and governance	CMIO or simulation director	Every 2 months	Review metrics, address emerging issues, and authorize changes
AI rounds coordination	Student super-user	Every 4–6 weeks	Facilitate structured peer review of recent AI-generated notes

Key Takeaway Assigning clear roles and recurring review cycles helps prevent project drift and ensures that your AI tool continues to evolve in response to real-world clinical needs and educational goals.

Sidebar: What Is a Hackathon?
A hackathon is an intense, time-limited event, often 8–48 hours, where multidisciplinary teams rapidly prototype solutions to real-world challenges. You don't need to write code to add value. Typical roles include the following:

- **Clinician voice or subject-matter expert:** Identify and frame the clinical problem.
- **UX/workflow designer:** Map user journeys, and propose intuitive interfaces.
- **Project lead/data analyst:** Coordinate tasks, interpret metrics, and craft the final presentation.

Many hackathons pair participants with faculty or industry mentors who offer technical advice and ensure clinical relevance.

Why Participate?

Even without programming skills, you'll sharpen your ability to translate clinical needs into project goals, practice leadership and teamwork under time pressure, and expand your network of peers and mentors. Deliverables, such as slide decks or posters, can become powerful additions to your CV.

Getting Involved

1. Monitor your school's student innovation channels (listservs, Slack, or bulletin boards) for upcoming events.
2. Sign up early and form a diverse team: Pair with data-savvy classmates or engineering students.
3. Focus on your strengths, clinical insight, and workflow design, and lean on mentors for technical support.

Even a single hackathon sprint will boost your confidence in guiding AI-driven solutions and lay the groundwork for future innovation.

Emerging Technologies and Next Steps

With your AI workflow integrated into daily routines and supported by governance structures, it's time to look ahead. What's next for AI in clinical care—and for you as a future leader in digital health?

Next-Generation Technologies
AI is rapidly evolving beyond single-modality tools. New multimodal models can interpret images, text, and physiological data simultaneously. These systems are already being tested in radiology, where they generate both the narrative report and annotated image findings in a single step [9]. Similarly, adaptive AI tools adjust their decision thresholds in real time as they encounter new clinical data. For example, decision-support systems now refine their risk predictions with each new lab result or patient admission.

Another frontier is real-time analytics. These AI tools monitor continuous data streams and alert care teams the moment vital signs signal sepsis or when ECGs show arrhythmias. Such applications illustrate the future of ambient intelligence in hospital care.

Regulatory Readiness and Ethical Awareness

As these technologies advance, regulatory frameworks are also changing. The FDA's AI/ML Action Plan outlines a path for software-as-a-medical-device clearance and emphasizes transparency, monitoring, and model updates [10]. At the same time, HIPAA regulations are evolving to address the unique risks posed by AI in data handling, especially around de-identification, data sharing, and algorithmic bias. Staying informed about these policies will prepare you to navigate both clinical and compliance challenges.

How to Stay Involved and Grow

You don't need to wait for residency to deepen your role. Consider these next steps:

- **Run a hackathon or join a pilot:** Collaborate with your simulation center, innovation lab, or faculty mentor to test AI tools in a supervised environment. These short-term projects often generate actionable insights and strong mentorship ties.
- **Participate in national networks:** Join professional organizations like the **AMIA Student Working Group**, the **Society of General Internal Medicine's Health IT Interest Group**, or your campus **Digital Health Circle**. These groups offer webinars, research mentorships, and access to national conversations in AI policy and clinical design.
- **Contribute to real-world data projects:** NIH-funded AI labs, public health schools, and open-source communities frequently recruit students to assist with data annotation, quality review, or protocol testing. These experiences strengthen your understanding of model development and validation.
- **Build your voice:** Publish a student editorial or blog post. Share your capstone results, reflect on your simulation experience, or explore ethical dilemmas in medical AI. Platforms like *Doximity*, *Medium*, or your institution's newsletter offer valuable exposure—and a searchable record of your thought leadership.
- **Mentor peers:** Once your project is complete, offer to co-lead a journal club or teach a simulation workshop. Becoming a peer educator not only consolidates your own learning but also strengthens your identity as an innovator and future clinician-educator.

Key Takeaway Staying engaged through clinical pilots, professional networks, and reflective publishing helps you evolve from project participant to field contributor. These activities lay the foundation for sustained leadership in digital medicine.

In the next chapter, we explore how to frame your AI project as a scholarly product, whether for presentation, publication, or residency application.

Sidebar: Real-Time Analytics in Health Care

What It Is: Real-time analytics refers to the continuous monitoring and analysis of clinical data as it is generated rather than in batches or after the fact. In practice, this means algorithms scan incoming streams of vital signs, lab results, and device outputs to detect critical patterns immediately.

Key Components

- **Data stream integration:** Inputs from monitors, EHR entries, and medical devices feed directly into the analytics engine.
- **Automated alerting:** When predefined thresholds or predictive models flag risk, such as early signs of sepsis, a notification is sent instantly to the care team.
- **Dashboard visualization:** Clinicians view live dashboards summarizing patient trends, enabling rapid triage and intervention.

Clinical example: An AI-driven sepsis monitor analyzes heart rate, temperature, and white-blood-cell counts in real time. If it detects a high likelihood of sepsis, it alerts the rapid-response team within seconds rather than waiting for periodic chart reviews.

Why it matters: By identifying deterioration or critical events the moment they occur, real-time analytics can accelerate clinical decision-making, reduce response times, and ultimately improve patient outcomes.

How to get involved: Ask your simulation or informatics department for demonstrations of their real-time dashboard tools. You can often participate in mock drills that simulate real-time alerts, giving you firsthand experience with this technology.

Closing Vignette and Reflection

Now that you've explored sustainability strategies and next-generation AI applications, consider what it looks like to present a successful project at the institutional level.

Imagine standing beside your faculty mentor at a department Grand Rounds, presenting the outcomes of your pilot. Dr. Patricia Tietjen begins the session with a slide showing measurable improvements: Documentation time decreased by 9 minutes per note, and clinical accuracy rose from 70% to 88% after prompt refinements. When the chief medical officer asks about long-term costs, Dr. Tietjen outlines a basic budget model showing that time saved by clinicians offsets the software and support fees within 4 months.

A faculty member from the quality-improvement team asks how the project will be maintained. Dr. Tietjen describes a governance structure that includes a CMIO sponsor, an IT integration lead, two simulation-based education faculty, and rotating student "super-users" who lead monthly reviews of AI-generated output. She then walks the audience through the next steps in the rollout: training the first new user cohort, integrating the workflow into a second clinical ward, and tracking quarterly metric reviews.

By presenting performance metrics alongside a transparent accountability plan and clear implementation timeline, the team secures leadership approval to expand the initiative.

Reflection Prompt

Before scaling up this AI workflow, identify one strategic change you would recommend. Would you revise a performance threshold? Reallocate budget priorities? Expand or modify the oversight committee?

Briefly explain how your proposed adjustment would improve a specific project outcome, such as model accuracy, adoption rate, or stakeholder trust. Your response should link the proposed change to measurable impact and reflect the priorities of clinical, administrative, or patient stakeholders.

Conclusion

By this point in your AI journey, you've gained practical skills in workflow integration, quality monitoring, and stakeholder alignment. You've explored how to embed your tool within clinical operations, sustain momentum through governance structures, and anticipate future innovations. These skills form the foundation for responsible, scalable AI use in health care. But to truly lead in this space, you must also know how to communicate your results clearly, credibly, and persuasively. In the next chapter, you will learn how to transform your AI pilot into a scholarly product. Whether you aim to submit a conference abstract, publish a student editorial, or present your findings to hospital leadership, Chap. 15 will guide you through the strategies, formats, and audiences that define success in academic and professional dissemination.

Instructor's Guide: Chapter—Reporting, Scale-Up, and Sustainability

Chapter Overview and Learning Objectives

Goal

1. Distill pilot results into clear, concise reports.
2. Tailor communications for clinicians, IT, compliance, and academic audiences.
3. Develop a feasible scale-up and budget plan.
4. Embed AI processes into sustainable governance and feedback loops.
5. Explore emerging AI technologies, and identify pathways for enhancing student engagement.

By the end, students will be able to present their findings, plan and sustain an AI initiative, and position themselves for future innovation.

Before Teaching

- **Materials Provided in Text**
  - Chapter student text and four case vignettes with gold-standard notes.
  - Shared log template (table in Chap. 13 Instructor's Guide).
  - Blank calendar worksheet (12-week roadmap grid in Chapter text).
  - Sidebars: Gantt chart example, sandbox definition, real-time analytics.
- **Tech Setup**
  - Access to generative AI interface for demonstrations.
  - Screen-sharing or projector for live walkthroughs.
  - Links to CDC Clear Communication Index and FDA AI/ML Action Plan (cited in text).

Section-by-Section Teaching Tips

Synthesizing Your Findings

- **Activity:** Provide students with baseline vs. refined metric data (from Chapter examples). In pairs, draft a one-page brief using the Shared Log Template as reference.
- **Discussion:** Compare briefs against SQUIRE 2.0 criteria; emphasize clarity and actionable recommendations.

Transition: "With your data organized, now tailor your message to each audience."

Communicating Results to Diverse Audiences

- **Role-Play:** Assign groups as clinicians, IT, compliance, or academic peers. Each group reviews a sample memo (from 14.1 drafts) and provides feedback on relevance and clarity.
- **Debrief:** Use the CDC Clear Communication Index (sidebar) to score each presentation.

Transition: "Once you've honed your presentations, plan how to broaden the impact."

Planning for Scale-Up

- **Workshop:** Using the Blank Calendar Worksheet, map three key milestones (e.g., sandbox integration, first cohort training, pilot evaluation), and assign roles (student, IT lead, CMIO mentor).
- **Budget exercise:** Have students calculate cost–benefit using the example formula from Section "Planning for scale-up" (time saved × clinician rate vs. software cost).

Transition: "Having set your roadmap and budget, ensure these processes endure."

Ensuring Long-Term Sustainability

- **Group exercise:** Draft a simple responsibility matrix on the board, assigning oversight roles as described in the governance sidebar.
- **Mock "AI Rounds":** Conduct a brief session where students present one recent AI output, compare it to the gold-standard note, and agree on a prompt tweak.

Transition: "With sustainability embedded, let's look ahead to emerging tools."

Emerging Technologies and Next Steps

- **Mini lecture:** Review sidebars on multimodal AI and real-time analytics.
- **Brainstorm:** In small groups, list one hackathon or innovation-lab proposal based on these technologies.

Transition: "Finally, envision presenting your full project to stakeholders."

Closing Vignette and Reflection

- **Read-Aloud and Discussion:** Share the Grand Rounds vignette. Ask: "What strategic adjustment did Dr. Tietjen make?"
- **Reflection:** Students write a paragraph in response to the prompt and exchange it with a peer for feedback.

Assessment and Reflection

- **Collect:** One-page briefs, role-play feedback notes, completed roadmap worksheets, responsibility matrix, and reflection paragraphs.
- **Quiz Ideas**
  - Define SQUIRE 2.0 and its purpose.
  - Explain a sandbox and API.
  - List three deployment criteria.
  - Describe one governance role.
  - Name an emerging AI technology and a related student activity.

Note to Instructor
Keep activities tightly linked to the student text and provided materials, so learners can focus on applying concepts rather than hunting for external resources.

References

1. Ogrinc G, Davies L, Goodman D, Batalden P, Davidoff F, Stevens D. SQUIRE 2.0 (Standards for QUality improvement reporting excellence): revised publication guidelines from a detailed consensus process. BMJ Qual Saf. 2016;25(12):986–92. https://doi.org/10.1136/bmjqs-2015-004411.
2. Agency for Healthcare Research and Quality. Quality improvement essentials toolkit. U.S. Department of Health & Human Services; 2017. Retrieved from https://www.ahrq.gov/sites/default/files/wysiwyg/professionals/quality-patient-safety/quality-resources/tools/qi-essentials-toolkit/qiessentials.pdf.
3. Centers for Disease Control and Prevention. CDC Clear Communication Index. U.S. Department of Health & Human Services; 2019. Retrieved from https://www.cdc.gov/ccindex/index.html.
4. Tufte ER. The visual display of quantitative information. Graphics Press; 2001.
5. Milat AJ, King L, Bauman A, Redman S. The concept of scalability: increasing the scale and potential adoption of health promotion interventions into policy and practice. Health Promot Int. 2013;28(3):285–98. https://doi.org/10.1093/heapro/dar097.
6. Damschroder LJ, Aron DC, Keith RE, Kirsh SR, Alexander JA, Lowery JC. Fostering implementation of health services research findings into practice: a consolidated framework for advancing implementation science. Implement Sci. 2009;4:50. https://doi.org/10.1186/1748-5908-4-50.

7. Batalden PB, Davidoff F. What is "quality improvement," and how can it transform healthcare? Qual Saf Health Care. 2007;16(1):2–3. https://doi.org/10.1136/qshc.2006.022046.
8. Provost LP, Murray SK. The health care data guide: learning from data for improvement. Jossey-Bass; 2011.
9. Topol EJ. High-performance medicine: the convergence of human and artificial intelligence. Nat Med. 2019;25(1):44–56. https://doi.org/10.1038/s41591-018-0300-7.
10. U.S. Food and Drug Administration. Artificial intelligence/machine learning (AI/ML)-based software as a medical device action plan; 2021. Retrieved from https://www.fda.gov/media/145022/download.

Chapter 15
Next Steps—Professional Growth and Lifelong AI Integration

Goals

1. Frame AI literacy as an ongoing professional competency.
2. Identify key certification and micro-credential pathways in clinical AI.
3. Develop a continuous learning plan using online courses, communities, and hackathons.
4. Understand ethical, legal, and accountability considerations for long-term AI use.
5. Explore research, interprofessional collaboration, and emerging career roles in AI medicine.

Chapter Overview (Revised)

In the previous chapter, you learned how to sustain an AI project within a clinical setting. Now, it is time to shift your focus toward long-term professional growth. As generative AI becomes increasingly embedded in healthcare delivery, AI literacy will no longer be optional. It will be a foundational skill that clinicians must continuously refine throughout their careers.

This chapter will help you chart that ongoing development. Whether you plan to specialize in clinical informatics, contribute to an innovation lab, or simply apply AI tools at the bedside, you will likely encounter new credentials, certification programs, or training pathways. Organizations such as the American Medical Informatics Association (AMIA) and the Healthcare Information and Management Systems Society (HIMSS) now offer micro-credentials. These are credentials from short, focused programs that validate your technical and ethical readiness to lead in this space.

You will also learn how to set professional learning goals using the SMART framework, which encourages objectives that are Specific, Measurable, Achievable,

© The Author(s), under exclusive license to Springer Nature Switzerland AG 2025

C. Quinn, *Generative AI for the Medical Student*,
https://doi.org/10.1007/978-3-032-01613-3_15

Relevant, and Time-Bound (see Sidebar: SMART Goals). These goals will help you stay focused during transitions, such as entering residency or joining a health system.

Finally, this chapter explores strategies for continuous learning beyond medical school. These include joining professional networks, enrolling in online courses, and contributing to research or innovation communities. The goal is to ensure that your AI competencies evolve in step with the field, so your expertise expands with each career milestone rather than plateauing at graduation [1, 2].

With your long-term learning strategy in view, let's begin by examining how formal credentials can validate your AI proficiency and strengthen your clinical credibility.

Sidebar: Setting SMART Goals
What Are SMART Goals?

SMART goals provide a clear framework for setting objectives that are:

- **Specific:** Clearly defined and focused (e.g., "Complete the 'AI for Everyone' course").
- **Measurable:** Quantifiable, so you can track progress (e.g., "Attend two AI Rounds").
- **Achievable:** Realistic given your resources and constraints.
- **Relevant:** Aligned with your overall career and learning priorities.
- **Time-Bound:** Set within a concrete deadline (e.g., "within six months").

Why They Help

By using the SMART structure, you transform vague aspirations into actionable plans. You'll know exactly what you need to do, how to measure success, and when you need to finish, keeping you motivated and accountable as you develop your AI skills.

Example

Instead of "Learn more about AI," a SMART goal would be:

"By December, I will complete Coursera's 'AI for Everyone' course and attend at least two AI journal-club sessions to strengthen my understanding of AI applications in clinical practice."

Certification and Credentialing in Clinical AI

Once you've defined your learning goals, the next step is to earn formal credentials that demonstrate your AI skills to potential employers, mentors, and collaborators. These certifications validate your technical and ethical readiness to engage with clinical AI in real-world settings.

Start with programs like the **Professional Certificate in Clinical Informatics** offered by the **American Medical Informatics Association (AMIA)**. This 6-month online course introduces core competencies in AI, data standards, and digital implementation strategies for patient care [3]. It is designed for early-career clinicians and is often pursued during medical school or residency.

Other organizations, such as the **Healthcare Information and Management Systems Society (HIMSS)**, offer credentials like the **Certified Professional in Healthcare Information and Management Systems (CPHIMS)**. This credential includes AI-focused modules and can be earned through an online exam and applied project. HIMSS often provides discounted exam fees for students and trainees [4].

Board-certified physicians may also see AI topics integrated into Maintenance of Certification (MOC) requirements. Several American Board of Medical Specialties (ABMS) member boards have begun embedding informatics and AI safety updates into recertification frameworks to ensure clinicians remain fluent in emerging technologies [5].

For more targeted skill validation, explore **micro-credentials**. These are short, skill-specific digital badges that demonstrate proficiency in areas such as clinical prompt engineering, bias auditing, or de-identification strategies. Micro-credentials typically require the completion of a task, short module, or mini-project, such as a 2-week bias mitigation challenge. Many are free or low-cost and can be added to your resume or LinkedIn profile [6].

Sample Pathway You might enroll in AMIA's certificate program during your final year of medical school and then supplement that foundation postgraduation by adding an AI module to your MOC schedule. Along the way, you could earn two micro-credentials, clinical prompt design and data privacy, to demonstrate practical skills beyond traditional coursework.

As you accumulate these credentials, you position yourself not just as a user of clinical AI but as someone capable of leading initiatives, guiding ethical implementation, and mentoring peers. In Section "Continuous professional development with AI", we will explore how to build a portfolio that showcases these accomplishments and supports your ongoing professional development.

Sidebar: Key Professional Associations in Clinical AI
American Medical Informatics Association (AMIA)

Founded in 1981, AMIA is the leading professional organization for informatics in health care, biomedicine, and public health. Its mission is to transform health and health care through trusted science, education, and practice of informatics. AMIA offers training, research forums, and the Professional Certificate in Clinical Informatics to help clinicians integrate AI and data science into patient care.

Website: https://www.amia.org

(continued)

Healthcare Information and Management Systems Society (HIMSS)

Established in 1961, HIMSS is a global advisor and thought leader supporting the transformation of health through information and technology. HIMSS provides professional certifications (such as CPHIMS), educational events, and policy advocacy to advance the use of AI, analytics, and digital health solutions across care settings.

Website: https://www.himss.org

Continuous Professional Development with AI

After earning credentials, your next challenge is sustaining growth. Continuous development ensures your AI skills remain current, practical, and aligned with real-world clinical demands. This section outlines building a structured learning portfolio and participating in professional communities that foster innovation and accountability.

Begin by creating an AI learning portfolio. This is a shared folder or digital notebook where you store evidence of your progress. Include project summaries, annotated prompt examples, abstracts from any posters or presentations, and certificates from completed courses or workshops. This living document helps showcase your initiative during residency interviews, grant applications, or institutional reviews.

To strengthen your knowledge base, enroll in no-code, beginner-friendly courses. Options include *AI for Everyone* by Andrew Ng on Coursera and the *AI for Healthcare* certificate series on edX [7, 8]. These programs require no programming experience and can be completed at your own pace. Many medical schools now offer internal webinars or electives on digital health. Reach out to your institution's medical education office, or check your school's learning portal to gain access.

Peer learning also plays a key role. Join or launch an "AI Rounds" group, where participants present a recent article, demo a new tool, and discuss clinical relevance. If your school hosts hackathons, participate—even if you do not code. Clinicians contribute by defining use cases, designing workflows, or presenting clinical narratives to technical teams (see Sidebar: What Is a Hackathon?).

To stay accountable, set a SMART goal such as: "Complete two AI journal club sessions and finish the 'AI for Everyone' course within six months." By combining structured learning with community engagement, you build habits that will sustain your expertise long after medical school [9].

Next, we'll explore how to apply these evolving skills with a strong foundation in ethical reasoning and responsible AI use.

SIDEBAR: Continuous Professional Development with AI—Student Checklist

☐ Create a digital AI learning portfolio (e.g., Google Drive or Notion).
☐ Upload summaries of each prompt-optimization project.
☐ Include certificates from completed workshops or online courses.
☐ Add abstracts or slides from any AI case studies, posters, or presentations.
☐ Enroll in a no-code AI course (e.g., "AI for Everyone" on Coursera).
☐ Complete the "AI for Healthcare" certificate on edX.
☐ Explore your school's learning portal for recorded webinars or AI electives.
☐ Join or start an AI Rounds or journal club with peers.
☐ Participate in a health-related hackathon as a clinical lead or workflow designer.
☐ Set a SMART goal for your next 6 months of AI learning.
☐ Track your goal progress and update your portfolio monthly.

Ethical Practice and Accountability

Ethical awareness is as essential as clinical skill when integrating AI into patient care. As AI tools become more embedded in clinical workflows, you must stay up to date with the evolving regulatory and ethical landscape. This includes the FDA's AI/ML Action Plan for the approval and postmarket oversight of AI-driven devices [10], HIPAA's privacy safeguards for patient data [11], and the AMA's augmented intelligence guidelines, which emphasize human oversight, transparency, and equitable deployment [12].

Transparency begins at the bedside. Every clinical note that incorporates AI should clearly document its use. Include the tool's name and version, summarize its output, and explain your clinical judgment. This approach strengthens patient trust and creates a defensible audit trail. For example:

> AI Tool (ChatHealth v2.1) recommended differential diagnosis: pulmonary embolism; clinician review confirmed and ordered CT angiogram.

You must take extra precautions when using AI beyond its original design parameters and indications. This is known as off-label use. This might include using a language model intended for drafting notes to generate differential diagnoses instead. In these cases, always obtain informed consent and clarify that a licensed clinician retains final decision-making authority. A simple phrase such as:

> This note includes AI-generated suggestions reviewed by Dr. Tietjen, who retains final responsibility for clinical decisions.

—helps clarify accountability and protect patient autonomy.

Ethical use also demands attention to fairness. Be alert to potential algorithmic bias, especially if the training data underrepresents certain populations. Evaluate outputs critically and seek explainability features where available. If the AI's reasoning is opaque, ask: would I still make the same decision without it?

As a learning activity, review your institution's current policy on clinical AI tools. If none exists, draft a one-page documentation guideline with sample phrases and consent language tailored for AI-assisted care.

Finally, ethical reflection can spark scholarly contribution. Document your experience using AI in clinical care, participate in AI-focused journal clubs, or collaborate on a quality improvement project. As a future clinician, your insights will shape not only how AI is used—but how responsibly it is integrated into patient care.

Beyond ethics, we'll see in the next section how scholarship lets you contribute original insights to the field.

Try This: 5 Ways to Share Your AI Insights Without a Full Research Study

You don't need a grant, lab, or IRB to contribute meaningfully to the conversation about AI in health care. Here are five accessible ways to turn your observations into scholarship:

1. Write a Case Report

   Document a real-world example of AI influencing diagnosis, treatment, or workflow. Follow ICMJE guidelines to structure your narrative professionally.
2. Contribute to a Student-Run Journal

   Submit an opinion piece, brief review, or commentary to your medical school's student publication or a peer-reviewed outlet with a dedicated trainee section.
3. Present at Journal Club

   Share an AI-related article at your next QI or informatics journal club. Include a short slide on clinical implications or future research directions.
4. Post a Professional Reflection

   Write a 300-word LinkedIn post about a recent AI elective, a challenge using a generative tool, or lessons learned during a rotation.
5. Submit a Blog Post to Your Institution's Innovation Office

   Most medical schools and hospitals have innovation centers eager for student perspectives. Ask if you can submit a blog or guest commentary.

Research and Scholarship Opportunities

Formal research is not a prerequisite for integrating generative AI into your clinical routine. However, for students aspiring to careers in academic medicine, clinical informatics, or digital health innovation, research experience can be a powerful accelerator. Institutional Review Board (IRB)-approved studies offer a training ground for designing protocols, understanding regulatory guardrails, and generating scholarship that strengthens residency applications.

For those interested in data-driven quality improvement, large, de-identified datasets like *MIMIC-IV* allow you to explore AI prompt performance in real-world scenarios without compromising patient privacy. Under the US Common Rule, many such studies qualify for exemption, streamlining the review process while still producing actionable insights [13].

Publishing your findings doesn't require a full randomized trial. A well-structured case report describing an AI-assisted diagnosis, workflow improvement, or unexpected model output can serve as an accessible on-ramp. Follow ICMJE standards for authorship and reporting to structure manuscripts and conference abstracts professionally [14]. Even small-scale analyses—such as comparing prompt outcomes across clinical settings—may qualify for institutional funding or NIH R03 seed grants, which offer up to $50,000 to support early-stage work [15].

If publication feels out of reach, there are still meaningful ways to share your insights. Submit a reflective blog post to your school's innovation office, contribute to student-run journals, or post thoughtful commentary on platforms like LinkedIn. These informal contributions can build your reputation as a thoughtful user of clinical AI.

Alternatively, if your interests lean more toward practical application than scholarly output, present lessons learned at local journal clubs, simulation-center workshops, or resident teaching sessions. You'll still develop valuable skills in critical appraisal, scientific communication, and faculty engagement—all without committing to the demands of a full research protocol.

To bring research and ethics into practice, it is essential to collaborate across disciplines.

Sidebar: What Is an Institutional Review Board (IRB)?
An **IRB** is a committee that reviews research involving human subjects to ensure ethics and participant safety. Even when using only de-identified data, you must check whether your project qualifies for exemption or expedited review.

Why It Matters

- Protects patient privacy and welfare.
- Ensures compliance with federal regulations and institutional policies.

How to Work with the IRB

1. **Draft Your Protocol:** Write a concise summary of your study's purpose, data sources (e.g., de-identified records), and methods.
2. **Submit for Review:** Use your institution's online IRB portal to upload the protocol, consent forms (if needed), and any supporting documents.
3. **Receive Determination:** The IRB will decide if your study is exempt, expedited, or requires full review—and you will receive formal approval or feedback.
4. **Maintain Compliance:** If your project changes (new data sources, additional analyses), submit an amendment. Report any unexpected issues or data breaches immediately.

Tip for Students: Many schools offer IRB workshops or templates—check your research office website, and attend an IRB orientation session before your first submission.

Interprofessional and Cross-Sector Collaboration

Turning your AI curiosity into meaningful contributions begins not with leadership but with observation, service, and humility. Join clinical informatics electives or seminars where data scientists, software engineers, and informaticists demonstrate how they convert clinical problems into technical solutions. Volunteer to assist with case reviews or workflow mapping—your medical lens adds real value, even early in training [16].

Engage in quality improvement settings like morbidity-and-mortality (M&M) conferences or institutional QI teams. One particularly accessible resource is the *IHI Open School*, the Institute for Healthcare Improvement's global learning platform offering free courses on patient safety, systems design, and clinical leadership [17]. These forums can help you recognize how AI could streamline handoffs, prevent errors, or improve resource allocation.

Finally, expand your network by joining student chapters of professional organizations such as the American Medical Informatics Association (AMIA) or HIMSS. Attend local chapter events, volunteer at conferences, or attend special interest group meetings. These informal but high-yield opportunities connect you with mentors and open the door to collaborative AI projects—even before you hold a formal role.

When you embed yourself in multidisciplinary teams, you see how ethical, technical, clinical, and administrative inputs must align for AI to work in real-world care. This collaborative mindset enhances your training and prepares you for emerging roles across the healthcare AI ecosystem.

Career Pathways and Emerging Roles

As artificial intelligence transforms health care, new hybrid career paths are emerging—ones that combine clinical expertise with technological innovation. Among the most prominent is the role of the clinical informaticist: a physician trained to optimize data systems and serve as a bridge between frontline providers and health IT teams. These professionals help ensure that AI tools integrate smoothly into clinical workflows and meet safety, usability, and regulatory standards [18].

Another rising profile is that of the AI-enhanced physician, clinicians who routinely apply generative AI models to streamline documentation, interpret complex data, or support diagnostic reasoning. Far from replacing clinical judgment, these tools serve as cognitive extenders that amplify physician effectiveness.

Some trainees take the entrepreneurial route, becoming digital health innovators. They may join hospital innovation hubs or found AI-driven startups tackling problems like emergency triage, remote monitoring, or personalized treatment planning. Others enter nontraditional fellowships, such as the AMIA-sponsored clinical informatics programs or health tech residencies that place physicians inside tech firms or academic-industry collaborations.

To prepare for these paths, begin exploring during medical school or residency. Join an AI-focused student interest group, pursue electives in data science, or contribute to clinical AI research projects. These early experiences can help you identify whether your future lies at the bedside, in the boardroom, or at the bleeding edge of digital health innovation.

Sidebar: AMIA Clinical Informatics Fellowship

In academia, the rise of AI medicine departments offers opportunities to pursue academic career tracks that combine clinical duties with AI research and teaching. To prepare, create a skills map that catalogs your clinical strengths, such as diagnostics or procedural care, and pairs them with project management competencies like prompt engineering, data interpretation, and stakeholder communication. This roadmap will guide your next steps, whether you aim for a leadership role in informatics, a hybrid clinical-tech appointment, or an entrepreneurial venture.

Skills Mapping Template

Clinical strength	AI/tech skill	Application
Clinical decision-making	Prompt refinement	Design triage chatbot prompts
Communication	Stakeholder presentation skills	Pitch AI tool to hospital innovation council
Workflow familiarity	Usability feedback	Contribute to EMR integration design

How to Use This Table

This **Skills Mapping Template** helps you identify how your current clinical competencies can be paired with AI-related abilities to unlock new roles in healthcare innovation.

1. Column 1: Clinical Strength
   Start by listing specific strengths or interests from your medical training (e.g., diagnostic reasoning, empathy, documentation, or team leadership).
2. Column 2: AI/Tech Skill
   Pair each strength with an emerging AI-related capability—this might include prompt writing, bias auditing, data interpretation, or software testing.
3. Column 3: Application
   Describe a real-world task, workflow, or project where these skills could be combined to deliver value.

You may expand the table with your own combinations to guide residency choices, elective selection, or fellowship goals.

Finally, frame your long-term plan with SMART goals and curated resources.

Sidebar: AMIA Clinical Informatics Fellowship

The **AMIA Clinical Informatics Fellowship** is a 2-year, ACGME-accredited program designed to train physicians in the science and practice of medical informatics, covering AI fundamentals, data standards, system implementation, and evaluation to improve patient care. Fellows complete rotations in clinical, operational, and research settings; participate in didactics; and undertake an independent informatics project under faculty mentorship.

Why It Benefits Medical Students

- **Deepens expertise:** Provides structured exposure to AI and digital health in real-world clinical environments
- **Career advancement:** Completes subspecialty training recognized by board certification in clinical informatics
- **Mentorship and networking:** Connects you with informatics leaders and multidisciplinary teams

(continued)

How to Apply

Applicants typically register through the ERAS system and participate in the AMIA Clinical Informatics Fellowship Match, opening each October. Visit the AMIA Match page for requirements, timelines, and program listings.

Learn more and apply: https://amia.org/membership/academic-forum/amia-clinical-informatics-fellowship-match

Your Lifelong AI Learning Plan

Transitioning from career exploration to personal development, chart your AI learning roadmap with clear SMART goals for 1, 3, and 5 years (see SMART Goals Sidebar). For example, in PGY-1, aim to "Join and present at least two AI journal clubs"; by year 3, set a goal to "Publish an AI-assisted case report"; and by year 5, target "Lead an AI quality-improvement project." These goals should be Specific, Measurable, Achievable, Relevant, and Time-Bound [19].

Populate your plan with a curated resource list: Subscribe to *Journal of Medical Internet Research—AI*, attend HIMSS and AMIA conferences, and join online communities such as the AI in Healthcare LinkedIn group or specialized Slack channels in your field. Many subspecialty societies (for instance, the Radiological Society of North America) also offer AI tracks—note these in your calendar.

Reflect on your evolving journey with the prompt:

What will your AI journey look like at residency, fellowship, and beyond?

Documenting this narrative and reviewing your goals annually ensures your AI expertise grows in parallel with your clinical responsibilities.

SMART Goal Worksheet

Time frame	SMART goal
1 year	Complete "AI for Everyone," and attend 2 AI journal clubs
3 year	Publish a case report, and mentor junior students in prompt design
5 year	Lead an AI quality improvement initiative, or join an informatics fellowship

Instructions for Students

Use this worksheet to draft Specific, Measurable, Achievable, Relevant, and Time-Bound goals related to your ongoing AI development. You may revise the suggested examples or create your own based on your clinical interests, residency plans, and emerging opportunities.

Conclusion

As generative AI becomes increasingly woven into clinical training and care delivery, your role as a future physician includes more than technical proficiency. It demands ethical discernment, continuous learning, and a commitment to transparency and patient-centered practice. This chapter has equipped you with the foundational tools to engage AI critically, understanding how to document its use, safeguard privacy, obtain informed consent, and evaluate its promise and limitations. Ultimately, responsible AI integration is not a matter of passive adoption but of active, accountable participation. The habits you build now—reflective practice, ethical vigilance, scholarly curiosity—will shape your clinical development and the future culture of medicine itself.

Instructor's Guide for This chapter—Professional Growth and Lifelong AI Integration

Chapter Overview and Learning Objectives

Goals

1. Frame AI literacy as an enduring professional competency.
2. Identify certification and micro-credential pathways in clinical AI.
3. Cultivate continuous professional development strategies.
4. Uphold ethical practice and accountability in AI use.
5. Explore research, collaboration, and emerging career roles.
6. Develop a SMART-based lifelong AI learning plan.

This chapter prepares students to integrate generative AI into their professional trajectory through credentials, ethics, scholarship, collaboration, and personal planning.

Before Teaching

- **Student Materials (Ensure Availability)**
  - Chapter 15 student text
  - Sidebars: SMART Goals, AMIA & HIMSS Overview, Hackathon, Sandbox, IRB
  - **Blank SMART-Goal Table Worksheet** (template provided at the end of guide)

- **Technology and Access**
  - Screen-sharing to demonstrate free resources (Coursera's AI For Everyone; edX AI for Healthcare)
  - Institutional LMS or lists of virtual seminar and online community links
- **Preparation**
  - Confirm student access to AMIA/HIMSS site details; prepare alternate free resources if needed.
  - Create a standardized mock chart entry for AI documentation exercise.
  - Review IRB portal demo pages to orient students.

Section-by-Section Teaching Tips

Chapter Goals and Overview

- **Kickoff:** Read goals; ask students which resonates with their interests.
- **Tip:** Emphasize lifelong nature of AI learning.

Transition: "With your objectives clear, explore formal credentials next."

Certification and Credentialing in Clinical AI

- **Activity:** In pairs, explore AMIA and HIMSS websites (or alternative free webinars) to note one certificate requirement and trainee discount.
- **Debrief:** Share findings and discuss low-barrier entry points for students without memberships.

Transition: "Credentials set a foundation—sustain your growth with ongoing development."

Continuous Professional Development with AI

- **Worksheet:** Distribute the Blank SMART-Goal Table; students draft a 1-year goal.
- **Peer review:** In small groups, exchange goals and apply the reflection rubric to provide feedback.

Transition: "Alongside learning, uphold ethical standards in AI use."

Ethical Practice and Accountability

- **Demo:** Show the mock chart entry documenting AI tool, version, and clinician interpretation.
- **Exercise:** In groups, draft a one-sentence informed consent addendum for AI use using the IRB sidebar.

Transition: "Ethics and consent pave the way for scholarly contribution."

Research and Scholarship Opportunities

- **Overview:** Briefly review IRB steps using sidebar; clarify exemption vs. full review.
- **Brainstorm:** Individually jot one case-report idea; discuss feasibility and required support.
- **Resource tip:** Provide links to IRB templates and department research office contacts.

Transition: "Scholarship benefits from teamwork—let's connect with collaborators."

Interprofessional and Cross-Sector Collaboration

- **Discussion prompt:** How to volunteer with informatics or quality teams—list first steps (email template provided).
- **Role-Play:** Students practice a 2-minute introduction to request observational time with an informaticist or IHI Open School mentor.

Transition: "Collaboration reveals diverse career opportunities."

Career Pathways and Emerging Roles

- **Presentation:** Highlight AMIA Fellowship sidebar; contrast fellowship vs. industry internship.
- **Group task:** Create a mini "skills map" on chart paper pairing a clinical interest with a complementary AI skill.

Transition: "Finally, let's build your long-term AI learning plan."

Your Lifelong AI Learning Plan

- **Worksheet:** Complete SMART-Goal Table for 1-, 3-, and 5-year milestones.
- **Reflection:** Write a response to: "What will your AI journey look like at residency, fellowship, and beyond?"
- **Group synthesis:** Small groups share key goals and discuss alignment with chapter objectives.

Final Synthesis and Debrief

- **Group discussion:** Each group presents one key takeaway per chapter goal and suggests one action step.
- **Instructor prompt:** Facilitate cross-group dialogue on common themes and next steps.

Assessment and Reflection Rubric

Reflection Exercise Rubric (apply to SMART-Goal and final prompt):

Criterion	Excellent (3)	Satisfactory (2)	Needs improvement (1)
Specificity	Goals clearly defined and focused	Goals somewhat clear	Goals vague or broad
Measurability	Includes quantifiable metrics	Partially measurable	No clear metrics
Relevance	Directly aligned with career goals	Some alignment	Misaligned or unclear
Timeline	Deadlines for 1/3/5 years provided	Partial timelines	No deadlines
Insight	Reflection shows deep understanding	Moderate insight	Minimal or superficial insight

Quiz Mapping
- Define micro-credential: 15.2.
- List SMART criteria: 15.3 and sidebar.
- Explain IRB exemption: 15.5.
- Describe ethical documentation: 15.4.
- Name an AI career role: 15.7.

Note to Instructor Ensure all resources and worksheets are accessible before class. Encourage low-barrier engagement and peer support rather than formal authority.

References

1. Frenk J, Chen L, Bhutta ZA, Cohen J, Crisp N, Evans T, et al. Health professionals for a new century: transforming education to strengthen health systems in an interdependent world. Lancet. 2010;376(9756):1923–58. https://doi.org/10.1016/S0140-6736(10)61854-5.
2. Wartman SA, Combs CD. Medical education must move from the information age to the age of artificial intelligence. N Engl J Med. 2018;379(16):805–6. https://doi.org/10.1056/NEJMp1801885.
3. American Medical Informatics Association. (2023). Professional certificate in clinical informatics. Retrieved from https://www.amia.org/training/certificate.
4. Healthcare Information and Management Systems Society. (2023). Certified Professional in Healthcare Information and Management Systems (CPHIMS). Retrieved from https://www.himss.org/resources/cphims.
5. American Board of Medical Specialties. (2022). Continuing certification: maintenance of certification requirements. Retrieved from https://www.abms.org/member-boards/continuing-certification/.
6. Mozilla Foundation. (2019). Open badges specification 2.0. Retrieved from https://openbadges.org/specification/2.0/.
7. Coursera. AI for everyone. n.d.. Retrieved from https://www.coursera.org/learn/ai-for-everyone.
8. edX. Artificial intelligence for healthcare professional certificate. n.d.. Retrieved from https://www.edx.org/professional-certificate/ai-healthcare
9. Wenger E. Communities of practice: learning, meaning, and identity. Cambridge University Press; 1998.
10. U.S. Food and Drug Administration. (2021). Artificial Intelligence/Machine Learning (AI/ML)-based software as a medical device action plan. Retrieved from https://www.fda.gov/media/145022/download.
11. U.S. Department of Health & Human Services. (2018). Health Insurance Portability and Accountability Act (HIPAA) privacy rule. Retrieved from https://www.hhs.gov/hipaa/for-professionals/privacy/index.html.
12. American Medical Association. (2020). Policy H-480.940: augmented intelligence in health care. Retrieved from https://policysearch.ama-assn.org/policyfinder/detail/augmented%20intelligence?uri=%2FAMADoc%2FHOD.xml-H-480.940.xml.
13. U.S. Department of Health & Human Services. (2018). Protection of human subjects. 45 CFR 46. Retrieved from https://www.hhs.gov/ohrp/regulations-and-policy/regulations/45-cfr-46/index.html.
14. International Committee of Medical Journal Editors. (2022). Recommendations for the conduct, reporting, editing, and publication of scholarly work in medical journals. Retrieved from http://www.icmje.org/icmje-recommendations.pdf.
15. National Institutes of Health. (2022). Small grant program (R03). Retrieved from https://grants.nih.gov/grants/funding/r03.htm.
16. Institute of Medicine. Health professions education: a bridge to quality. National Academies Press; 2003.
17. Institute for Healthcare Improvement. IHI open school. n.d.. Retrieved from http://www.ihi.org/education/ihiopenschool/Pages/default.aspx.
18. Saltz JH, Kuo MH. Clinical informatics and the future of artificial intelligence in healthcare. JAMA. 2020;324(4):319–20. https://doi.org/10.1001/jama.2020.9282.
19. Doran GT. There's a S.M.A.R.T. way to write management's goals and objectives. Manag Rev. 1981;70(11):35–6.

Conclusion

By pursuing the goals of Chap. 15, you've connected AI's technical underpinnings to real-world clinical practice and built a roadmap for lifelong growth. Through the exercises in the other chapters, you have mastered prompt engineering, stakeholder engagement, ethical safeguards, quality-improvement cycles, and reflective goal-setting. These competencies form the toolkit you'll carry into rounds, research, and leadership roles.

AI will never replace your clinical judgment; it amplifies it. Treat generative models as partners that flourish under your critical oversight and human values.

Two Commitments to Carry Forward

- **Stay curious:** Review and revise your SMART goals each year, pursue new badges or certificates, and dive into AI communities.
- **Honor trust:** Document AI use clearly, secure informed consent, and champion equity and transparency in every interaction.

Your Next Steps (Set Reminders)

1. In 6 months, revisit one SMART goal and note your progress.
2. Join an AI journal club or a student chapter of AMIA/HIMSS.
3. Teach a peer a prompt-engineering technique or lead a mini–AI pilot.

By weaving generative AI into your evolving practice, you'll enhance patient care and help define the future of medicine.

© The Editor(s) (if applicable) and The Author(s), under exclusive license to Springer Nature Switzerland AG 2025

C. Quinn, *Generative AI for the Medical Student*,
https://doi.org/10.1007/978-3-032-01613-3

Reflection Prompt

"Which skill from this book will you prioritize in the coming year, and how will you hold yourself accountable?"

Go forth with competence, integrity, and compassion. Your patients and the profession depend on physicians like you who lead with innovation.

Glossary

Acronyms and Initialisms

ABMS	American Board of Medical Specialties
ACGME	Accreditation Council for Graduate Medical Education
AGI	Artificial General Intelligence
AI	Artificial Intelligence
AI/ML	Artificial Intelligence/Machine Learning
AMIA	American Medical Informatics Association
AHRQ	Agency for Healthcare Research and Quality
API	Application Programming Interface
CFR	Code of Federal Regulations
CMIO	Chief Medical Information Officer
CoT	Chain-of-Thought (prompting technique)
CNN	Convolutional Neural Network
CME	Continuing Medical Education
CPHIMS	Certified Professional in Healthcare Information and Management Systems
DDSS	Diagnostic Decision Support System
EHR	Electronic Health Record
EMR	Electronic Medical Record
FDA	US Food and Drug Administration
GLLMM	Generative Large Language Multimodal Model
GNC	Gaussian Naïve Classifier (example) [if used]
HIPAA	Health Insurance Portability and Accountability Act
HIMSS	Healthcare Information and Management Systems Society
IHI	Institute for Healthcare Improvement
IRB	Institutional Review Board
IT	Information Technology

© The Editor(s) (if applicable) and The Author(s), under exclusive license to Springer Nature Switzerland AG 2025

C. Quinn, *Generative AI for the Medical Student*,
https://doi.org/10.1007/978-3-032-01613-3

IVR	Immersive Virtual Reality
LLM	Large Language Model
LMS	Learning Management System
LSTM	Long Short-Term Memory (neural network)
MIMIC-IV	Medical Information Mart for Intensive Care, Version IV
ML	Machine Learning
NLP	Natural Language Processing
OSCE	Objective Structured Clinical Examination
PDSA	Plan–Do–Study–Act (quality-improvement cycle)
PHI	Protected Health Information
QI	Quality Improvement
RAG	Retrieval-Augmented Generation
ReAct	Reasoning and Acting (prompting framework)
RLHF	Reinforcement Learning from Human Feedback
RRT	Rapid Response Team
SBAR	Situation, Background, Assessment, Recommendation (hand-off format)
SP	Standardized Patient
STAR	Smart Tissue Autonomous Robot
USMLE	United States Medical Licensing Examination

Key Terms

Attention Heat Map A visual overlay showing which words or image regions a model focuses on when generating an output.

Bias (AI) Systematic skew in AI outputs due to imbalanced or unrepresentative training data.

Data Drift Shifts in input data patterns over time that reduce an AI model's accuracy unless prompts or models are updated.

Deep Learning Advanced machine learning using layered neural networks to recognize complex patterns in data.

Digital Twin A dynamic virtual replica of a patient or system used for simulation and analysis.

Hallucination (AI) When a generative model produces plausible-sounding but incorrect or fabricated information.

Hackathon A time-limited event (often 24–48 hrs) where multidisciplinary teams rapidly prototype solutions; roles include clinician expert, designer, and data analyst.

Haptic Feedback Tactile sensations in virtual simulations that mimic the sense of touch or resistance.

Infogram A visual diagram or infographic summarizing a process or data flow.

Micro-credential A focused digital badge or certification recognizing mastery of a specific skill, such as prompt engineering.

Prompt Engineering The craft of designing and refining input prompts to guide generative AI toward desired, accurate outputs.

Real-Time Analytics Continuous processing of incoming data streams to provide immediate insights or alerts.

Retrieval-Augmented Generation (RAG) An AI approach that fetches relevant documents from external databases before generating responses, enhancing factual grounding.

Self-Attention A transformer mechanism enabling the model to weigh different parts of the input sequence when creating representations.

SMART Goals Goals that are Specific, Measurable, Achievable, Relevant, and Time-Bound, used for structured learning plans.

Transformer A neural network architecture using self-attention to process sequences in parallel, foundational to modern language and vision models.

Virtual Instructor (VI) An AI-driven simulated teacher used in remote or virtual clinical training.

Virtual Patient (VP) A computer-generated simulation of a patient scenario for medical education and assessment.

Sandbox A safe, isolated environment where AI models can be tested without risking production systems or patient data.

Index

© The Editor(s) (if applicable) and The Author(s), under exclusive license to Springer Nature Switzerland AG 2025
C. Quinn, *Generative AI for the Medical Student*,
https://doi.org/10.1007/978-3-032-01613-3

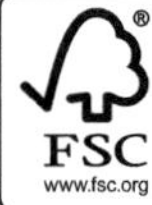

MIX
Papier aus verantwortungsvollen Quellen
Paper from responsible sources
FSC® C105338

If you have any concerns about our products,
you can contact us on
ProductSafety@springernature.com

In case Publisher is established outside the EU,
the EU authorized representative is:
Springer Nature Customer Service Center GmbH
Europaplatz 3, 69115 Heidelberg, Germany

Printed by Libri Plureos GmbH
in Hamburg, Germany